The Heredity of Behavior Disorders in Adults and Children

The Heredity of Behavior Disorders in Adults and Children

Steven G. Vandenberg
University of Colorado
Boulder, Colorado

Sandra Manes Singer
University of Southern Indiana
Evansville, Indiana

and

David L. Pauls
Yale University
New Haven, Connecticut

PLENUM MEDICAL BOOK COMPANY
New York and London

Library of Congress Cataloging in Publication Data

Vandenberg, Steven G. (Steven Gerritjan), 1915–
   The heredity of behavior disorders in adults and children.

   Includes bibliographies and index.
   1. Mental illness—Genetic aspects. 2. Developmental disabilities—Genetic
aspects. 3. Behavior genetics. I. Singer, Sandra Manes. II. Pauls, David L. III. Title.
[DNLM: 1. Genetics, Behavioral. 2. Mental Disorders—familial & genetic. 3. Social
Behavior Disorders—familial & genetic. WM 100 V227h]
RC455.4.G4V36   1986   616.89′042   86-15095
ISBN 0-306-42191-7

© 1986 Plenum Publishing Corporation
233 Spring Street, New York, N.Y. 10013

Plenum Medical Book Company is an imprint of Plenum Publishing Corporation

Printed in the United States of America

To our families, for both their genetic and
environmental influences

Foreword

Current trends in morbidity suggest that by the beginning of the twenty-first century, psychiatric illness may become the most pressing problem in public health in many of the advanced countries. As ably demonstrated by Vandenberg, Singer, and Pauls, the principal identifiable etiology of the major psychiatric disorders is heredity; if progress is to be made in prevention and treatment of these disorders, it may have to come from improved understanding of their inheritance.

A relentless increase has been observed in the frequency of mood disorders, primarily major depression but also manic-depressive illness, appearing earlier and more frequently in each age cohort born since (approximately) 1940. Because major depression is a recurrent disorder, whose episodes increase in frequency with age, the number of observed depressions can be expected to increase dramatically as these people reach middle and old age.

The rate of suicide has also increased enormously, according to birth cohort. Starting with people born around 1935, the rate of suicide between 15 and 19 years of age has increased more than 10 times from the earliest to the most recent birth cohorts. What is not clear is if there will be a compensatory reduction in suicide rate as this cohort ages, because people likely to commit suicide will have done so earlier, or if this presages a general increase in suicide, comparable to the increase in mood disorders and perhaps a function of them. Now, suicide is classically more frequent, starting in middle age and increasing into old age. It is not possible to compare the rate in middle and old age for the most recent cohort with those of other cohorts, because they will not reach middle age until the beginning of the twenty-first century, but it is ominous that the age-specific rates for the next most recently born cohorts show a marked increase in suicide rate up to age 44, the latest age for which data are available.

One can confidently predict that Alzheimer's disease will show a great increase in prevalence because of the general improvements in longevity. Accumulated evidence shows that this disease is largely a familial disorder. The age of onset is variable, but so late as to have obscured the familial nature of the illness until large numbers of families had multiple members living until very old age (over 85), and until appropriate corrections for variable age of onset were entered into the familial prevalence estimates.

Alzheimer's disease offers an example of a rapid increase in a genetic disorder produced by nongenetic events, in this case improved life expectancy. The increase in affective illness and suicide is also too rapid to have been produced by gene frequency changes, and points to the role of environmental factors, broadly conceived, in these disorders. To consider the genetics of these illnesses is impossible unless nongenetic events are well accounted for. This fact has led to complex mathematical modeling of transmission of illness, perhaps better known in psychiatry than in other areas of human biology. But the astute reader of the accounts in this volume will appreciate that the same complex conceptualization is required in numerous medical disorders, such as hypertension, in which there is an intricate mix of genetic and environmental factors, with perhaps many of these discrete factors each capable of producing disease independently. From this perspective, behavior genetics has been in the forefront of the genetics of chronic disease, and the present work can well serve the student of such disorders.

What has been absent until the appearance of this book has been a synthesis of the genetics of the numerous disorders that principally affect behavior, that is, cognition and affective state as well as observable actions. This approach requires a broader perspective than that of academic psychiatry, which has unexplainably excluded the mental retardations over the past few generations, and has only recently taken a serious interest in adult onset dementias such as Alzheimer's or Huntington's. Unfortunately for the psychiatric student of genetics and behavior, these areas are precisely those in which the most striking advances have been made in identifying specific genetic defects, which is a conceptual quantum leap forward from a demonstration that unspecified genetic factors must be playing a role in the production of a disorder.

How can the genetic defect be pinned down? There are two meth-

ods: gene mapping and the identification of the inherited pathophysiological defect. In the past few years, advances in molecular genetics
have greatly enhanced the power of both methods. Gene mapping is
greatly improved by the orders of magnitude increase in known gene
polymorphisms in man, since the demonstration of the first restriction
fragment-length polymorphism (RFLP) by Kan and Dozy, in 1978. Although their demonstration was of a DNA variation associated with
the abnormal globin gene in sickle cell anemia, a gene of obvious
pathophysiological interest, the most notable use of RFLPs in behavioral disorders has been in gene mapping, as an application of the
theorem advanced by Botstein, White, Skolnick and Davis in 1980 that
150 properly located polymorphisms would allow the entire human
genome to be scanned. Using random single-copy probes, Gusella *et al.*
mapped the gene for Huntington's disease to a small region of chromosome 4, in 1983. This was a landmark study, demonstrating the power
of RFLPs in pedigrees to map a gene for illness when there is no *a priori*
knowledge of where the gene might be. High-resolution two-dimensional electrophoresis of proteins is another method of identifying
polymorphisms at the molecular level, perhaps less well known than
the RFLP method, but still identifying new polymorphisms in expressed genes that were previously unknown. Applications to behavior
genetics are at present most tentative. Chromosome-banding polymorphisms represent yet another new method, which has been used in
behavioral genetics to tentatively locate a gene for specific reading
disability on chromosome 15.

As important as these advances are, they only specify the region
where the defect is to be found but do not specify what the pathophysiological event is. In the mental retardations, we have two examples of
firmly established etiologic events whose gene location is known but
whose pathophysiology remains obscure: Down's syndrome and the
fragile site of the X-chromosome. But there are a large number of cases
of severe retardation in which the pathophysiology has been identified,
starting with Fölling's 1934 observation that the urine of two retarded
brothers had a phenolic smell, leading him to discover phenylketonuria as a genetic disease. There is no comparable example of a proven
inherited defect in the traditional psychiatric disorders; it is only in the
context of a general overview of all the inherited behavior disorders
that this missing knowledge in psychiatric genetics becomes apparent.
There is, however, the finding in Alzheimer's disease of specific degeneration of certain cholinergic neurons in the nucleus basalis, which
may prove to be an inherited pathophysiological event if family studies
of autopsy materials can be performed.

The molecular genetic methods can also serve to investigate pathophysiology. Starting with pro-opiomelanocortin, a neuropeptide which is the precursor of ACTH and other peptides important in behavior, human genomic DNA fragments have been isolated and RFLPs identified for substances important in nervous system function, including enzymes of neurotransmitter synthesis, neuropeptides, and receptor molecules. Pathophysiological hypotheses on the role of these structural genes can be reliably tested using pedigree-linkage methods, since a single RFLP scans an entire region around the gene.

The comprehensiveness of this book, which presents all these areas in a knowledgeable and systematic manner, is to be commended. It can serve as a textbook of both genetics and behavior, including well-considered discussions of psychiatric diagnosis, biology of illness, and role of life events, in psychiatry. In genetics it goes beyond mathematical genetics, in which synthesis with psychiatry has been traditional, into molecular genetics and pathophysiology, in which applications to genetics of psychiatric illness are only just beginning. One of the obstacles to these latter applications is that it is so very difficult for a molecular geneticist to think like a psychiatrist or even like a population geneticist, and vice versa. The present text is a timely facilitator for those investigators who are ready to cross the boundaries of their discipline and thus pursue the science of inherited behavioral disorders.

ELLIOT S. GERSHON, M.D.

Chief, Neurogenetics Branch
National Institute of Mental Health

Preface

Fifteen years ago, in the preface of a book with a similar topic, David Rosenthal wrote:

> For many years I have been continually surprised how little most mental health devotees know about the possible hereditary contributions to the phenomena they are studying and treating. Moreover many do not want to know. These include not only most clinical psychologists, but psychiatric social workers, nurses, social scientists, counselors, physicians and others who must deal with mentally disturbed persons. (Rosenthal, 1970, p. ix)

Our personal assessment of the present situation is that some progress has been made since then. Workers in the mental health professions are more likely to acknoweldge that "genes exist" and that nature as well as nurture can influence behavior. However, the level of understanding of how, and to what extent, inherited factors exert this influence is still very limited. For example, many newer textbooks in psychiatry and abnormal psychology include the fact that heredity may play a role in the expression of schizophrenia. However, the coverage of this topic is often limited to a single sentence that merely states the premise, with no detail.

This book is an attempt to provide some of those missing details. Rosenthal helped to introduce the concept of the influence of heredity on abnormal behavior to professionals in the health and helping fields, and to social scientists in general. The years between the publication of his book and the present have been a period of fruitful research in human genetics. One thing that has become obvious as a result of this research is that the pathways from genes to behavior are quite complex. In the pages that follow, we attempt to shed some light on how these complicated processes exert their influence on individual behavior disorders. Two recurrent themes will be encountered: the critical importance of accurate diagnosis, and possible etiological heterogeneity. For any genetic analysis, correct, reliable diagnoses are necessary. Much progress has been made in the last 10 years in refining diagnostic procedures. However, as we will note at various points, much work still remains to be done. Additional knowledge is needed too about the second related issue, that of possible heterogeneity within certain diagnostic categories. Many examples can be given from medical-genetic disorders in humans that demonstrate etiological/genetic heterogeneity (e.g., the wide variety of anemias now known to exist). So it should be expected that subtypes of mental disorders will likely be discovered that have independent etiologies. These subtypes will no doubt have considerable overlap of symptoms and, in fact, may be clinically indistinguishable yet be the result of very different underlying causes. Thus, the work discussed in the following pages should be interpreted with the understanding that the conclusions drawn from existing studies may change as more accurate subtyping of disorders is accomplished.

As we write, we are aware of the fact that new, powerful techniques in biochemical genetics, including recombinant DNA techniques and improved methods of determining genetic linkage, may soon provide us with more specific details about genetic factors than we have today. It is likely that, as more information becomes available, the details about how heredity affects behavior will become increasingly relevant to both the treatment and prevention of behavior disorders. We hope this book will be an introduction to this area for those with little previous experience and will serve as a point of reference for others who already have some knowledge of the field.

We gratefully acknowledge the help of our colleagues who have offered advice on several sections. The chapter on specific reading disabilities was notably strengthened by our exposure to the treatment of this topic by Dr. Terryl T. Foch in her dissertation.

Many hours of typing and manuscript preparation were contributed by Lori DeVillez, Ronda Hall, and Susan Hunt. We also thank the staff of the Science Library at the University of Colorado, especially David M. Fagerstrom and Susan Anthes. Finally, the encouragement and editorial assistance of Janice Stern, Lisa Honski, and Anthony Franchina at Plenum were most helpful.

STEVEN G. VANDENBERG
SANDRA M. SINGER
DAVID L. PAULS

Contents

CHAPTER 1

Heredity and Mental Disorders

In this book we shall be reviewing the evidence for hereditary factors in behavior disorders in adults and children. These will include both the very serious ones, such as schizophrenia, and milder ones, such as stuttering. The importance of mental health can hardly be over-emphasized. At a meeting of the Committee on Interstate and Foreign Trade of the House of Representatives in 1953, when the problem of mental illness first became a high priority issue in national government, the following remarks were made:

> 1. Mental illness is the nation's No. 1 health problem. More than half of all hospital beds in this country are occupied by the mentally ill. The number of mentally ill patients in the United States exceeds the number of patients suffering from any other type of illness. Mental ill health represents our greatest health problem in cost. Conservative estimates based on incidence studies have shown that approximately 50% of patients who are treated in general practice have psychiatric complications. If the present birth rate remains constant, if the number of mentally ill who are hospitalized remains constant, and if the cost for hospitalizing the mentally ill remains constant, each year's crop of new babies will, because of the percentage of them who will go to mental hospitals, cost the taxpayers . . . $800 million before they die. 2. At least 6% of the total population, 9,000,000 people, suffer from a serious mental disorder. Of 980,000 disability discharges from the Army during the period December 1941 through December 1945, 43% were for neuropsychiatric reasons. 3. Of the 500,000 resident patients in our State mental hospitals, one-quarter have been hospitalized for more than 16 years, one-half for more than 8 years, and three-fourths for more than 2.5 years. (Committee on Interstate and Foreign Commerce, 1953, pp. 1030–1134)

An early report prepared by Fein in 1958 for the Commission on Mental Illness and Health entitled "Economics of Mental Illness" estimated the annual *direct* cost of care at $1.7 billion which, the author noted, was a low estimate that did not include construction and maintenance of buildings, private patient costs, or costs of medical treatment for physical complaints really due to psychological problems. These latter were then put at between $2 and $3 billion a year. Total annual *indirect* cost associated with loss of patient earnings is not easily measured but this too would add substantially to the figures.

We have now entered the decade of the 1980s, and the cost of mental illness is staggering. Estimates are presently over $17 billion yearly and are projected to increase over time.

To many laypersons, the tremendous cost of mental illness may be surprising and somewhat perplexing. What is the element that is so costly? Mental illness as a rule does not require expensive surgical procedures, and the drugs commonly used to treat the disorders are quite inexpensive compared to those needed to treat many other illnesses. The answer to what makes the treatment of mental illness such a costly phenomenon is chronicity, and ironically, the more psychologically disabling forms of mental disorders are the most chronic forms. Thus, schizophrenia is often a lifetime disorder with the usual age of onset in the early 20s. Therapy emphasizing drug treatment can keep the disorder under control more or less successfully for certain periods of time, and a few lucky individuals may experience complete remission of symptoms at some point in their lives. However, there is no known cure for schizophrenia. Thus, many schizophrenics require lifetime treatment. In the past, most schizophrenics had a shortened life span; tuberculosis was a particular problem. This early mortality (often before the age of 30) probably was a direct result of the poor health conditions that prevailed in most mental health institutions until very recently. But improved institutional care and modern medicines have eliminated this particular side effect of schizophrenia, and many schizophrenics are now living to old age. We could extrapolate that, as the life span of the average individual continues to increase, so will the cost of treatment for chronic mental disorders.

One might object that the number of persons in mental hospitals has drastically declined since the advent of antipsychotic drugs and community mental health centers. Thus, we should have experienced a drop in costs. Although there was a short-lived trend in that direction during the 1960s, the number of patients treated in state hospitals actually rose from 802,216 in 1966 to 836,326 in 1971, according to Chu and Trotter (1974). In 1976, data from a U.S. Public Health Survey

Table 1. *The Most Common Causes in Adults (15–44 years) for Hospitalizations in the U.S., 1976. In Rank Order*

1. Genito-urinary
2. Accidents
3. Gastrointestinal
4. Respiratory
5. Mental
6. Musculoskeletal
7. Neoplasm
8. Circulatory
9. Nervous system or sense organs

Note. From *Vital Statistics of the United States*, 1976, p. 479, by U.S. Department of Health, Education and Welfare. Rockville, Md: Public Health Service.

revealed that mental illness is the fifth most common cause of hospitalization among adults in the age range of 15 to 44 years (see Table 1). The one encouraging factor that emerges from a review of recent mental health statistics is that the hospital stay of the average person treated for mental illness has declined. Therefore, there are fewer long-term residents than in earlier times, and although many patients are admitted for treatment a number of times during the course of their illness, each stay is likely to be shorter than it would have been even a few years ago. This trend is illustrated in Figure 1. Unfortunately, as we are now realizing, a considerable proportion of those released are not ready for discharge and frequently suffer bad experiences. This was a particularly widespread practice in the 1960s and 1970s. Discharged patients were so often reduced to roaming the streets and suffering the ostracism of communities that did not want to accept them, that by the mid-1970s steps had been taken to change this pattern of premature release.

In the preceding discussion we have emphasized the economic cost of mental illness because in these present times of belt-tightening economies, it is easy for agencies that fund research to cut back on that funding. However, if viewed from the proper perspective, research money for chronic, severe forms of mental illness is money very well spent. A successful form of treatment for schizophrenics alone, for example, would probably reduce mental health costs by billions of dollars yearly, and the funds spent for such research would be repaid many times over in a very short period of time. But infinitely more

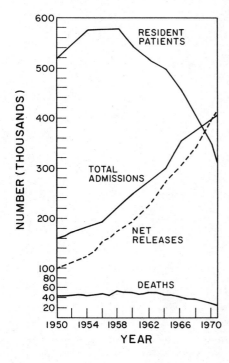

Figure 1. Number of resident patients, total admissions, net releases in U.S. state and county mental hospitals. *Note.* From *Vital Statistics of the United States*, 1975, by U.S. Department of Health, Education and Welfare. Rockville, MD: Public Health Service.

important than any economic concern is the reduction in the years of pain and misery for patients and their families. Their suffering warrants, by itself, every effort at finding ways to reduce or eliminate this dread disorder.

Our primary aim in writing this text is to review the evidence for the influence of heredity on behavior disorders and thus to round out the narrow concept that many researchers have that these disorders are solely the result of environmental stress. Because most readers will already be somewhat familiar with the environmental view and because countless volumes have been written from that perspective, we will generally not discuss the importance of environmental influences on behavioral disorders. However, this does not imply that we are dismissing environmental factors as unimportant; it is merely that the focus of this volume is on hereditary influences.

Our second reason for presenting the material in this book is to emphasize the fact that hereditary factors are not immutable; that is to say, if a mental disorder is determined partially or even completely by genetic factors, the disorder could still be expected to respond as readily to proper treatment as a disorder that is caused by environmental factors. The best example of this is the dietary treatment of phenylketonuria that is used to prevent the severe mental retardation that formerly was the main symptom of this inherited single-gene disorder. Phenylketonuria is only one of a number of abnormalities of metabolism with serious behavioral consequences. Many geneticists feel that in the very near future the biochemical abnormalities underlying numerous inherited disorders will be treatable in such a way as to ameliorate the symptoms or to completely correct the abnormal condition. In the meantime, knowledge of inherited influences permits us to counsel couples about their risk of having a child afflicted with a particular disorder; to perform amniocentesis screening for fetal evidence of abnormality in time for a couple to elect therapeutic abortion if they choose; and be prepared to provide proper medical and psychological intervention as early as possible for an affected individual. We continue to be amazed at the number of well-educated individuals who have the mistaken idea that if a trait is under genetic influence it cannot be altered. We hope this volume will play a part in dispelling that notion.

Finally, our third aim is to contribute to the body of knowledge regarding the *epidemiology* of behavior disorders. We feel that these disorders constitute a public health problem of the first order. As MacMahon (1978) noted, familial resemblance (in mental illness) is "no more than time–place clustering with measurement units somewhat different from those to which the epidemiologist is accustomed". (p. 4). Many forms of mental illness do "run in families." That is probably one of the most interesting aspects of these disorders. For too many years this fact has not been emphasized, in part because of the social stigma attached to mental disorders. Even today many families will drift away from a mentally ill relative, virtually disown that person, and rarely talk about or acknowledge the existence of that individual. Epidemiological studies of mental illness need to focus on the family as a unit of transmission. To this end, we have included family frequency data whenever available in our discussion of each disorder included in this text.

As noted earlier, although we obviously espouse a notion of behavioral disorders that emphasizes the importance of inherited factors, we are truly committed to a model that always includes contributory environmental influences. In some instances, the genetic factors seem to account for much of the variance in the expression of the disorder (e.g., schizophrenia). In others (mild depression), environmental stress is seen to be of central importance in many cases. This situation, unfortunately means that the models that ultimately will explain the various forms of mental illness will probably be complex ones, but that seems only reasonable. Human behavioral disorders *are* complicated in their expression, to the point that diagnosis is often problematic even for highly trained individuals. One only needs to consider the enormous economic and social proportions of the problem of mental illness, however, to realize that we must continue to search for solutions.

CHAPTER 2

The Diagnosis of Psychopathology

Current ideas about ways of classifying mental abnormality into different diagnostic entities gradually began to assume their present form in the 19th century. These ideas were contributed by many individuals, but Kraepelin (1896) is often credited with the first modern synthesis. Details are given in several books on the history of psychiatry, such as those by Alexander and Selesnick (1966) or Zilborg (1941). Mental deficiency was eventually distinguished from mental illness, and both from behaviors defined as criminal or morally deviant. Perhaps *mental illness* is an inappropriate term at times, especially when the "patient" resents treatment or displays behavior that is more unconventional than deleterious to self and others. However, mental illness is not entirely the myth it was often claimed to be in the 1960s and early 1970s (Szasz, 1961).

It is common sense to assume that before one can help it is necessary to know what is wrong. Or to put it in more elegant terms: successful therapy requires accurate diagnosis. Unfortunately, mentally ill persons display such a variety of unusual behaviors that it is often difficult to recognize many regular patterns. For that reason psychiatry has lagged behind other medical specialties in devising a precise diagnostic system for the clinician. And, of course, accurate diagnosis is a *sine qua non* for the researcher into possible hereditary factors. A sample consisting of people having several different disorders, all of which superficially appear to be the same, can hardly yield any clear-cut pattern of inheritance.

In the next section of this text we will trace the history of mental

7

disorders and take up in more detail the difficulties inherent in diagnosis of these disorders.

HISTORICAL PERSPECTIVE

Mankind has attributed abnormal behavior to a variety of causes.
At one time or another the devil, atavism, pride, sexual excesses, se-
clusiveness, the moon, parental sins visited on the child, negative
childhood experiences, or bad breeding have all been held responsible.
We shall not attempt to trace the waxing and waning of these ideas
here, except to note that in the West, in the last 100 years there has
been a gradual erosion of the very generally held belief that heredity is
primarily responsible for abnormal behavior. An increasing emphasis
on environmental influences was caused by many factors. Changes in
political ideas led to increased public rather than private charity. This
produced an expansion of social work that resulted in reform of pris-
ons, workhouses, poorhouses, asylums for the insane and feeble mind-
ed, and educational systems. Because attention was often focused on a
better future for children, the period has sometimes been called the
Age of the Child. The generally optimistic attitude prevailed that, if
environmental conditions were improved enough, most insanity and
crime could be prevented. Among the thinkers responsible for these
ideas, perhaps foremost was Jean Jacques Rousseau, who believed in
the inborn goodness of the natural child and the inherently evil nature
of society. Later influential figures were August Comte, who introduced the concept of a scientifically organized society; Karl Marx, who
believed the reorganization of the economic structures of society
would inevitably lead to the emergence of a new, high-order civiliza-
tion; and Sigmund Freud, who posited that the ventilation of repressed
childhood anxieties would cure even severe behavioral abnormalities.
Another factor in the shift of emphasis from hereditary to environmental influence was the tendency of experimental psychologists during
the early part of the 20th century to focus on behavioristic studies of
animal learning. The emphasis on learning, due in part to the British
associationist tradition of a "blank slate" at birth, led to a rejection of
hereditary explanations for human behavioral traits. Thus, early be-
liefs that heredity played some role (either exclusive or contributory)
in the etiology of abnormal behavior were replaced to a large degree in
the first half of the 20th century by theories espousing the importance
of experiential events in determining the expression of human
behaviors.

It is only in recent years that the tide of opinion is turning again toward heredity. We now must guard against a tendency to go too far in this direction. Exclusion or even neglect of environmental hypotheses would be just as detrimental as the previous overemphasis of them. What we must strive for is the much more difficult accomplishment of an integration of viewpoints.

The presentation that follows will not attempt such an integration, however. Rather, it will emphasize those findings that suggest hereditary factors, although environmental influences and the interplay between heredity and environment will be mentioned when these factors are included as part of what is primarily genetic research. Unfortunately, little detailed knowledge exists about how specific environmental factors affect a particular diagnostic entity.

DIFFICULTY OF ACCURATE DIAGNOSIS

Emil Kraepelin (1896, 1921) was one of several 19th-century psychiatrists who gradually established modern psychiatric diagnostic categories. A major contribution to the diagnostic system was Kraepelin's recognition of *dementia praecox* as a separate entity. (*Dementia praecox* was later renamed schizophrenia by yet another pioneer in psychiatric classification—Eugen Bleuler). Kraepelin distinguished schizophrenia from manic-depressive illness. He based this distinction on differences in lifetime patterns of illness. Schizophrenia has an earlier onset than manic-depressive illness, tends to be accompanied by delusions and hallucinations, and often is a lifetime condition. Manic-depressive illness is episodic. During symptom-free intervals, the affected individual functions quite normally. As a result, there is generally not as much deterioration of the personality as one observes in schizophrenia. Also, in manic-depression there is often no distortion of reality other than feelings of worthlessness.

Bleuler (1911/1950), using a Freudian point of view, introduced psychodynamic concepts into his theories about the origin of the psychoses. One consequence of this was to weaken the sharp distinction Kraepelin felt existed between schizophrenia and manic-depression. As a result, new categories were proposed, including one in particular—schizoaffective disorder. As the name implies, this disorder was seen as a blend of symptoms of schizophrenia and manic-depressive illness.

Whatever the nature of patients in those earlier times, at present it is indeed occasionally difficult to distinguish between schizophrenia and manic-depressive disorders. The thoughts of a severely depressed or manic person can take bizarre forms. When regarding oneself an evil person, which sometimes occurs in depression, an individual's thoughts may begin to border on the delusional thinking that characterizes schizophrenia.

The reader who is not acquainted with the vicissitudes of various forms of mental illness may gain some insight by reading case histories and personal accounts by former patients. In so doing, it becomes quite apparent that the variation of symptomatology from one case to another is perplexingly large. Landis and Mettler (1964) have collected a number of excerpts, many from historical figures, whereas Stone and Stone (1966) and Kaplan (1964) have edited selections from literary works dealing with abnormal personalities. Most of these selections were written by recovered individuals or someone close to a patient. As brief illustrations, consider the following, written by or about individuals all diagnosed as suffering from symptoms of mania and/or depression.

In a chapter entitled The Sick Soul in his book *The Varieties of Religious Experience,* James quoted from a manuscript written by a depressed person.

> Whilst in this state of philosophic pessimism and general depression of spirits about my prospects, I went one evening into a dressing-room in the twilight to procure some article that was there; when suddenly there fell upon me without any warning, just as if it came out of the darkness, a horrible fear of my own existence. Simultaneously there arose in my mind the image of an epileptic patient whom I had seen in the asylum, a black-haired youth with greenish skin, entirely idiotic, who used to sit all day on one of the benches, or rather shelves against the wall, with his knees drawn up against his chin, and the coarse gray undershirt, which was his own garment, drawn over them enclosing his entire figure . . . . *That shape am I,* I felt, potentially. Nothing that I possess can defend me against that fate, if the hour for it should strike for me as it struck for him. There was such a horror of him, and such a perception of my own merely momentary discrepancy from him, that it was as if something hitherto solid within my breast gave way entirely, and I became a mass of quivering fear. After this the universe was changed for me altogether. I awoke morning after morning with a horrible dread at the pit of my stomach, and with a sense of insecurity of life . . . . I remember wondering how other people could live, how I myself had ever lived, so unconscious of that pit of insecurity beneath the surface of life . . . . I mean that the fear was so invasive that had I not clung to scripture-texts . . . . I think I should have grown really insane. (James, 1902, pp. 160–161)

Another quotation from a manuscript by a depressed patient emphasizes physical sensations.

> I was seized with an unspeakable physical weariness. There was a tired feeling in the muscles unlike anything I had ever experienced. A peculiar sensation appeared to travel up my spine to my brain. I had an indescribable nervous feeling. My nerves seemed like live wires charged with electricity.

My nights were sleepless. I lay with dry, staring eyes gazing into space. I had a fear that some terrible calamity was about to happen. I grew afraid to be left alone. The most trivial duty became a formidable task. Finally mental and physical exercises became impossible; the tired muscles refused to respond, my "think apparatus" refused to work, ambition was gone. My general tired feeling might be summed up in the familiar saying "What's the use." I had tried so hard to make something of myself, but the struggle seemed useless. Life seemed utterly futile. (Reid, 1910, pp. 612–613)

In contrast to the first two descriptions, the symptoms described next are much milder. This material was drawn from a case study included in *Psychopathology, A Case Book*, by Spitzer, Skodol, Gibbon, and Williams (1983), another excellent source for the reader who wishes to learn more about the intricacies of diagnosis.

Mary Griffith had a fragile air about her. Looking frightened, she sat with her coat on, her body perfectly still except for her hands twisting nervously on her lap and her quivering lower lip. Her eye contact was minimal, and her speech verged on a whisper.

Mary was 25 years old and had just begun her senior year in college. She had come seeking help for "depression" after she had seen a notice advertising a program for "coping with depression." Asked to recount how her life had been going recently, Mary began to weep. Sobbing, she said that for the last year or so she felt she was losing control of her life and that recent stresses (starting school again, friction with her boyfriend) had left her feeling worthless and frightened. Because of a gradual deterioration in her vision, she was now forced to wear glasses all day. "The glasses make me look terrible," she said, and " don't look people in the eye much any more." Also, to her dismay, Mary had gained 20 pounds in the past year. She viewed herself as overweight and unattractive. At times she was convinced that with enough money to buy contact lenses and enough time to exercise she could cast off her depression; at other times she believed nothing would help. She also complained of difficulty falling asleep, loss of energy, and not feeling interested in anything anymore.

Mary saw her life deteriorating in other spheres, as well. She felt overwhelmed by schoolwork and, for the first time in her life, was on academic probation. Twice before in the past seven years feelings of inadequacy and pressure from part-time jobs (as a waitress, bartender, and salesclerk) had caused her to leave school. She felt certain that unless she could stop her current downward spiral she would do so again—this time permanently. She despaired of ever getting her degree.

In addition to her dissatisfaction with her appearance and her fears about her academic future, Mary complained of a lack of friends. Her social network consisted solely of her boyfriend, with whom she was living. Although there were times she experienced this relationship as almost unbearably frustrating, she felt helpless to change it and was pessimistic about its permanence. (Spitzer *et al.*, 1983)

Some individuals suffer not only from depression but also have periods of mania. Below are portions taken from the well-known autobiographical account of Clifford Beers (1905, 1920).

My emotions on leaving New Haven were, I imagine, much the same as those of a condemned and penitent criminal who looks upon the world for the last time. The day was hot, and, we drove to the railway station, the blinds on most of the houses in the streets through which we passed were seen to be closed. The reason for this was not then apparent to me. I thought it was an unbroken line of deserted houses, and I imagined that their desertion had been deliberately planned as a sign of displeasure on the part of their former occupants. As citizens of New Haven I supposed them bitterly ashamed of such a despicable inhabitant as myself. (p. 34)

I know of no better way to convey to the reader my state of mind during these first weeks of elation than to confess—if confession it is—that when I set upon a career of reform I was impelled to do so by motives in part like those which seem to have possessed Don Quixote when he, madman that he was, set forth, as Cervantes says, with the intention "of righting every kind of wrong, and exposing himself to peril and danger, from which in the issue he would obtain eternal renown and fame". . . . What I wish to do is to make plain that one abnormally elated may be swayed irresistably by his best instincts, and that while under the spell of an exultation, idealistic in degree, he may be not only willing, but eager to assume risks and endure hardships which under normal conditions he would assume reluctantly, if at all. (pp. 85–88)

During the latter part of that first week I wrote many letters, so many, indeed, that I soon exhausted a liberal supply of stationery. . . . It was not at my own suggestion that the superintendent gave me large sheets of manila wrapping paper. These I proceeded to cut into strips a foot wide. One such strip, four feet long, would suffice for a mere billet-doux; but a real letter usually required several such strips pasted together. More than once letters twenty or thirty feet long were written; and on one occasion the accumulation of two or three days of excessive productivity, when spread upon the floor, reached from one end of the corridor to the other—a distance of about one hundred feet. My output per hour was something like twelve feet with an average of one hundred and fifty words to the foot. Under the pressure of elation one takes pride in doing everything in record time, despite my speed, however, my letters were not incoherent. They were simply digressive, which was to be expected, as elation befogs one's "goal idea." (p. 89)

We might compare these descriptions with the following sample from a much longer poem by Christopher Smart (1950) (1722–1771), who supposedly suffered from a "religious mania." As these selections clearly indicate, when the symptoms include unusual associations and delusional elements, it is frequently difficult to decide whether the patient is schizophrenic or manic or depressed. Often, only careful observation of the patient over time will provide the necessary clue to correct diagnosis.

OF JEOFFRY, HIS CAT

For I will consider my Cat Jeoffry.
For he is the servant of the Living God, duly and daily serving him.

For at the first glance of the glory of God in the East he worships in his
way.
For is this done by wreathing his body seven times round with elegant
quickness.
For then he leaps up to catch the musk, which is the blessing of God
upon his prayer.
For he rolls upon prank to work it in.
For having done duty and received blessing he begins to consider himself.
For this he performs in ten degrees.
For first he looks upon his fore-paws to see if they are clean.
For secondly he kicks up behind to clear away there.
For thirdly he works it upon stretch with the fore paws extended.
For fourthly he sharpens his paws by wood.
For fifthly he washes himself.
For sixthly he rolls upon wash.
For seventhly he fleas himself, that he may not be interrupted upon the
beat.
For eightly he rubs himself against a post.
For ninthly he looks up for his instructions.
For tenthly he goes in quest of food.

For having consider'd God and himself he will consider his neighbour.
For if he meets another cat he will kiss her in kindness.
For when he takes his prey he plays with it to give it chance.
For one mouse in seven escapes by his dallying.
For when his day's work is done his business more properly begins.
For (he) keeps the Lord's watch in the night against the adversary.
For he counteracts the powers of darkness by his electrical skin and
glaring eyes.
For he counteracts the Devil, who is death, by brisking about the life.
For in his morning orisons he loves the sun and the sun loves him.
For he is of the tribe of Tiger.
For the Cherub Cat is a term of the Angel Tiger.
For he has the subtlety and hissing of a serpent, which in goodness he
suppresses.
For he will not do destruction, if he is well-fed, neither will he spit
without provocation.
For he purrs in thankfulness, when God tells him he's a good Cat.
For he is an instrument for the children to learn benevolence upon.
For every house is incompleat without him and a blessing is lacking in
the spirit. (p. 118)

Adding a final note to this brief consideration of the history of
diagnostic concepts, it is amusing to remember that the term *neurosis*
("nervous" illness) originally was introduced to suggest a physical abnormality of the nerves, whereas *psychosis* referred to a psychological
or mental (i.e., nonorganic) abnormality. Today these two terms have
virtually exchanged meanings. A neurosis is often thought to be a
learned condition without a biological basis, but more and more recent
evidence is suggesting that there may be a biochemical basis for the so-
called "major psychoses," schizophrenia and affective disorder.

THE DIFFICULTY OF ESTIMATING INCIDENCE OF TYPES OF
MENTAL ABNORMALITY

As mentioned previously, it is very difficult to make an accurate estimate of the frequency of various types of mental illness. However, before one can apply genetic models, it is often necessary to have a reasonable estimate of the frequency of a disorder in the population. One may base such estimates on two different types of data: number of admissions to mental hospitals and clinics in a year, or number of patients occupying these institutions at a given time.

There are a number of difficulties with both methods. Some mentally ill individuals will not be reported because they are kept at home. The precise diagnostic criteria used by various institutions will differ; there may be delays, errors, and omissions in the reporting itself; and finally, the grouping of various illnesses into major categories varies among countries and, in this country, among regions of the country. Because of repeated admissions of the same persons, the two methods do not yield the same estimates. Nevertheless, some rough figures may be useful. At the end of World War II, before the introduction of psychotropic drugs, Landis and Bolles (1950) reported that of 1,000 adults, 8 to 10 would be diagnosed as neurotic, 6 to 8, feebleminded, 6 to 8, criminal or delinquent, 6 to 8, psychotic, and 2, epileptic. They reported that in 1946, there were 11,677 first admissions for neurosis, 12,078 for manic-depressive conditions, 29,753 for schizophrenia, and 3,000 for epilepsy. Referring back to the graph in Figure 1, we can see that there was a total of about 400,000 admissions in 1971. Although such figures will be somewhat different today, there is still a ratio of about 2.5 to 1 for schizophrenia and manic-depression.

Table 2, gives the number of patient-care episodes for the years 1955, 1965, 1971, 1975, and 1977. We see a steadily mounting number, perhaps due to discharges and readmissions now that drugs can bring improvements that may quickly be lost when discharged patients discontinue their medication. In Table 3, we see the same data on a per 100,000 basis. From the table it becomes clear that the state and county mental hospital population decreased from 1955 to 1977; the community mental health centers took up the difference, both in inpatient services and in outpatient services, whereas the proportion in private institutions remained about the same. The increase in the proportion in VA hospitals is perhaps due to the aging of World War II veterans plus some new patients who were veterans of the Korean and Vietnamese wars. The same source (p. 119 of the *1980 Statistical Abstracts in the United States*), suggests that in 1976 there were only

Table 2. Number of Patient Episodes for Mental Health Services in 1955,
1965, 1971, 1975 and 1977 (In Thousands)

	Inpatient services				Outpatient services		
	Mental hospitals				Community mental health services		
Year	State and county	Private	General hospitals	VA	Community mental health services	Community mental health services	Other	Total
1955	819	123	266	88	NA[a]	NA[a]	379	1675
1965	805	125	519	116	NA[a]	NA[a]	1071	2636
1971	748	127	543	177	130	623	1694	4042
1975	599	165	566	214	247	1585	3033	6409
1977	574	184	570	218	269	1742	3081	6640

[a]NA = not applicable, centers not yet existing.
Note. From Statistical Abstracts of the United States, 1980, p.121, by U.S. Department of Health, Education and Welfare. Washington, D.C.: Government Printing Office.

46,000 male and 18,000 female residents of psychiatric "long-term" institutions. This strengthens the interpretation that there must be many discharges and readmissions counted in Table 2.

Table 4 shows the number of patients in institutions for the mentally retarded during the period from 1960 to 1979. The decrease after 1970 may be due to the fact that individuals were cared for locally, although numbers are only given for this category for the year 1977.

Table 3. Rate of Patient Care Episodes for Mental Health Services per
100,000 population in the years 1955, 1965, 1971, 1975, 1977

	Inpatient services				Outpatient services		
	Mental hospitals				Community mental health centers		
Year	State and county	Private	General hospitals	VA	Community mental health centers	Community mental health centers	Other	Total
1955	502	76	163	54	NA[a]	NA[a]	233	1028
1965	420	65	271	60	NA[a]	NA[a]	559	1375
1971	365	66	266	89	64	305	829	2202
1975	283	78	268	101	117	750	1435	3032
1977	266	85	265	101	125	808	1429	3039

[a]NA = not applicable, centers not yet existing.
Note. From Statistical Abstracts of the United States, 1980, p. 121, by U.S. Department of Health, Education and Welfare. Washington, D.C.: Government Printing Office.

Table 4. Patients in Institutions for the Mentally Retarded in the years
1960, 1965, 1970, 1975, 1978, and 1979ª

	Year	Residents at start of year	Residents at end of year	New admissions	Rate for 100,000 population
	1960	158,682	163,730	14,701	91.9
	1965	181,549	187,273	17,300	97.7
State	1970	189,956	186,743	14,985	92.6
institutions	1975	166,689	159,041	13,424	75.2
	1978	161,562	152,476	14,286	70.4
	1979	155,114	147,729	17,308	67.6
Community facilities	1977	17,396	62,397	17,398	29.1

ªFigures for deaths and live releases omitted.
Note. From *Statistical Abstracts of the United States*, 1980, p. 121, by U.S. Department of Health, Education and Welfare. Washington, D.C: Government Printing Office.

Also noted in the U.S. 1980 Statistical Abstracts is the fact that 11,000 male and 78,000 female residents were in "long-term" institutions for the mentally handicapped for the year 1976. Note that the estimate of 188,000 is similar to the figure given for 1970 in Table 4 or to the sum of the figures for state institutions for 1978 (or 1979) *plus* the figure for community facilities in 1977. Thus, there appears to be no big change in the incidence of severe mental retardation from 1960 through 1979 but perhaps a marked shift toward the use of local facilities.

CRITICISMS OF METHODS FOR MAKING PSYCHIATRIC DIAGNOSES

Currently there are two diametrically opposed camps that offer criticisms of the way in which diagnostic categories are assigned to the various forms of mental illness. One of these groups feels that the medical model is inappropriate. They view mental illness as a sociocultural phenomenon and, for that reason, are adverse to any diagnostic process. Taken to the extreme, it is this group that speaks of the "myth of mental illness" (Szasz, 1961). On the other hand, there are many professionals who advocate less reliance on clinical interviews, projective tests, and the sociocultural aspects of diagnosis, and an increased emphasis on biochemical and neurophysiological signs of a disorder.

In a third variation of these criticisms leveled at psychiatric diagnostic methods, Buchsbaum and Haier (1983) would like to reverse the traditional medical model approach in which one attempts only after the fact to find laboratory procedures that separate patients into the traditional diagnostic categories. They argue that, even in the best psychiatric research studies, agreement about the diagnosis is seldom above .75 (which accounts for just 50% of the variance). Therefore, it may be more appropriate if, at least in research, laboratory results were used as the point of departure against which the success of medication, the patient's history and family background, symptoms and the like are evaluated. It seems likely, they argue, that different diagnostic groupings would result from this method and that some of those groupings might be closer to the underlying biological facts. Thus, Buchsbaum and Haier are *not* saying that the medical model is wrong, just that it is not being utilized correctly.

They believe that the lack of consistency to date in the biochemical research directed at finding differences between psychiatric disorders may reflect too much error in the original diagnoses. Groupings of patients based on laboratory tests may at first seem somewhat far removed from the obvious concern one has for symptoms, but after suitable analyses by clustering techniques the test results may well prove to be very predictive of patients' responses to treatment.

Further, Buchsbaum and Haier note that often "physical illness can complicate the psychiatric picture not only by requiring . . . treatment, which may interact with psychiatric medication, but which may mimic mental illness." Jefferson and Marshall (1981) have summarized the various physical illnesses that can produce symptoms resembling psychiatric disorders. These include cardiovascular, respiratory, gastrointestinal, renal, and endocrine malfunctions as well as certain effects of the aging process. One wonders how often such causes of chronic abnormal behavior are overlooked. In addition, it is becoming more apparent that psychological symptoms may often arise from treatment of physical illness, especially with some of the powerful drugs that are used in today's pharmacotherapy. The habitual use of recreational drugs may also contribute to the incidence of mental illness that is a direct result of a known physiological agent. However, Buchsbaum and Haier do caution that even in physical medicine there is rarely a perfect correlation between laboratory tests and a disease entity. Some tests exclude a number of affected individuals (false negatives).

Other tests err toward false positive results, so the final diagnosis in medicine in general remains a matter of weighing several types of evidence in a probabilistic manner rather than in a fully deterministic way. Given the delicate complexity of the workings of the brain, it is even less likely that we will, in the near future, have fully accurate laboratory tests upon which to base diagnosis of mental illness.

METHODS FOR DIAGNOSING BEHAVIOR DISORDERS: RATING SCALES AND CLASSIFICATION SYSTEMS

With the application of modern statistical methods, in particular factor analysis, there have been many efforts to make the diagnostic procedure more precise.

Several rating scales have been developed that require judging whether or not a particular behavioral syndrome is displayed by the patient or how strongly and/or how often it occurs. Some of the best-known scales of this type are by Wittenborn (1955, 1962), Lorr, Klett, and McNair (1963), Overall and Gorham (1962), Lorr, Klett, McNair, and Lasky (1963), Crown and Crisp (1966, 1970), and Endicott and Spitzer's Schedule for Affective Disorders and Schizophrenia, or SADS (1978). Such rating scales are usually "scored" in such a way as to result in a diagnostic profile of each individual evaluated. One of the most interesting efforts to develop a rating scale of this type was a cooperative analysis of ratings of about 1,200 psychiatric patients from the following countries: Columbia, Czechoslovakia, Denmark, India, Nigeria, China, U.S.S.R., the United Kingdom, and the U.S.A. In this international study of schizophrenia organized by the World Health Organization, a computer program, Catego, was used to derive a clearer clinical definition of the disorder (Cooper, 1970; Cooper et al., 1972; Sartorius, 1976; WHO, 1973). This program took 350 items from the Present State Examination to form 140 symptoms that, in turn, defined 35 syndromes; these syndromes were grouped into 6 descriptive categories that finally constituted 2 main classes—schizophrenia and psychotic depression (see Figure 2). Using this method, it was possible to count the frequency of certain units of behavior in various types of patients.

Figure 3 shows the results of three types of disorders. Although there were differences between countries in the frequency with which particular symptoms were noted, there was a surprising level of overall similarity that suggests that a considerable degree of agreement about diagnosis can be achieved by using a checklist of symptoms. Of course, care must be taken to insure that the checklist is clinically accurate and reliable. Because of this positive evidence, the development of such scales is increasing, and the consistent use of particularly good scales in making diagnoses could be very helpful to future research in mental illness.

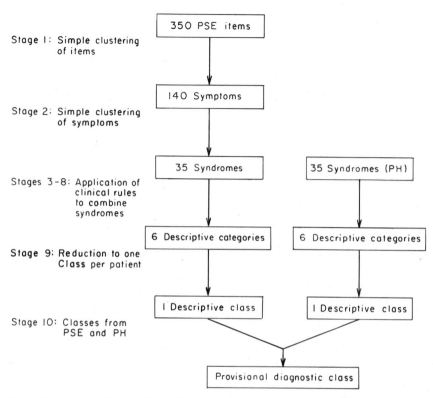

Stage 1: Simple clustering of items

Stage 2: Simple clustering of symptoms

Stages 3-8: Application of clinical rules to combine syndromes

Stage 9: Reduction to one Class per patient

Stage 10: Classes from PSE and PH

Figure 2. Summary chart of CATEGO Program. *Note.* From *Report of the International Pilot Study of Schizophrenia* by the World Health Organization, 1973, Geneva: World Health Organization.

Probably more helpful to the diagnostic process than rating scales for specific behavior disorders have been the ambitious attempts to catalog and describe a wide spectrum of disorders with sufficient clarity to allow a researcher or therapist to make diagnoses of many forms of mental illness in a systematic, reliable manner from patient to patient. This type of diagnostic system has been incorporated in the ICD-9-CM (*The International Classification of Diseases,* ninth edition), used by medical professionals in many countries throughout the world.

Another very rigorous and exacting classification system has been devised by Feighner *et al.* (1972) specifically for research purposes. Adherence to the diagnostic criteria in this system by researchers in the field of mental health will insure greater comparability of results across research efforts. For that reason, many of the researchers in the forefront of the field today are using Feighner criteria in selecting pa-

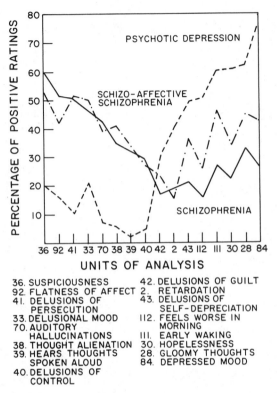

Figure 3. Percentage of positive ratings on selected units of analysis for all schizophrenia, psychotic depression, and schizo-affective schizophrenia. In this figure, percentage refers to the number of patients on whom the units were positive in relation to the total number of patients in the group. *Note.* From *Report of the International Pilot Study of Schizophrenia* by the World Health Organization, 1973, Geneva: World Health Organization.

tients for research. This approach has been elaborated upon by Spitzer, Endicott, and Robins (1975b, 1978) in their Research Diagnostic Criteria (RDC). The RDC in turn led to the construction of one of the structured interviews mentioned previously, the Schedule for Affective Disorders and Schizophrenia.

Perhaps the best-known of all the diagnostic systems in the United States is that of the *Diagnostic and Statistical Manual of Mental Disorders* of the American Psychiatric Association (1980). This manual, now in its third edition, is commonly referred to as the DSM-III and was first published in 1978. It is considered by many practitioners and researchers to be the most comprehensive document of its kind. In addition to outlining detailed, generally unambiguous criteria for the major forms of abnormal psychiatric conditions (see Table 5 for a list of disorders included in DSM-III), this system provides information regarding associated features that are often but not invariably part of the disorder: usual age of onset of symptomatology, prognosis or outcome of the disorder, common complications, predisposing factors, prevalence, sex ratio, and familial patterns. Finally, when certain disorders need to be distinguished from others, differential diagnostic criteria are provided.

The DSM-III was designed to be a so-called "multiaxial classification system." This is a modern concept, based on the fact that to treat a mental disorder most effectively, other aspects of an individual's life must be taken into account. Therefore, not only is the primary mental disorder identified in the system, but the presence of any accompanying personality disorders or developmental deficiencies are also noted. In addition, information is coded for each individual on such dimensions as physical disorders and psychosocial stress.

The code is based on five axes; Axes I and II include all the mental disorders: personality disorders and specific developmental disorders are coded on Axis II, whereas all the others are on Axis I. Axis III is for physical disorders and conditions. Axis IV codes severity of psychological stressors and Axis V, the highest level of adaptive functioning past

Table 5. Categories in the DMS-III *Classification of Mental Disorders*

Organic mental disorders	Dissociative disorders (or hysterical
Dementias arising in the senium and	neuroses, dissociative type)
presenium	Psychosexual disorders
Substance induced disorders	Gender identity disorders
Other organic brain syndromes	Paraphilias
Substance use disorders	Psychosexual dysfunction
Schizophrenic disorders	Other psychosexual disorders
Paranoid disorders	Factitious disorders
Psychotic disorders not elsewhere	Disorders of impulse control not else-
classified	where classified
Neurotic disorders	Adjustment disorder
Affective disorders	Psychological factors affecting physical
Major affective disorders	condition
Other specific affective disorders	Personality disorders
Atypical affective disorders	V-codes for conditions not attributable
Anxiety disorders	to a mental disorder that are a focus
Somatoform disorders	of attention or treatment
	Additional codes

Note. Adapted from *Diagnostic and Statistical Manual of Mental Disorders* (3rd ed.), pp. 15–19, by American Psychiatric Association, 1980, Washington, DC: American Psychiatric Association.

year. Two examples given in the DSM-III (pp. 30–31) of how this code is used are:

Axis I: 296.23 major depression, single episode, with melancholia
        309.93 alcohol dependence, in remission
Axis II: 301.60 dependent personality disorder (provisional, rule out
        borderline personality disorder)
Axis III: Alcoholic cirrhosis of liver
Axis IV: Psychosocial stressors: anticipated retirement and change in
        residence with loss of contact with friends Severity: 4—moderate
Axis V: Highest level of adaptive functioning past year: 3—good

Axis I: 295.92 schizophrenia, undifferentiated type, chronic V62.89
        borderline intellectual functioning (provisional)
Axis II: V71.09 No diagnosis on Axis II
Axis III: Late effects of viral encephalitis
Axis IV: Psychosocial stressors: death of mother Severity: 6—extreme
Axis V: Highest level of adaptive functioning past year: 6—very poor

USE OF PSYCHOLOGICAL INVENTORIES

Two somewhat different strategies can be distinguished in the development of psychological questionnaires for use with psychiatric patients. One can start with known psychiatric categories and attempt to develop items that will differentiate patients from normal controls. This is the strategy used in constructing the Minnesota Multiphasic Personality Inventory (MMPI), as described later. The second strategy is to develop scales that will cover the full range of personality variation in a normal population. One can either base the scale upon a personality theory, such as the typologies proposed by Jung (1923) or the needs and presses theory of Murray (1938). Or one may start "from scratch" by surveying the concepts of personality commonly found in the literature, developing questions that reflect those ideas, and then eliminating redundant, unclear, or contradictory items. An extreme example of the latter approach is provided by Cattell's development of a questionnaire based upon the compilation by Allport and Odbert (1936) of personality traits found in a dictionary. The questionnaire is described in detail by Cattell, Eber, and Tatsuoka (1970).

General personality tests with particularly impressive statistical properties are the Comrey Personality Scales (Comrey, 1970) and the Jackson Personality Research Form (Jackson, 1967, 1978). The Comrey test, which includes a validity check and a response bias measure, has the following eight scales: trust versus defensiveness, orderliness versus lack of compulsion, social conformity versus rebelliousness, activity versus lack of energy, emotional stability versus neuroticism, extraversion versus introversion, masculinity versus femininity, and empathy versus egocentrism. Jackson's test is based on the system of needs developed by Murray (1938). It measures 20 needs such as harm avoidance, play, social recognition, and the like.

By far the best-known psychological inventory of personality, the Minnesota Multiphasic Personality Inventory (MMPI) was constructed in 1940 by Hathaway and McKinley. Ten "clinical" scales were developed to measure various personality constructs, and 4 "validity" scales were designed to detect patterns of responses suggestive of improper or uncooperative test-taking behavior. These scales are listed in Table 6. The format of the approximately 550 items is basically a true/false self-reporting of attitudes, emotions, and behaviors that the authors believed were relevant to the diagnosis of mental illness. The items in the original version of the MMPI were drawn from a wide variety of clinical categories, as shown in Table 7.

Since its inception, there has been a veritable avalanche of studies reported that have used the MMPI. In 1975, for example, Dahlstrom, Welsh, and Dahlstrom included 6,000 references in their MMPI handbook. It probably would be impossible to summarize all the studies, but Graham (1977) and Greene (1980) provide useful condensations of

Table 6. MMPI Validity and Clinical Scales

Scale name	Number	Abbreviation
Validity		
Cannot say		?
Lie		L
F		F
K		K
Clinical		
Hypochondriasis	1	Hs
Depression	2	D
Hysteria	3	Hy
Psychopathic deviate	4	Pd
Masculinity-femininity	5	Mf
Paranoia	6	Pa
Psychasthenia	7	Pt
Schizophrenia	8	Sc
Hypomania	9	Ma
Social introversion	0	Si

Table 7. Categories of MMPI Items

Category	Number of items
General health	9
General neurologic	19
Cranial nerves	11
Motility and coordination	6
Sensibility	5
Vasomotor, trophic, speech, secretory	10
Cardiorespiratory	5
Gastrointestinal	11
Genitourinary	6
Habits	20
Family and marital	29
Occupational	18
Educational	12
Sexual attitudes	19
Religious attitudes	20
Political attitudes, law and order	46
Social attitudes	72
Affect, depressive	32
Affect, manic	24
Obsessive, compulsive	15
Delusions, hallucinations, illusions, ideas of reference	31
Phobias	29
Sadism, masochism	7
Morale	33
Lie	15
Total	504

Note. Adapted from "A Multiphasic Personality Schedule (Minnesota): I. Construction of the Schedule by S. R. Hathaway & J. C. McKinley, 1940, *Journal of Psychology, 10.*

some of the literature. It became clear rather early that the diagnostic precision of single scales was poor. This may be due in part to the fact that some constructs, such as psychasthenia and hysteria, have gone out of fashion. One construct, hypochondriasis, generally is not viewed as useful in diagnosing mental illness. On the other hand, it appears that the total pattern of a person's scores on the various scales, the "profile," does provide diagnostic information. In addition, a number of new scales have been developed for specific purposes. Some of the "content" scales developed by Wiggins (1966) seem to be especially promising (see Table 8). Note that most of these scales do not suggest a specific diagnosis but rather indicate various symptoms. Data on item and scale scores and profiles for 50,000 medical patients have been summarized by Swenson, Pearson, and Osborne (1973).

Besides general personality tests, a large number of tests or scales designed to "measure" more limited personality constructs exist. For example, a British questionnaire developed specifically to help diagnose psychiatric disorders is the Middlesex Hospital Questionnaire (Crown & Crisp, 1966, 1970). It has six scales: anxiety, phobic anxiety, obsessional neurosis, depression, somatic complaints, and hysteria. Crisp, Jones, and Slater (1978) have published the results of a validity study. Both a Hebrew version (Dasberg & Shalif, 1978) and a Dutch version (Dasberg, unpublished) have been developed.

Eysenck's Personality Inventory (Eysenck & Eysenck, 1977) was devised primarily to discriminate among psychotics, neurotics, and normals. In its present form, it has four scales: introversion versus extraversion (E); neuroticism versus emotional stability (N); a scale (P) that is sometimes said to measure "psychoticism" and at other times is referred to as measuring "psychopathy," that is, antisocial attitudes, including criminality; and a "lie" scale to detect a response style intended specifically to create a good impression.

The General Health Questionnaire, developed by a British psychiatrist (Goldberg, 1972),

> should give information only about the current mental state, so that the respondent should score high if the questionnaire is completed during a period of illness, but low if it is completed during a period of health. The questionnaire will therefore neither be a measure of long-standing attributes of personality such as Eysenck's neuroticism nor make assessments of the patient's liability to fall ill in the future. (p. 15)

Table 8. Wiggins' Content Scales

Abbreviation	Name
SOC	Social maladjustment
DEP	Depression
FEM	Feminine interests
MOR	Poor morale
REL	Religious fundamentalism
AUT	Authority conflict
PSY	Psychoticism
ORG	Organic symptoms
FAM	Family problems
HOS	Manifest hostility
PHO	Phobias
HYP	Hypomania
HEA	Health

A total of 139 items in the original questionnaire fell into the following 8 categories: general health and central nervous system (17 items); cardiovascular, neuromuscular, and gastrointestinal (18 items); sleep and wakefulness (19 items); observable behavior—personal behavior (22 items); observable behavior—relations with others (20 items); subjective feelings—inadequacy, tension, temper, and the like (25 items); and subjective feelings—mainly depression and anxiety (19 items). The validity of the total score was investigated in several studies reported by Goldberg (1972). There were 17 misclassifications in one study of 200 general practice patients; another study of 91 outpatients revealed 10 misclassifications. A shorter version of the questionnaire (a total of 60 items) has subsequently been developed. The Menninger Health Sickness Rating Scale (Luborsky, 1962), which attempts to assess an individual's mental health, is probably also more a measure of a "state" than of a "trait."

The single item in the General Health Questionnaire that discriminates best between patients and controls is indicative of failure to concentrate (Goldberg, 1972). However, when Broadbent, Cooper, FitzGerald, and Parkes (1982) used a questionnaire specifically designed to assess "cognitive failures," they found that absentmindedness, forgetting names, not remembering a passage just read, and other such "failures" were relatively common in the normal group in their study. Scores on their questionnaire correlated only minimally with the Eysenck "lie" scale and with a defensiveness measure from the Gough Adjective Checklist (Gough & Heilbrun, 1965), slightly with the Eysenck neuroticism scale, and not at all with Eysenck's E and P scales. It would be interesting to know whether scores on these questionnaires would increase shortly before the occurrence of a psychiatric illness.

Hoffer and Osmond (1961) developed a questionnaire for use with schizophrenic patients. The questionnaire consists of 145 true/false items designed to assess visual, auditory, olfactory, touch, and taste aspects of delusions and hallucinations as well as distorted time perception, unusual thoughts, and disturbed mood. Several of the questions are quite blunt and require a cooperative and truthful attitude on the part of the patient if valid information is to be obtained. It has been reported that as many as 30% of nonschizophrenics score above the established cutoff point (Buros, 1965). This may be partially attributable to the presence of similar (psychotic) symptoms in other types of patients such as those suffering from acute toxic conditions, mania, or brain damage.

Among scales measuring more narrowly defined entities are the

Leyton Obsessional Inventory (Cooper, 1970a), the Hamilton Depression Scale (Hamilton, 1960) and the Anxiety and Depression Scale developed by Hassanyeh, Eccleston, and Davison (1981). One of the newest self-report scales for depressive symptoms is the CES-D scale developed by Roberts and Vernon (1983) that reportedly correlates well with the Schedule for Affective Disorders and Schizophrenia described earlier. Bech (1981) has recently evaluated the validity and consistency of some of the most widely used depression scales.

Pollak (1978) has reviewed some of the personality tests measuring the obsessive-compulsive personality constellation. Hudson (1982) has published a collection of scales for use with persons without major psychiatric disorders, who seek help with personal or marital problems, whereas Ihilevich & Gleser (1982) constructed and validated a set of scales for evaluating progress toward mental health as a result of therapy.

Finally, mention should be made of the Global Assessment Scale (Endicott et al., 1976) that measures severity of behavior disorders by rating the patient's level of general functioning. The main purpose of this scale and its companion version, the Children's Global Assessment Scale (Rothman, Sorrells, & Heldman, 1976), is not to discriminate among diagnostic entities but rather to describe accurately the severity of disturbance.

PSYCHOLOGICAL PERFORMANCE TESTS USED FOR DIFFERENTIAL DIAGNOSIS

A wide variety of performance tests have been used in efforts to develop methods for differential diagnosis that might not be subject to deliberate or unwitting distortion by the patient, either to look better, or sometimes to look worse in order not to be discharged or denied help. Object-sorting tests were especially prominent for awhile, until the consensus seemed to be that brain-damaged patients performed similarly to schizophrenics. Various perceptual tests have also been investigated, such as the spiral aftereffect, the rod and frame test, size estimation, and size constancy.

Because disordered thinking is so common in schizophrenia, various attempts have been made to measure this systematically. Word association tests give results that differ from those of normals, but when the lower overall ability of schizophrenics is taken into account, the difference is generally no longer important. Other, more psycholinguistically sophisticated studies have not been successful either

(Broen 1969; Neale & Oltmanns 1980). Currently, measures of eye movements while scanning pictures or text, eyeblinks, evoked potentials, and other computer-driven and analyzed tasks are being studied. However, these newer techniques have not been tested enough to say anything definitive about their ability to assist in differential diagnosis.

The Nebraska version of the Luria battery of neuropsychological tests (Golden, Purisch, & Hammeke, 1979; Golden *et al.*, 1982) yields better results than other tests in discriminating brain-damaged from schizophrenic patients (Purisch, Golden, & Hammeke, 1978). A success rate of 88% was achieved using this method.

USE OF PSYCHOLOGICAL TESTS IN DIAGNOSING BRAIN DAMAGE

In comparison with the lack of progress in the differential diagnosis of psychoses and neuroses, there has been considerably more progress in the development of psychological tests for the detection and localization of brain damage. Although various new techniques are being developed for observing electrical activity in the brain, psychological tests are perhaps still the most useful means of determining the amount and type of brain damage. An example of a computer analysis of EEG data is described by Morihisa, Daffy, and Wyatt (1982). The three best-known test batteries are the Halstead-Reitan Neuropsychological Test Battery (Reitan & Davison, 1974), the Michigan Neuropsychological Test Battery (Smith, 1975), and the collection of tasks developed by Luria (see Christensen, 1974) and standardized by Golden, Purisch, and Hammeke (1979). Diamant (1981) has contrasted these two approaches and advocates an integration of both methods.

Probably because brain damage has traditionally been the domain of neurology, there is a long tradition of using circumscribed tasks to establish a precise inventory of intact and impaired psychomotor and perceptual functions. Because damage to different parts of the nervous system produces different patterns of impairment, a number of separate causes of neurological dysfunction have come to be recognized. Aside from head wounds or acute poisoning, these causes include strokes and a number of diseases. Among the diseases that cause brain damage are some, such as Alzheimer's disease, and other types of presenile dementia that are thought to have a hereditary basis. For a description of many of these, see Paulson and Allen (1970).

It is conceivable that the very specific tasks used in neurology may also prove useful in psychiatry, not only to exclude neurological disorder but also to aid in diagnosis of psychiatric patients. There is some evidence of larger cerebral ventricles—and hence an alteration in brain tissue—in some schizophrenics, although it is not known whether this is related to the cause—or the result—of schizophrenia (Weinberger & Wyatt 1982). We have already mentioned that Purisch, Golden, and Hammeke (1978) have even discriminated between brain-damaged and schizophrenic patients with the Nebraska version of the Luria test battery.

POSSIBLE DIAGNOSTIC USE OF BIOCHEMICAL TESTS

There has been an enormous amount of research aimed at finding biochemical differences between certain types of patients, such as manic-depressives or schizophrenics and either normal controls or other types of patients. Other patients are often included to control for the possible effects of hospital conditions such as restricted diet, limited exercise, and so forth. In some studies, they are included to control for the effects of therapeutic drugs. Although hope springs perennially, the results of all this biochemical research suggest it is unlikely that there will soon be available, for psychiatry, the kinds of biochemical tests that have been so effective in other areas of medicine. We say this in the conviction that (a) most major diagnostic categories are formed by heterogeneous types of patients; (b) variation in biochemical processes is sometimes the *cause* and sometimes the *result* of the mental illness; and (c) there are large individual differences in these processes that are themselves partly heritable but are not directly related to specific disorders.

Cowdry and Goodwin (1978) have suggested that multivariate analyses of patients' responses to various drugs may lead to a classification system different from the traditional one that is based mainly on behavioral symptoms.

Although we are not hopeful about the success of present diagnostic biochemical tests, a few recent proposals are included in later chapters. It is also possible that refinements of the diagnostic procedures involving interviews of patients and relatives plus evaluations of their life histories may produce further improvements in the diagnosis of psychoses and neuroses, which would allow possible differences to be seen more clearly. However, it appears that the major breakthroughs are most likely to result from genetic analyses, especially from studies of linkage of specific disorders to known genetic markers. Linkage studies present a different approach to the search for biochemical correlates of mental illness. We will briefly review the meaning of the term *linkage* as it is used in genetics in Chapter 4.

Despite the rather somber impression we have given from time to time in our discussion of diagnosis and of how difficult it remains to properly diagnose mental illness, one need only take a historical perspective to feel renewed optimism. As noted earlier in this chapter, it was not so very many years ago that mental illness was attributed to such things as evil spirits and the influence of the moon. We have made great progress from that point and will most likely continue to do so.

CHAPTER 3

Mental Retardation

HEREDITARY FACTORS IN MENTAL DEFICIENCY

The following discussion uses the definition of mental retardation suggested by the American Association on Mental Deficiency (Heber, 1959). It is "a disorder associated with significantly subaverage general intellectual functioning expressed concurrently with deficits in adaptive behavior and manifested during childhood."

Subaverage intellectual functioning is frequently defined as an IQ score of less than 70 on an intelligence test that has been standardized to have a mean score of 100 and a standard deviation of 15.

The debate regarding whether all mental deficiency is caused by environmental or hereditary factors continued well into the 20th century. Two prototypic lines of research helped to clarify the situation. The first was the elucidation of the etiology of phenylketonuria (PKU), and the other was the discovery of trisomy-21 associated with Down's syndrome.

Phenylketonuria (PKU)

In 1934, a Scandinavian physician, Fölling, observed that several severely retarded patients (including some sets of siblings) had a peculiar, characteristic odor about them. This finding prompted him to do extensive biochemical tests of these individuals, which in turn led to his discovery that these patients excreted large amounts of phenylpyruvic acid in their urine. Five years later, Jervis (1939) provided evidence that this disorder, which we refer to as PKU, was due to a single autosomal recessive gene. He did so by demonstrating that a person affected with the disease had received an abnormal gene from both parents, who were heterozygous for the disorder and were not affected. Heterozygosity in the parents was deduced from the presence of other affected relatives in their families. Subsequently, Jervis, Block, Bolling, and Krange (1940) and Jervis (1953, 1959) reported that the system of phenylketonuric individuals contained large amounts of amino acid, phenylalanine, which was not metabolized in the normal way into tyrosine (see Figure 4). They hypothesized that the abnormal amounts of phenylalanine acted to disrupt the development of the

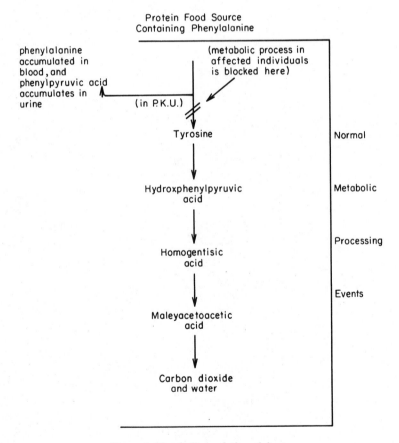

Figure 4. Metabolism of phenylalanine.

nervous system in affected children. These observations led to the conclusion that the defect was due to the inactivity of the liver enzyme, phenylalanine hydroxylase. This finding verified a prediction made by the English clinician, Garrod (1909), that "inborn errors of metabolism" would be found in which specific pathways could be traced from a mutant gene through the defective enzyme it produced to a given disease that was the final result of the abnormal genetic material. Although PKU is caused by the inactivity of phenylalanine hydroxylase, the mental retardation seen in these patients is a secondary phenomenon. Posen and Van Bogaert (1959) and Crome, Tymms, and Woolf (1962) showed that defective myelination of nerve cells in the brain caused by lower amounts of brain cerebrosides is present in PKU patients. The reduced myelin presumably is the major cause of the severe mental deficiency.

Soon after the identification of the cause of PKU, a treatment was proposed based on the premise that a diet low in phenylalanine begun soon after birth would eliminate a buildup of toxic substances in the system (Armstrong & Tyler, 1955; Bickel, 1954). The researchers reasoned that the mother provides normal nutrition for the fetus before birth, and it is only after birth that the infant starts to metabolize foods containing phenylalanine. This begins the insidious process that results in damage to the developing brain. In addition, Hsia, Troll, and Knox (1956) showed that heterozygotes ("carriers") could be detected by "loading" their systems with excess amounts of phenylalanine. This finding permitted more effective genetic counseling of relatives of affected persons and provided the final proof of the recessive nature of PKU.

Screening of newborns for PKU is now widespread. In most hospitals in the United States, a blood sample is taken within the first few days after birth. If excessively high levels of phenylalanine are found, further testing is done. For those individuals who are diagnosed as having phenylketonuria, commercial diets low in phenylalanine are readily available. This has led to a massive reduction in retardation due to PKU, which occurs on the average in 1 in 10,000 births and in the past accounted for 1% of institutionalized mental defectives. (An incidence of the defect of 1 in 10,000 is equivalent to a gene frequency of about 1 in every 100 individuals in the population.)

Despite this success, a number of research questions remain unanswered. For example, even though there has been a clear specification of the enzyme defect, the gene for PKU has only been tentatively assigned a location on chromosome 1, and other loci are involved in rarer types of hyperphenylalaninemias (Scriver & Clow 1980). Some

individuals with high phenylalanine blood levels who are not provided
with a special diet may escape serious mental retardation (Knox 1974)
and when put on the diet may suffer or even die from malnutrition
(Scriver & Clow 1980). Science still has not provided a good way to
prevent the often noted *in utero* damage to children by their treated
PKU mothers, and we do not know specifically how the cerebrosides
are affected, or whether there has been a selective advantage for the
heterozygote in our evolutionary past, which helped to maintain the
rather high frequency of the defective gene in the population. Mc-
Cullough (1978) has suggested that heterozygotes have less skin
melanin and are therefore are able to produce more vitamin D_3, thus
reducing the incidence of rickets. He did find a correlation between
PKU frequencies and availability of midwinter sunlight in European
countries, thus supporting this idea. Many other errors of metabolism
resulting in mental retardation have since been described and are listed
in Stanbury, Wyngaarden, and Fredericksen (1966), Carter (1970), and
McKusick (1978). Fortunately, most of these conditions are not as
prevalent as PKU, suggesting that the gene frequencies are lower, or
the frequency of spontaneous abortion is higher than for PKU.

Trisomy 21 and Other Aneuploidies

During most of its life, a cell shows a rather undifferentiated nucleus. It is only when the cell is getting ready to divide into two new
cells that individual chromosomes become visible. Because only a few
cells in any sample will be in that stage at any one time, a dividing cell
is difficult to find under a microscope. No really good photographs of
human chromosomes existed prior to 1956, and even the generally
accepted chromosome number was wrong, until Tjio and Levan (1956)
reported that humans had 46 chromosomes rather than the 48 previously reported in textbooks. Their procedure for producing photographs of human chromosomal material was based upon some effective techniques developed by plant geneticists which we will describe.

First, cells were cultured *in vitro* so that they could be made to
divide more frequently. White blood cells were utilized, as they are
easy to obtain. This type of culture is still used, although cells from
many other tissues including bone marrow or dermal skin tissues can
also be utilized. Then an alkaloid, colchicine, is added to the culture.
Colchicine has the useful property of arresting cell division at the stage

called *metaphase*, when each chromosome has doubled and is ready to move away from its partner. If one waits some hours after adding colchicine, large numbers of cells will be found in which all the chromosomes are visible. Those cells in which the chromosomes are suitably arranged for clearly photographing each one separately can then be selected. Third, a hypotonic salt solution is applied, causing the cells to expand so that the chromosomes move farther apart. A microscope is then utilized to search for a clear set of chromosomes in this preparation. Several such sets are usually photographed for each sample. After photographing, the developed prints are cut apart and the individual chromosomes arranged in a "karyotype" such as that shown in Figure 5. When other investigators applied this technique, they not only confirmed the normal chromosome number to be 46 but began to identify exceptions. This new technique also provided more details about human chromosomal material. It was found that various chromosomes were clearly of different size. For example, the male sex chromosome (Y) was found to be the smallest, whereas the female sex chromosome (X) was of average size.

Using these techniques Lejeune, Gautier, and Turpin (1959) discovered that nine children affected with mongolism (or Down's syndrome) each had 47, rather than 46, chromosomes. The extra chromosome was later identified as probably being a number 21 (thus the

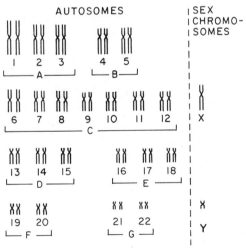

Figure 5. Schematic presentation of human chromosomes arranged in accord with the Denver convention.

designation *trisomy-21*). This finding helped explain why the condition is congenital (present at birth), and why it is presented in both members of identical twin pairs but rarely present in both fraternal twins or in siblings or other relatives of affected individuals. It is due to the failure of a newly formed pair of chromosome 21 to split apart. This phenomenon, referred to as *nondisjunction*, occurs during meiotic cell division, so that one sex cell (egg or polar body in females and sperm cell in males) receives two chromosomes and the other cell in the pair receives none. The absence of a chromosome 21 is more likely a lethal mutation; however three chromosomes 21 produce a viable zygote.

Down's syndrome is a frequently encountered form of moderate to severe mental retardation with a frequency rate of .15% of all newborns in the United States. Down's syndrome individuals usually express the upward and outward slant of eyelid fissures and epicanthal folds of the lids so characteristic of this disorder. A slackness of muscle tone, especially noticeable in the facial muscles is also common, as are white spots in the iris (Brushfield spots). There is a high risk for respiratory ailments, heart malformations, and leukemia among Downs's syndrome children that acts to reduce their expected life span drastically.

The incidence of Down's syndrome is highly correlated with maternal age. Penrose and Smith (1966) collected data on 9,441 births among mothers of various ages. They found that mothers older than 35 had given birth to about 56% of all the Down's syndrome children in the sample and to only 16% of all the normal children. This is a sharp contrast to mothers younger than 35, who gave birth to 84% of all the normal children in the sample. Because of age-related phenomena such as this, it has been suggested that nondisjunction increases with maternal age. To date, there is very little evidence that paternal age is directly correlated with the incidence of Down's syndrome. Therefore, most nondisjunction hypotheses suggest that the disorder is related to the effects of long-term exposure of the 300,000 to 400,000 ova that are present in the human female at birth to biochemical events that affect the body over the course of the normal adult reproductive period.

Human sex chromosomes, that is, those chromosomes that directly determine gender, normally assort in a single pair. Normal females and males are denoted by XX and XY pairs, respectively. However, Jacobs and Strong (1959) first reported an individual with an extra X chromosome (XXY); Ford, Jones, Polani, DeAlmeida, & Briggs (1959) first reported an individual with only one sex chromosome (XO), and Jacobs *et al.*, (1980) were the first to have reported an XYY. Another

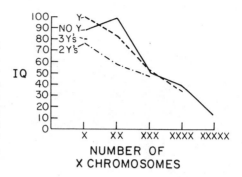

Figure 6. Mean IQ of individuals with varying numbers of X chromosomes. *Note.* Adapted from survey data collected in "Niveau intellectuel et polygonosome: Confrontation du caryotype et du niveau mental de 374 malades dont le caryotype comporte un exces de chromosomes X ou Y" by L. Moore, 1967, *Revue de Neuropsychiatrie Infantile.*

chromosomal anomaly, the XXY, was discovered by Sandberg, Koef, Ishihara, and Hauschka (1961). The XO anomaly produces a condition referred to as Turner's syndrome, and the condition produced when there is at least one Y and two or more X chromosomes is called Klinefelter's syndrome. Since chromosomal anomalies were first discovered in 1959, all possible combinations with up to five sex chromosomes have been reported. The degree of mental retardation in these cases seems roughly proportional to the amount of excess chromosomal material. This can be seen in Figure 6, which was prepared from survey data collected by Moor (1967). With regard to retardation, each extra X seems to do more harm than an extra Y chromosome. The phenomenon of abnormal chromosome number is called *aneuploidy.*

Precise identification of individual chromosomes within a group made up of others of approximately the same size was not possible before the advent of chemical staining techniques that reveal unique banding patterns associated with each chromosome (see Figure 7). Lubs and Walknowska (1977) summarized a number of different partial aneuploidies such as deletions or duplications of some bands on some of the chromosomes. Most of these produce a distinctive syndrome, usually involving some degree of mental and motor retardation and frequently producing a characteristic distortion of the facial features. In fact, the latter has proven to facilitate diagnosis in several cases. Since 1977, additional deletions and duplications have been reported. Even more minor abnormalities, such as variations in the width of bands, have been suggested. As it becomes practical to measure these variations with sufficient precision, researchers may find that there are hereditary characteristics that can be used as genetic markers in the search for relationships between behavioral traits and genetic loci that have already been located on a particular chromosome.

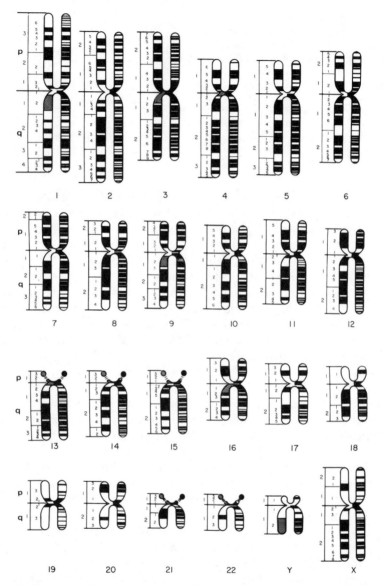

Figure 7. Chromosome banding patterns: (p) denotes the two upper arms of each chromosome; (q) denotes the two lower arms of each chromosome. *Note.* From "High Resolution of Human Chromosomes" by J. J. Yunis, March 1976, *Science, 191.* Copyright 1976 by the American Association for the Advancement of Science. Reprinted by permission.

X-linked Inheritance

Early reports of pedigrees showing an X-linked pattern of inheritance for mental retardation did not receive much attention, in part because many authors suspected that the observed excess of male retardates might be due to cultural factors such as an admission bias on the part of institutions or greater tolerance for low IQ in girls than in boys. But, in 1969, Davison noted that individuals with an IQ below 55 are male in disproportionate numbers and suggested that gene mutations carried on the X chromosome may contribute to such severe retardation. In 1974, Lehrke reported on several families that had evidence of retardation carried by females and expressed most often through their sons. (Allan, Herndon, & Dudley, 1944; Dunn, Renpenning, Gerrard, Miller, Tabata, & Federoff, 1963; Losowsky, 1944; Martin & Bell, 1943; Renpenning, Gerrard, Zaleski, & Tabata, 1962). He also described five additional large pedigrees that did not show father-to-son transmission of mental retardation. In these pedigrees, 105 out of 282 male offspring of suspected female carriers exhibited retardation, whereas very few female offspring were retarded. Further, Wolff, Hameister, and Roper (1978) reported transmission of mental retardation by a *normal* male to 4 of his 12 daughters but to none of his 12 sons! Except for the absence of any evidence that the father was retarded, this is a classical pattern for X-linked inheritance, wherein the father's X-linked condition was expressed in some of his daughters but in none of his sons, who by virtue of being male inherited a Y chromosome from their father rather than an X chromosome. One wonders what the intelligence of this father's siblings and parents was. It could be that the father was less intelligent than his family members, although his IQ might still have been in the normal range.

These descriptions of families that manifest X-linked inheritance of mental retardation suggested one reason for the considerable excess of males over females among the mentally retarded. In the past, it was frequently argued that this excess merely reflected a greater variability in intelligence in males, so that there would be more males than females at both extremes of the distribution. In other words, in comparison with females, there would be more males among the severely retarded and among the highly gifted. This sex effect was attributed to the fact that females have two X chromosomes. Possession of two X chromosomes could provide protection against a recessive gene leading to mental retardation; however, it is difficult to see how having two X chromosomes would reduce the incidence of very high intelligence because that would require that the gene or genes for *high* intelligence also be located on the X chromosome. If that were the case and if the genes for high intelligence were recessive, females would be highly gifted only if both X chromosomes carried the alleles—a much less likely event than for males to receive just one X chromosome with the recessive alleles. This idea of a rare, recessive allele providing some-thing beneficial to the individual is rather unusual. Rare recessives that are harmful seem to be the rule. (It should be noted, however, that a hypothetical X-linked spatial gene has been proposed to account for the sizable sex difference in spatial visualization ability in favor of males. However, it has also been suggested that the allele for good spatial ability has a frequency of .50 [Bock & Kolakowski, 1973], so it is possible to regard the other allele as one leading to poor spatial ability and also having a frequency of .50.)

In 1969, Lubs first described a fragile site located on the X chromo-some around the region referred to as "locus q 27" that may explain X-linked mental retardation. There have subsequently been several other reports of an association between retardation and the chromosomal abnormality referred to as "fragile X" (Deroover, Fryns, Parloir, & Van Den Berghe, 1977; Giraud, Ayme, Mattei, & Mattei, 1976; Harvey, Judge, & Wiener, 1977; Shapiro, Kuhr, Wilmot, Lilienthal, & Higgs, 1982; Sutherland & Ashforth, 1979; Van Den Berghe, Deroover, Par-loir, & Fryns, 1978). A fragile site is an area on a mitotic metaphase chromosome that does not stain as this area normally does. The cause of the phenomenon is not known. It may lead to breakage of the chro-mosomal material at that point, but this is not used as a criterion by everyone. Fragile sites have been reported on Chromosomes 2, 10, 11, 16, and 20, as well as on the X chromosome, although the fragile X has received the most attention. Sutherland (1977, 1979a, 1979b) showed that fragile sites were more likely to be observed with a particular cell-culturing medium, commonly refered to as "medium 199," which is deficient in folic acid. He proposed that higher pH values of the medi-um caused fragile sites to be revealed in a larger percentage of cells. This percentage varies widely among studies and also among indi-viduals in a single study.

Turner and Turner (1974) had suggested that there might be a correlation between the number of cells showing a fragile X and the degree of mental retardation. However, Sutherland's discovery of the effect of the culture medium indicates that any such observed correla-tions are likely to be artifacts or, at least, very unreliable. Neverthe-less, gross differences in percentage of fragile X chromosomes may be related to differences in mental ability, especially if one takes into account Mary Lyon's (1961) hypothesis. Lyon proposed that in females, in every cell, one of the two X chromosomes is inactivated; that this happens rather early, after only a small number of cell divisions; and that it is a matter of chance whether the maternal X or the paternal X is turned off. This hypothesis is consistent with observations of the incorporation of radioactive material during DNA replication, an indication that one of the two X chromosomes replicates late. This is the one that is thought to be inactive. Thus, according to the Lyon hypothesis, females are "mosaic" for the X chromosome. *Mosaicism* is a term used to describe the phenomenon in which cells differ in the expression of genetic material. Although mosaicism was rather difficult to demonstrate, it is now well established. The occurrence of inactivation after only a small number of cell divisions means that a whole organ system might be descended from a cell with a given X inactivated, so that all the cells in that system (the retina, for example) could have the same X turned off. If the Lyon hypothesis holds true for the fragile X, the degree of mental retardation would be dependent upon the percentage of cells with a normal X chromosome that is inactivated versus the percentage of cells in which a fragile X is inactivated.

In Uchida and Joyce's (1982) study of two sisters heterozygous for the fragile X, they found that it was the X chromosome containing the fragile site that was activated in 100 out of 126 cells in one sister and in 85 out of 120 cells in the other. For two controls with fragile X chromosomes but normal intelligence, the numbers of cells in which the fragile X was activated were 40 out of 78 and 10 out of 32.

The degree of mental retardation produced by the fragile X occasionally may be mild enough so that it may be overlooked unless there are other affected persons in the family. Perhaps the effect of the fragile X would be particularly likely to be overlooked in more gifted families, where a drop of 30 points from an average family IQ of 125, for example, would still leave an IQ of 95 (Nielsen, Tommerup, Poulsen, & Mikkelsen, 1981). It is not known whether the apparently wide range of retardation is entirely due to variation in average family intelligence, or whether the fragile X itself has a variable effect. Such a variable effect could be due to the fact that the number of cells showing the fragile X varies among patients, as does the percentage of those fragile Xs that are activated in females. Another interesting feature of the condition as noted to date is that retardation in females is found at a higher frequency than would be expected for a recessive trait. In the study noted previously of a kindred that was reported by Nielsen *et al.*, 4 of the 10 affected individuals were female. This proportion would suggest dominant transmission, but there are too many exceptions to this pattern to really entertain that hypothesis at this time.

The study of X-linked mental retardation is further complicated by reports suggesting heterogeneity. We have already mentioned the remarkable family reported by Wolff *et al.* (1978) in which the father was seemingly unaffected. An association between macroorchidism (clinical enlargement of the testicles in males) and X-linked retardation has been reported in several papers (Cantu *et al.*, 1976; Escalante, Grunspun, & Frota-Passod, 1971; Turner, English, Lindsay, & Turner, 1972; Turner *et al.*, 1975). It is not known to what extent the fragile X condition overlaps with the symptom of macroorchidism. Individuals in the early studies of X-linked retardation were not examined for either the fragile X or enlarged sexual organs (although extreme instances of the latter might well have been mentioned in the published reports if it had been present). Juberg and Massidi (1980) have reported on a male child and two maternal uncles with rudimentary scrotum, small penis, mental retardation, deafness, and similar facial features. They suggest that this is a unique type of X-linked retardation. Another form of X-linked retardation has been reported by Davis, Silverberg, Williams, Spiro, and Shapiro (1982), who found nine retarded males with progressive spastic quadriparesis in three generations of one family. Finally, Fried and Sanger (1973) have suggested that there may be linkage between the blood group allele X_g and a gene causing mental retardation.

As Kaiser-McCaw, Hecht, Cadlin, and Moore (1980) have emphasized, there remain many unanswered questions concerning X-linked mental retardation. The frequency and distribution in the population of fragile X sites are perhaps the most interesting unknown factors. If the fragile X syndrome could account for most of the excess males at the lower end of the IQ distribution, one would no longer expect to find an equivalent excess of males at the upper end of the distribution. A greater frequency of males than females with very high IQs has been suggested to account for the relative scarcity of female geniuses. If that explanation is no longer plausible, cultural explanations become more likely. However, questions concerning the variable effect of the fragile X and the mode of transmission cannot be answered until many more families have been studied.

PREVALENCE OF GENETICALLY RELATED FORMS OF MENTAL RETARDATION

A comprehensive list of genetic causes of mental retardation would include hundreds of disorders. Many of these forms are extremely rare, however. The Appendix contains a partial list of some of the better documented, more prevalent disorders.

While the number of known genetic causes of mental retardation keeps increasing, it is difficult to determine what proportion of the cases is attributable to hereditary factors. Estimates vary considerably. When Dupont (1980) analyzed the records of 1,500 mental retardates registered in Denmark, he found that genetic factors appeared to be involved in only 7% of the cases. Much larger percentages have been reported by other investigators, however. For example, analyses of preliminary data from a study of 650 retardates conducted at the University of Leuven (Van Den Berghe, Fryns, Parloir, Deroover, & Keulemans, 1980) indicated that 15.2% of the cases were due to chromosomal anomalies (including small deletions, translocations, etc.); 16.9% were due to single genes, and 5.7% may have been due to the influence of polygenic inheritance. Linna, Koivisto, and Herva (1980) reported that 27.5% of 1,000 cases of mental retardation appeared to be due to chromosomal abnormalities. Perhaps the much lower percentage of apparent genetic involvement in the Danish study is attributable to the fact that the data were based on older records collected before highly technical karyotyping and banding techniques were perfected.

Fryers (1981) summarized recent attempts to measure the prevalence of severe mental retardation in various countries. He discussed differences in rates in terms of the criteria used and the age structure of the population. Estimates varied from 2 to 5 per thousand.

Another Cause of Mental Retardation

In addition to single-gene abnormalities such as PKU, chromosomal anomalies such as trisomy-21, and X-linked causes of mental retardation there may be yet another explanation for a certain proportion of low intelligence that is not related to a disorder in the clinical sense of the word. If intelligence is approximately normally distributed, as it seems to be in the general population, the distribution would have two tails: one at the low end as well as one at the high end. Although further genetic discoveries may reduce the proportion of persons of low intelligence with no known hereditary abnormality, it seems plausible that there will always be some individuals who fall at the lower extreme of the distribution of intelligence—just as in the case of height or any other continuous variable, both extremes are represented in the population. To the extent that intelligence is influenced by heredity, this form of retardation will also be a product of gene action. However, even the most staunch hereditarians agree that intelligence is influenced by environmental factors as well. Thus, many researchers have begun to call mental retardation that is not associated with any obvious genetic anomaly or medical trauma, "cultural-familial" retardation. Relative to this hypothesized form of mental retardation, and currently at issue, is the question: what proportion of the variance in intelligence is genetic, and what proportion is influenced by environmental conditions? Opinions on this issue depend to some extent on the research approach used by the investigator. For example, calculation of correlations between parents and children and between other relatives, comparisons of identical and fraternal twin similarities, studies of adopted children and their biological and adoptive parents, research on the effects of inbreeding, and studies of identical twins reared apart are representative of techniques that have been used to analyze the strength of hereditary factors as they affect a given trait. Investigations of specific environmental factors have focused on such variables as birth order, child-rearing practices of the parents, nutrition, illnesses and injuries before, during, and after birth, including such known factors as rubella, maternal alcohol consumption, and anoxia at delivery.

A problem with the research done in this area is related to the fact that most of the studies to date have each considered only one of the possible environmental variables that might influence intelligence. Thus, it becomes very difficult to integrate the findings. Ideally, one would like to be able to state what proportion of the total variation in intelligence is attributed to heritable factors and to each of the suggested environmental variables. No data for such a complete analysis are now avaliable, nor are they likely to be in the near future. For that reason the relative importance of genetic and environmental factors in intellectual ability will continue to be debated.

Forms of Mental Retardation that are Associated with a Genetic Abnormality

I. Single-Gene Mutations Resulting in Mental Retardation

Included in this category are just a few of the more frequently described single-gene disorders. The number of identified disorders of this type is increasing rapidly. For example, it is hypothesized that there are between 114 and 330 different varieties of single-recessive gene conditions alone that are associated with mental retardation.

All of these disorders can be traced to a particular enzymatic abnormality. In some cases, the defect relates to the absence of certain necessary enzymatic products. In other disorders, the critical element seems to be related to a defect in a particular catabolic pathway. This results in abnormal levels of enzymatic by-products accumulating within a cell. Still other disorders involving single-gene mutations result from defects in transportation and absorption of biochemical substances to target organs. The degree of retardation associated with most of these disorders is usually severe or profound.

1. Phenylketonuria (autosomal recessive)
2. Homocystinuria (autosomal recessive)
3. Tyrosinemia (autosomal recessive)
4. Methylmalonic aciduria (autosomal recessive)
5. Maple-syrup-urine disease (autosomal recessive)
6. Galactosemia (autosomal recessive)

7. Mucolipidosis, Type I, Type II (autosomal recessive)
8. Hurler's syndrome (autosomal recessive)
9. Sanfilippo's syndrome (X-linked)
10. Hunter's syndrome (autosomal recessive)
11. Pompe's disease (autosomal recessive)
12. Menke's syndrome (X-linked recessive)
13. Hartnup's disease (autosomal recessive)
14. Wilson's disease (autosomal recessive)
15. Tuberose sclerosis (autosomal dominant with variable expressivity)
16. Tay-Sachs disease (autosomal recessive)
17. Lesch-Nyan disease (X-linked recessive)

Chromosome Abnormalities

It has been estimated that, on the average, 10% of all conceptions result in a zygote that carries a chromosomal abnormality. Most of these abnormalities arise from nondisjunction of chromosome pairs during meiotic cell division. The vast majority of these affected fetuses are spontaneously aborted. With exception of the sex chromosomes, complete absence of a chromosome results in almost certain death of the developing child. Deletion of parts of chromosomes is, however, occasionally compatible with survival. The degree of retardation associated with the autosomal disorders is usually severe or profound.

A. Autosomal Trisomic Conditions

1. Trisomy 21 (Down's syndrome)
2. Trisomy 18 (Edward's syndrome)
3. Trisomy 13 (Patau's syndrome)
4. Trisomy 8
5. Partial Trisomy 15

B. Autosomal Chromosome Deletions

To date, reports of mental retardation associated with deletions of chromosomal material have been made for the following chromosome numbers: 4, 5, 9, 13, 18, and 21. The best described of these conditions are Wolf's syndrome (affecting number 4) and Cri du Chat syndrome (affecting number 5).

III. Sex Chromosome Abnormalities

These anomalies are much more common than the autosomal disorders leading to mental retardation. Many individuals suffering from sex chromosome abnormalities have normal intelligence. However, a small proportion are retarded. The retardation is almost always mild, with the exception of those rare conditions in which more than two X chromosomes are present; in those conditions, retardation is more severe. The sex chromosome disorders include: (1) Turner's Syndrome (45 chromosomes: one X chromosome, no Y); (2) Klinefelter's syndrome (47 chromosomes: two X chromosomes and one Y); (3) XYY syndrome (47 chromosomes, retardation is present, it is minimal); and (4) XXX syndrome (47 chromosomes, retardation is often present).

CHAPTER 4

Methods for Studying Hereditary Factors in Humans

The success stories of scientific breakthroughs discussed in the previous chapter concerned mental retardation, a concept that until 15 to 20 years ago was as undifferentiated as the concept of mental illness. Today a growing number of specific etiologies for many kinds of mental retardation are recognized. This has raised the hope that the same process of new discoveries will take place with mental illness (i.e., that specific genetic entities will be identified). Currently, there is considerable research activity focused on elucidating possible genetic factors in mental illness. In this chapter, we will first review several research paradigms appropriate for the study of hereditary factors in humans. Next we will review some analytic approaches useful for the examination of specific hypotheses about genetic mechanisms. In this review, we will concentrate on the methods and the assumptions, rather than on specific numerical results.

As indicated in the previous chapter, a genetic element of a disorder is assumed if an enzyme or structural protein is abnormal or absent. Certain other biochemical aberrations are presumptive evidence of genetic influence even in the absence of family data. Unfortunately, for most behavior disorders, the biochemical studies done to date have not yet provided evidence for any genetic abnormality. In the absence of biochemical data, there are at least four other types of evidence that suggest that genetic factors are responsible for a disease of unknown etiology: (1) a higher concordance rate among monozygotic (MZ) twins than among dizygotic (DZ) twins; (2) a higher incidence of the trait among biological offspring of affected individuals than among biological offspring of unaffected individuals, when those individuals have been reared in adoptive homes where the parents did not have the trait under investigation; (3) a significant aggregation of the illness within families; and (4) genetic linkage of the illness with an identifiable allele at a marker locus.

RESEARCH PARADIGMS

The Twin Study Method

The twin method consists of comparing the number of MZ and DZ twin pairs in which both members are affected (i.e., the pair is concordant) to the number of MZ and DZ twin pairs in which only one member is affected (i.e., the pair is discordant). The method is primarily used to obtain preliminary evidence that genetic factors are important in the disorder being studied. The method can also be used to provide an estimate of the proportion of the total variance observed for a particular disorder in the population that is due to genetic segregation. We will discuss later how this can be done.

Monozygotic (MZ, one-egg, identical) twins result from the splitting of a single fertilized cell and therefore are genetically identical; if differences between MZ twins occur, they can be due to genetic mutations or different environmental influences experienced by the two developing individuals. Because genetic mutation of this type would be an extremely rare event, the differences are usually assumed to be environmentally induced. Dizygotic (DZ, two-egg, fraternal) twins result from two separate fertilized ova and therefore are no more closely related genetically than two siblings born at different times. Any differences between DZ twins are attributed to both genetic and environmental factors. Presumably, if DZ twins are more alike than two siblings, it could be due to shared environment. It should be emphasized that environmental influences can begin at conception so that any environmental differences experienced prenatally could also influence behavior.

The twin study method has been used widely in the genetic study of behavior. The results of many studies have been interpreted to suggest that genetic factors are important in a variety of behavioral disorders. When comparing MZ and DZ twin pairs, if the resemblance between MZ twins is greater (i.e., the concordance rate is higher) than that between DZ twins for a particular trait, the difference is assumed to be due to the fact that MZ twins are genetically identical and DZ twins share on average only 50% of their genes. Based on that assumption, it is possible to make a rough estimate of the genetic contribution to the variation observed for the trait.

This estimate will be inflated if MZ twins have a more common environment than do DZ twins and if that environment in some way influences the trait being studied. To control for that possible bias, MZ twins reared apart can be studied. If we assume that twins reared apart do not share similar environments, then the degree of similarity between them should reflect solely their genetic identity. That is, if the trait is entirely due to genetic factors, then the two twins should have the same phenotype 100% of the time. If the trait is entirely of postnatal environmental origin, then the twins should not have the same phenotype any more frequently than any two individuals reared in dissimilar environments. However, the obvious problem with the use of MZ twins reared apart is that it is a rare phenomenon. Thus, the possibility of accumulating data on any substantial number of MZ twins reared apart, with the added restriction that at least one of them is affected by a behavioral disorder, is limited.

In summary, twin studies may yield data suggesting genetic involvement, but twin research is limited in its scope because it is not a complete methodology. It is most useful as a preliminary test of hypotheses that suggest some genetic or common environmental involvement in the trait being studied. However, MZ-DZ twin comparison studies alone are incapable of proving the existence of genetic factors for any traits that might have a major environmental component in their etiology. Allen (1976) suggested that the greatest weakness in most twin studies, particularly those where the trait is psychological, is their dependence on the assumption that shared MZ and DZ environments are comparable. Results of several studies do suggest that there is no evidence of relevant differences. Thus the assumption is presumed acceptable by many, but it is necessary to interpret the results of twin research with this possible limitation in mind.

Adoption and/or Separation Study Method

Adoption or separation studies have also been employed to give evidence for a genetic factor. If a trait is genetic, then children should resemble their biological relatives more closely than they do their adoptive relatives. In addition, separation studies can provide the opportunity to see the extent to which the environment influences the trait in question. If the children resemble their adoptive parents and siblings to any extent, that resemblance in theory is due to environmental similarities. It may then be possible to identify specifically some of the environmental and genetic influences on the trait being studied.

Adoption studies present unique difficulties. Very often, adoptive children are placed in homes that closely resemble the homes of their biological parents. Hence, when comparisons are made between child and biological parent, the similarity may result from this selective placement and not from genetic contribution (Singer & Hardy-Brown, 1984). This may be less of a problem for serious psychiatric problems than for traits like IQ; however, it is a difficulty that needs to be noted. Another complication of separation studies is that it is often difficult to get adequate data on the biological parents. Because these studies tend to be retrospective, information necessary for diagnoses must often be obtained from old obstetric records of the mother. Frequently, the information is not adequate. Also, in order to do a good genetic analysis, information from both parents is necessary. Unfortunately, information on the biological father is often missing completely.

If information about one biological parent is inadequate, adoption studies will not provide enough information to permit the examination of the possible mode of transmission. Unless information is available about other biological siblings of the adoptive children, nothing can be said about specific genetic factors involved in the transmission of the trait. Hence, adoption studies can demonstrate that genetic factors may be important but cannot reveal specific information about mode of inheritance (e.g., dominant, recessive, single-gene, or polygenic). Such studies are also difficult to conduct and are not commonly done. Even when conducted, they can still give ambiguous results.

In addition to classical adoption studies, there are two other types of data that fall into the general category of separation studies that can provide information on the presence of cultural transmission in addition to, or instead of, genetic transmission. Nance and Corey (1976) have advocated the use of children of adult MZ twins and these twins' spouses. Because MZ twins are genetically identical, the children of MZ twins by different spouses are genetically half-sibs but are socially and environmentally comparable to first cousins. Nance and Corey (1976, 1977) have suggested the use of such data to estimate various genetic and environmental components important to the etiology of the trait being studied. Finally, Cloninger, Rice, and Reich (1979a) have developed general formulas using path analysis to aid in the analysis of data from a variety of types of broken or extended families, including half-siblings and biologically unrelated children reared as siblings. They show that analyses of multiple types of sibs can help in the study of genetic and cultural inheritance.

Family Study Method

Studies of biological families also yield data suggesting genetic involvement. The family study method consists of comparing rates of illness in families ascertained through an affected individual (the proband) with rates in the general population or with rates in families ascertained through unaffected persons (controls). If the risk in families ascertained through an affected person is significantly greater than the risk in the population or in the control families, this suggests that the trait is familial. However, as with twin studies, if a major environmental component is important in the etiology of the trait in question, results drawn from family studies will be unable to prove the existence of genetic factors. Genes and familial environment are confounded in determining similarities among relatives and cannot be separately quantified without prior specific identification. For this reason, geneticists stress the distinction between familial and nonfamilial environmental factors as well as the possibility of confounding familial environmental similarity with genetic similarity among relatives (Cavalli-Sforza & Feldman, 1973; Cloninger, Rice, & Reich, 1978; Kidd & Matthysse, 1978; Rao, Morton, & Yee, 1976; Cloninger, Rice, & Reich, 1979a,b). The familial environmental factors that come readily to mind include those that tend to be shared by all members of a family, such as religion, language, health habits, and diet. Actually, most environmental factors show some familial aggregation, but the degree of their concentration in families varies considerably. Among the environmental factors having a familial concentration, some, especially the cultural ones, are often transmitted from parent to child in a pattern similar to a genetic relationship. In practice, it may be very difficult to distinguish cultural from genetic transmission.

Data from families can, however, be used to demonstrate that vertical transmission occurs, and as we will discuss later, these patterns of transmission can be compared to those expected under a variety of specific genetic hypotheses. In this way, data from families can be used to identify specific modes of genetic transmission.

Genetic Linkage Method

The methods discussed thus far are the usual first steps one takes in demonstrating that genetic mechanisms influence behavioral traits. If a significant genetic component can be established, a next step is to attempt to determine the mode of inheritance of that genetic component. As we discuss later, there are several different modes of inheritance. One of the simplest models of genetic transmission is that the trait is largely controlled by a single genetic locus. One of the strongest forms of evidence for a simple genetic factor is the demonstration of genetic linkage. To understand how this is accomplished, a quick summary of Mendelian principles is necessary.

Mendel formulated two laws that are the basis of genetics: the law of segregation and the law of independent assortment. The law of segregation states that if an individual is carrying two alternative forms (alleles) of a particular gene pair (i.e., the individual is *heterozygous* rather than *homozygous*), each form will be transmitted independently and with equal probability to all gametes produced by that individual. For example, the genotype of a heterozygous individual is denoted Aa as a particular locus. Thus, we expect two types of gametes to be produced with equal frequency, A and a.

The law of independent assortment states that the alleles at two separate genetic loci will segregate independently so that if an individual has genotype AaBb, the expectation is that the gametes AB, Ab, aB, and ab will occur with equal frequency. If those gametes are not consistently produced with equal frequencies, then the two loci are not assorting independently, and they are said to be linked. Nonindependent assortment occurs when two loci are located fairly close together on the same chromosome. For example, Figure 8(a) shows two loci located on the same chromosome. During the production of gametes, the two homologous chromosomes segregate, and we would expect that A and B should always segregate together, as well as a and b. The two combinations are referred to as the parental types. On occasion, individuals with the arrangement of genes shown in Figure 8(a) will produce gametes containing the alleles A and b, and a and B. This is due to a phenomenon called "recombination." The likelihood that this will occur increases with the distance between the two genes along the chromosome. Recombination usually occurs during the first meiotic division, when each set of the parental chromosomes is being duplicated. The process is illustrated in Figure 8(b). The interchange of paternal and maternal chromosomal material is due to crossing over of two of the chromatids (Figure 8(c)). The four types of gametes that are

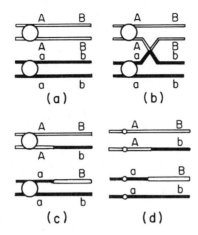

Figure 8. Recombination: (a) position of gene pairs AB and ab on chromosome; (b) the process of crossing over, leading to new exchange of genetic material and new gametic material.

produced are shown in Figure 8(d). Crossing over occurs in man during the formulation of both types of gametes: spermatozoa and ova. The incidence of the phenomenon has been found to differ somewhat between the sexes. Its more frequent occurrence in females is probably due to the fact that whereas sperm are formed during most of the lifetime of the male, eggs are formed during only one period very early in development of the female.

Genetic linkage is detectable, at least in theory, if a known genetic marker locus is sufficiently close to a locus segregating for alleles affecting the trait under study so that nonrandom segregation of alleles at the two loci results in an association of phenotypes within a family. The demonstration of genetic linkage requires family studies showing that alleles at two separate loci are physically close on the same chromosome. Family data are used to estimate how frequently the alleles at the two loci are transmitted by a person to his or her children in new combinations that are different from those in which they were transmitted to that person by his or her parents. The degree of linkage is measured as the recombination fraction (the frequency of such new combinations) and can range from zero (complete linkage) to 0.5 (independent assortment). The minimum recombination frequency of zero is found for alleles that are always transmitted in the same combinations from generation to generation. The maximum recombination frequency of 0.5 is found for alleles (at two separate loci) that have the same likelihood of being transmitted in new combinations as in the same combination from generation to generation. This maximum recombination frequency occurs for alleles at loci far apart on the same chromosome and, of course, for alleles at loci on different chromosomes. Hence, maximum recombination is just another way of phrasing Mendel's second law of independent assortment. Linkage is the violation of that law.

Statistical significance for a particular recombination fraction is determined on the basis of the null hypothesis of independent assortment by measuring the difference in the probability of observing linkage rather than independent assortment in a given family. Finding statistically significant deviation from independent assortment for alleles at a known marker locus and at an hypothesized locus for a complex disorder provides convincing evidence that there is a major gene contributing to the disorder; it is highly unlikely that any other explanation could mimic linkage with a marker locus.

As a simple example, consider a well-characterized genetic marker like the ABO blood group system that has four alleles that can be identified—A1, A2, B, and O. In this system A1, A2, and B are said to be co-dominant, whereas O is recessive. If a locus for a behavioral disorder occurs nearby, then within a given family the disorder will tend to be transmitted to children with a particular blood marker allele. For example, if the affected father is heterozygous for A1 and B (AB blood type) and the normal mother is homozygous for O (which yields blood type O), the affected children will be predominantly A1 O (blood type A), if the allele for the disorder was on the chromosome with the A1 allele; or the affected children will be predominantly B O (blood type B), if the allele for the disorder was on the chromosome with the B allele. In this case, the exact linkage phase in the father is unknown, making the data on his children less clear. If the father's father had also been affected and had blood type A, the data would be clearer because the nonrecombinant chromosome would be the one with the A1 allele and the allele for the disorder. In different families, a different allele at the marker locus may be co-transmitted with the allele for the disorder. Within a family, whenever a recombination occurs, the new combination is the one preferentially transmitted to the offspring of the individual who inherited the recombinant gamete. It is the very particular nature of the co-segregation that results from genetic linkage that permits us to accept linkage over alternative hypotheses whenever this nonrandom segregation is observed.

Some methodological problems in detecting linkage in human data include small family sizes, the inability to control matings, and the small prior probability that the two loci are linked. The method has had limited applicability chiefly because of the small number of sufficiently polymorphic genetic markers that were available for humans. This is changing rapidly because of the advance in genetics brought about by recombinant DNA techniques. A new class of polymorphisms has been identified. This class of polymorphisms is referred to as "restriction fragment length polymorphisms" (RFLPs) because they are visualized as inherited variations in the length of defined fragments of DNA when it is digested with specific restriction enzymes. Though technically quite sophisticated, the methods are logically quite simple. As stated by Kidd (1982), one essential component is the existence of enzymes (usually from bacteria) that recognize specific DNA sequences of four to six base pairs and break the DNA at those sites. With the use of these techniques, many polymorphisms have recently been identified. These restriction endonucleases thus digest DNA into precise segments defined by the sequences in the DNA and the particular restriction enzyme. Electrophoresis can then separate these fragments according to molecular weight, resulting in an apparently homogeneous smear of DNA when total cellular DNA from an individual is used. The second critical component of the method is the ability to identify in this smear the piece (or pieces) containing a particular gene. Because a given gene exists in identical DNA sequences in all cells of the individual, all fragments of the DNA from a single chromosome will be at identical positions in this smear. The only requirement is a method by which to visualize the position of that fragment containing the gene of interest. What is needed is an appropriate "stain." Recombinant DNA technologies allow us to "stain" any piece of DNA containing a sequence that has been isolated and cloned. These cloned sequences act as probes for the position of the homologous cellular DNA. A variety of different human probes has now been assembled, and more probes are rapidly being developed.

Any probe is capable of identifying a genetic variant in the DNA sequence it recognizes or in the surrounding sequence, provided that the genetic variants result in fragments of different molecular weight when digested by some restriction enzyme (Botstein, White, Skolnick, & Davis, 1980). Difference in length (weight) of fragments may result from the absence of a particular cleavage site in some chromosomes because of a mutation that either destroyed a preexisting sequence or created a new one. In addition, inversions of DNA sequences can alter the spacing between restriction sites and lead to fragments of different lengths. Similarly, insertions or deletions of genetic material between restriction sites would result in fragments with different molecular weights. In the few years since the first such human polymorphism was discovered in 1978 (Kan & Dozy, 1978), this class of polymorphisms has come to surpass in importance all of the previous forms of genetic markers. As of August, 1983, over 150 RFLPs had been defined (Skolnick, Willard, & Menlove, 1984), at least in a preliminary way. These provide markers sufficient to map approximately 45% of the human genome. Because new RFLPs are being discovered at an ever-increasing rate, it should be possible to construct a linkage map of the entire human genome within the decade. Therefore, genetic linkage is becoming increasingly important because it can be used as a tool to study the inheritance, and hence indirectly both the etiology and pathogenesis, of human behavioral disorders.

Despite the increased availability of polymorphic markers, genetic linkage studies will still have certain methodological problems having to do with the disorder in question. The phenomenon of reduced penetrance or a variable age of onset will reduce the power of the statistical methods that have been developed to test for linkage (*penetrance* is a term employed to account for the absence of the trait in the phenotype, even though it is believed to be coded for in the genotype). Most of the earlier methods of linkage analysis assume high penetrance for the trait being studied and are not appropriate for the more complex traits. However, the computer program LIPED developed by Ott (1976) performs the complex statistical analyses allowing for incomplete penetrance required in some linkage studies. Moreover, it has been modified to allow for sex- and age-dependent penetrance values (Hodge, Morton, Tideman, Kidd, & Spence 1979). Methods have also been developed that permit the use of multiple linked loci in studying complex traits. With these improved methods and the likely discovery of many more polymorphic markers, genetic-linkage studies may, in the future, make a major contribution to our understanding of the causes of behavior disorders.

Two additional methods now allow us to assign genes at a particular chromosome, determine the distance between them, and specifically map their location. The techniques for staining chromosomes produce bands allowing for more accurate identification of each chromosome but, in addition, the banding makes it possible to detect deletion or duplication of small segments of the chromosome. Whenever a specific deletion or duplication is accompanied by a particular genetic anomaly, we may be confident that the anomaly most probably is localized in that segment.

Another method uses hybrid cells. It is possible to culture cells containing one set of human chromosomes and one set of chromosomes of another species, for instance, mouse. Such cells do *not* contain the full complement of chromosomes: certain human chromosomes are selectively lost. It is ultimately possible to obtain cell lines that have just one human chromosome remaining. By testing which biochemical processes are still operating, these can be assigned to the remaining human chromosome. Using different cultures, it is possible to narrow down the assignment of a process to one chromosome, and sometimes even to a certain segment. Although, at present, these methods are particularly designed for biochemical abnormalities, a number of genetic diseases are due to such abnormalities, and it is hoped that more will be found.

APPROACHES TO DATA ANALYSIS

Before reviewing the methods for analyzing data collected in the approaches outlined previously, the issue of heterogeneity needs to be discussed.

Genetic Heterogeneity

Whether one is primarily interested in the psychological or the biological aspects of a behavioral disorder, it is essential to consider that the disorder being studied may be heterogeneous. Heterogeneity can be present at several different levels. When a syndrome subdivides into distinct classes by onset, course, or response to treatment, a corresponding heterogeneity in etiology is a possibility that must be considered. For example, it is likely that infantile autism is a behavioral syndrome with multiple etiologies (Rutter, 1974). It is known that the syndrome can develop in association with (and presumably as a result of) conditions as pathologically diverse as congenital rubella (Chess, Korn, & Fernandez, 1971) and infantile spasms (Taft & Cohen, 1971). However, infantile autism can also develop in the absence of any environmental agents such as these. Any genetic factors that might exist for autism will almost certainly be different in these etiologically different classes. As a first step, as in any genetic study, recurrence risks in families of autistic children should be calculated separately according to environmental factors present (e.g., the mother's having had rubella while carrying the child) and compared to risks in families with no known causes for the disorder. Matthysse and Kidd (1976) discuss many of the general principles that should be considered for any behavioral disorder, though their examples are drawn from adult-onset schizophrenia.

It has been firmly established that an apparently homogeneous syndrome may be heterogeneous, with quite different etiologies producing nearly indistinguishable symptoms. For example, the mucopolysaccharide storage diseases encompass defects of at least nine different enzymes. Initially, all affected children were considered to have "gargoylism." Now the symptoms for most of the defects are recognized to be different, largely as a result of biochemical/genetic differences having been demonstrated. Often, the multiple causes of a "single disease" become easily identifiable as new phenotypic levels are defined: what is apparently homogeneous at the level of gross behavioral symptomatology becomes obviously heterogenous as physiological and/or biochemical aberrations are used to redefine the phenotype. There are many other examples of genetic heterogeneity, in which the same phenotype can be caused by one of several independent defects at different gene loci. Hemophilia, congenital deafness, and anemia are examples of this phenomenon (McKusick, 1978).

Unfortunately, various forms of heterogeneity may be found. For example, several different genetic types may exist, and each may have its own separate array of environmental precipitants. Diabetes may be such a disorder, with different modes of inheritance for susceptibilities to juvenile-onset diabetes, to the maturity-onset type of diabetes of the young, and to maturity-onset diabetes. Additional genetic heterogeneity may be present within each of these types. In addition, different environmental agents are thought to be involved for each type (Ganda & Soeldner, 1977). The anemias are a second well-documented example of multiple etiologies. There are several different genetic types (McKusick, 1978). Some, such as B-thalassemia and hereditary spherocytosis, have pathological processes largely unaffected by environmental variation. Others, such as favism, are quite susceptible to environmental variation. There are also nongenetic anemias caused by environmental factors, such as iron deficiency.

Genetic studies of behavioral disorders—whether twin, family, linkage, or adoption studies—have been hampered by the imprecision and variability in diagnostic criteria. In fact, much variation in results among different studies might be explained solely by the differences in diagnostic methods.

There are several sources of unreliability in diagnosis; however, we shall consider only two examples. The first is the method of collecting information necessary for making diagnostic distinctions. In doing genetic studies, it is desirable to obtain comparable information from all family members. The development of structured interviews and their use has facilitated this goal. However, in studies of disorders that usually begin in childhood, it is often difficult to obtain comparable information because this means interviewing adults about their behavior some 20 to 40 years ago. Such retrospective elicitation is necessary because of the transitory nature of symptoms in many childhood behavioral disorders. Often the disorder is outgrown completely. In other cases, the symptomatology changes over time. It may be very difficult to determine if an adult being studied actually had the appropriate symptoms during childhood, but accurate diagnoses are a necessity in genetic studies. It is clear that work needs to be done in this area. Improved methods of retrospective diagnoses would result in the diagnostic precision needed to progress in this field. A second source of unreliability in diagnosis is in the rules for using symptomological data to classify patients. The systematically collected information on symptoms needs to be used in a precisely defined way to assign valid diagnoses. The problem of validity is one, of course, that can be finally resolved only with a complete understanding of the etiology of any disorder, but it must still be considered in early research on the disorder.

New diagnostic methodologies that take into account these sources of variation and improve reliability considerably (such as the DSM-III described in Chapter 2) are now being applied to genetic studies. Improved definitions of diagnostic categories and the greater accuracy with which patients can be assigned valid diagnoses will undoubtedly improve future genetic studies. But much work remains to be done. For example, follow-up studies are needed to determine whether any relationships exist between childhood and adult behavioral disorders. Such studies would facilitate the development of diagnostic criteria that would allow more accurate diagnoses. When the use of uniform diagnostic criteria becomes widespread, the resulting diagnostic uniformity will not only reduce heterogeneity within a given study but also allow meaningful comparisons between studies.

After diagnostic criteria have been used to define the phenotype as rigorously as possible, there are additional ways to minimize possible heterogeneity within the data set prior to any genetic analysis. These are (1) imposing controls in the sample data to eliminate possibly relevant nongenetic variables; and (2) collecting data from a population as genetically homogeneous as possible. The first is a standard part of research design in many behavioral studies; we wish to elaborate on the second.

Genetic homogeneity is more likely in a sample from the same ethnic group than in a completely random sample; it is even more likely to exist in an inbred isolate and is yet more likely to be found in a single family pedigree. Even in situations that are relatively homogeneous, such as a single locus underlying most variation in susceptibility, genotypic heterogeneity may exist among affected individuals; that is, some are heterozygous, and some are homozygous. In such cases, the frequency of homozygosity may be increased by special ascertainment criteria for families. Matthysse and Kidd (1976) have shown that inclusion of a family in a sample through two affected children rather than just one changes the expected genotype distribution of the family markedly in that the probability of affected individuals being homozygous is increased considerably.

Selecting for additional affected individuals among remote relatives in multigenerational data should also enhance etiologic homogeneity and greatly simplify interpretation of biochemical data. However, if those same pedigrees are to be used for a statistical analysis to estimate genetic parameters, the bias introduced by the ascertainment through multiple affected members must be estimated and removed. Morton and Kidd (1979) have developed one method for removing the bias from a likelihood procedure for parameter estimation. Their method is impractical for much general use because it requires extensive computer simulation, but their results do show the necessity of considering the "high-density" ascertainment bias.

If homogeneity is achieved by collecting data from a population with a restricted gene pool (e.g., an isolate or a single pedigree), one drawback is that the results obtained might not extrapolate to the same phenotype in other populations. That should not be a deterrent for special ascertainment strategies, however. If it is possible to identify a specific etiology for a homogeneous group selected with a unique ascertainment technique, it may be possible to establish clinical differences that could then be used to identify additional cases of this type from a general population of patients. Moreover, the residual cases would also be more homogeneous than the original total population.

Another strategy for enhancing homogeneity has been suggested by Buchsbaum and Rieder (1979). If a biochemical abnormality has been suggested as associated with a particular trait, then selecting subjects on the basis of that biochemical phenotype rather than a behavioral phenotype might enhance homogeneity. After the biochemically defined sample has been selected, evaluations may then be done to see if a higher than expected number of these subjects have a behavioral disorder. As these authors point out, this strategy allows the investigator to determine whether a spectrum of symptoms (i.e., symptoms that may vary somewhat from individual to individual) is associated with the biochemical abnormality.

Genetic Hypotheses

It is clear that much work is needed before we will completely understand the genetics of behavior. It is not, however, a hopeless task. In fact, psychiatric and behavioral disorders in humans present many of the same problems to researchers as do other "nonbehavioral" genetic disorders. In those, too, it is often the case that the etiologies are poorly understood, and the specific pathogenesis for each disorder is largely unknown. However, because there are so many behavioral disorders that display a strong familial pattern, it is reasonable to assume that some, perhaps the majority, are under some genetic control. We have already reviewed the general research designs that yield data allowing tests of specific genetic hypotheses. We now will review the ways in which those data may be analyzed.

Each hypothesis to be tested is based on some genetic model. The most general hypothesis is simply the presence of some genetic influence. For example, if there is *no* genetic factor involved in the etiology of a disorder, then the concordance rates for groups of MZ and DZ twins should not be different (assuming as noted earlier, that the shared environment of the two types of twins has the same effect on the phenotype). If this hypothesis can be rejected (e.g., the concordance rate is higher for MZ then DZ twins), we can assume that genetic factors are etiologically important. The next step is to try to estimate just how important they are. This step requires some assumptions about a specific genetic model. Genetic models for behavioral traits serve as hypotheses that relate genes and genotypes (i.e., the combinations of different forms of those genes), their frequencies in the population to the phenotypes (i.e., specific characteristics of individuals), and the distributions of phenotypes within the population and within individual families. Thus, using a genetic model for analyzing a specific trait can provide considerable insight into the etiology of the disorder.

Before describing some of the more complex models that have been developed in the last 10 years we will briefly review the simplest ones.

Single Gene Conditions (Mendelian Ratios)

Gene action follows regular patterns that have clearly specifiable outcomes for offspring of affected individuals. Thus, when it has been established that a specific disorder is under genetic control, the probability that a child will be affected, given that a relative is affected, can be calculated. The simplest cases are those in which the disorder is due to a single *autosomal* gene that is *dominant*. Here the chance that a given child of an affected heterozygous individual will be affected is 50%.

Recessive inheritance, on the other hand, is the type in which a phenotypically normal heterozygous carrier has a 50% chance of transmitting the unexpressed abnormal allele to any one of the children, where it will remain unexpressed, unless it happens to be paired with another copy of this abnormal allele from the other parent. If that parent is also heterozygous and thus unaffected, there is the same 50% chance of transmission of the abnormal allele. The risk of an affected child from such a mating is therefore .25. The other possible outcomes are .50 that any child will be an unaffected carrier and .25 that it will receive two normal alleles.

When an abnormal gene is located on the X chromosome, the resultant condition is said to be X-linked. For an X-linked recessive gene, the principles outlined before would also hold, but a male, because he has just one X chromosome would be affected if that one X carried the abnormal gene. A female, however, could only be affected if she had two abnormal Xs. As noted in Chapter 3, males can only transmit an abnormal X allele to female offspring because to have a male child they would have to have contributed their Y chromosome instead. In the case of a dominant condition, all daughters of affected males would be affected; in the case of a recessive X-linked condition, all daughters of such males would be carriers. Therefore, it often appears that the disease skips a generation. These patterns of inheritance become more understandable when placed in the context of the diagrams in Figure 9.

When a condition is caused by alleles at a single genetic locus, the law of segregation predicts that a certain percentage of offspring and/or relatives will either carry the gene or be affected. This expectation of risk is conditional on the genotypes of the parents. Therefore, if you know the parental genotypes, predictions can be made regarding the risk to certain types of relatives that are based on the law of segregation. These ratios are referred to as "Mendelian ratios."

Unfortunately, in most behavioral disorders, Mendelian ratios are not observed. Therefore, it seems reasonable to assume that the underlying genetic mechanisms are complex, involving more than one genetic locus. It is important to note, however, that although the etiologic factors important for the manifestation of a specific behavior or abnormality may be many and have complex interactions, the underlying genetic mechanism could still be very simple. It is possible for a single gene to give rise to patterns within families that are very

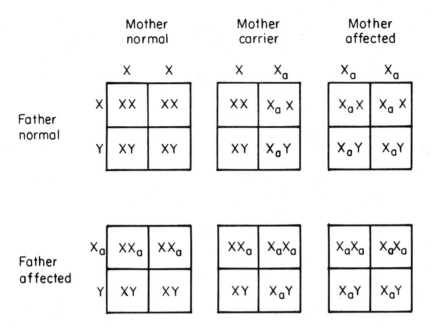

Figure 9. Possible genetic outcomes for a hypothetical X-linked recessive trait.

similar to patterns related to the segregation of many genes. In fact, there are many different genetic models that lead to predictions of risk that are of this non-Mendelian type. We will review only three and show how different types of data can be used to learn about the different modes of inheritance.

Multifactorial-Polygenic Inheritance

A collection of genes all influencing a single trait is referred to as a "polygenic system." When a polygenic system and additional non-genetic factors influence the expression of a disorder, it is referred to as a "multifactorial-polygenic trait."

The assumptions that characterize the classical multifactorial-polygenic model are as follows: (1) a non-Mendelian quantitative trait, P, may be partitioned as $V_P = V_A + V_E$, where V_A denotes the variance due to the segregation of transmitted factors that contribute to the expression of the trait, and V_E denotes random environmental influences on the variance of the trait; (2) all factors (both genetic and environmental) have an equal and additive effect on the variance of the trait; and (3) the covariance (A,E) is assumed to be zero (i.e., it is assumed that there is no interaction between the genetics and environmental factors).

For traits that are continuously distributed, like IQ, this is an attractive model. Unfortunately, many behavioral disorders are qualitative, not quantitative traits, and for these the preceding model is seemingly not applicable. Although there may be gradations of severity within the disorder, there are still definite categories of "affected" and "unaffected." A multifactorial model for qualitative traits as first described by Crittenden (1961) and Falconer (1965) provides a means to apply this model to these qualitative traits. They postulated an underlying "liability" scale that satisfies all of the aforementioned criteria. *Liability* is defined as the sum of all events both genetic and environmental that contribute to the expression of the trait. They postulate that a threshold on this liability scale, presumably a reflection of some physiological phenomenon, divides the distribution into affected and unaffected individuals. Any individual with a sufficient number of factors for the trait (whether genetic or environmental) will exceed the threshold, display an abnormal phenotype, and be classified as affected.

In order to understand a multifactorial-polygenic trait, it is first helpful to be able to estimate how much of the phenotypic variance is due to the segregation of alleles at all of the genetic loci. The proportion of the total variance in a population that is due to genetic variation is referred to as the *heritability* of the trait. Two kinds of genetic variance can be distinguished: (a) that which is due to the additive effects of each single gene; and (b) that which is due to the nonadditive effects due to the particular combination of genes received by each individual. The proportion that includes the first kind of variance in the numerator is referred to as heritability in the narrow sense; the proportion that includes the second plus the first in the numerator is defined as heritability in the broader sense. The latter includes the effects of dominance of one allele over another for each gene pair, plus epistasis (the effect of a given gene at any locus on all other genes). The distinction between *broad* and *narrow* heritability is particularly important when studying twins because identical twins have all their genes in common (hence, they share all the nonadditive genetic variance), whereas fraternal twins *on the average* share only 50% of their genes (so that they share only the additive variance plus some small and varying amount of the nonadditive variance). The genetic resemblance between parents and children is the same as that between fraternal twins.

The formulas used in most earlier studies for determining the proportion of phenotypic variance to be attributed to a genetic factor for characteristics believed to be inherited in an all or none fashion, such as cleft palate or schizophrenia, were similar to the one proposed by Holzinger (1920):

$$H = \frac{C_{MZ} - C_{DZ}}{100 - C_{DZ}} \tag{1}$$

where C_{MZ} is the percentage concordance in MZ twins, and C_{DZ} is the percentage concordance in DZ twins.

When studying hereditary factors in continuous traits, formula (1) has been modified to permit comparison of MZ and DZ intraclass correlations. An intraclass correlation differs from a Pearson product moment correlation between variables x and y in that it is completely arbitrary which twin is assigned to x and which one to y. For that reason it would be necessary to enter each pair both ways: John as x and James as y, and vice versa. Actually, the intraclass correlation is more easily calculated as the ratio of the variance among pairs of twins divided by the total variance. This method has been severely criticized, however, and various modifications have been proposed.

Because identical twins share all of their genetic variance, whereas fraternal twins only share half their genetic variance, Falconer (1960) has proposed:

$$2(r_{MZ} - r_{DZ}) \tag{2}$$

as an estimate of heritability in the broader sense. Although the formula has a certain elegant look of simplicity, this measure is complicated by a large set of assumptions one must make for it to be valid. One assumption is that all similarities between MZ twins are due to their identical genes and that all differences are environmental. Another is that MZ and DZ twins share equally similar environments. In reference to the latter assumption, it is not necessary to assume that the influences are all of the same magnitude for all pairs, only that the two distributions of common environmental effects are similar for both types. The evidence from several studies (e.g., Smith, 1965; Zazzo, 1960) suggests that this assumption may be unwarranted. For example, MZ twins tend to spend more time together and to share more friends than do DZ twins. An argument can be made, however, that this is a reflection of the hereditary difference in a fraternal pair, which leads them to seek out somewhat different environments.

Although this suggestion is plausible, it is difficult to prove. It resembles the chicken or the egg question. Some investigators who deny the greater similarity of environments within MZ twin pairs point to possible differential prenatal conditions, such as the undernourishment or oxygen deprivation of one MZ twin relative to the other, conditions that are more frequently experienced by MZ twins than singletons, or even DZ twins. Others mention family favoritism, dominance of one twin over the other, or division of roles as causes of dissimilar environments between MZ twins. It is quite plausible that MZ twins may react differently to environmental pressures in spite of the original external similarities between them. No attempt has yet been made to use estimates of the similarity of twin environments obtained by direct observation to improve estimates of heritability. However, it seems eminently possible to do so.

In general, the heritability estimate obtained from the typical twin study will be *too high* if it is true that members of identical twin pairs are more similar because of factors associated with a common environment than fraternal twins who are relatively less affected by these factors. By the same token, the estimate would be *too low* if identical twins are made less similar by the common environment than are fraternal twins. Both processes may be at work for some or all pairs and may largely cancel out, but it is not possible to quantify these possibilities. Scarr-Salapatek (1979) and Vandenberg (1976) have reviewed the evidence and suggest that the range of "twinness" (the special dyadic relationship) is not very different for the two types of twins.

The comparability of MZ and DZ sex and age distributions for variables where these factors may have an effect must also be assumed. In fact, the classical twin study assumes that the total variance of all the MZ individuals equals the total DZ variance, whereas both should be estimates of the variance in the total population. The total MZ variance in some twin studies has exceeded the total DZ variance for reasons that are not clear. This discrepancy may be explained by such things as the possibility that fewer male DZ pairs than MZ pairs participated in twin studies. It is also possible that very dissimilar DZ pairs are less likely to participate in twin studies.

A group of British investigators (Eaves, 1969, 1977; Jinks & Fulker, 1970) advocate the use of the additional information contained in the between-pair variance of both types of twins. One advantage of this method is that it leads quite naturally to a test of the basic assumption that the MZ and the DZ twins come from the same population. One tests this by asking whether the values for the two types of individuals have the same means and variances. It is also possible to go one step further and test whether there is a sex difference by looking at the four

Table 9. Analysis of Variance for Twin Data

Sums of squares	df	Expected mean squares
MZ pairs		
Between	$n_{MZ} - 1$	$\sigma^2_{W_{MZ}} + 2\sigma^2_{B_{MZ}}$
Within	n_{MZ}	$\sigma^2_{W_{MZ}}$
DZ pairs		
Between	$n_{DZ} - 1$	$\sigma^2_{W_{DZ}} + 2\sigma^2_{B_{DZ}}$
Within	n_{DZ}	$\sigma^2_{W_{DZ}}$

$^a n_{MZ}$ and n_{DZ} are the number of MZ and DZ twin *pairs*, respectively.

groups: male MZ, female MZ, male DZ, and female DZ. Using a model of this sort, if any significant differences are found, one can either make a correction for the difference or take into account the sex difference when calculating heritability.

In this particular model, the first step is an analysis of variance that is performed as shown in Table 9. Notice that the expected mean square for the between-pairs data is not just a measure of variances between pairs (σ^2_B) but rather $\sigma^2 + \sigma^2_B$ or $(\sigma^2_W + 2\sigma^2_B)$, where σ^2 equals the total variance and σ^2_W equals the variance within twin pairs. The results of this partitioning of the variance can now be used in testing various hypotheses.

A simple model with one genetic and two environmental factors is shown in Table 10. The additive genetic variance is V_{G_A}, and V_{E_C} and V_{E_W} are environmental variance. Between-family environmental variance, V_{E_C}, is assumed to be due to factors that influence both members of a twin pair equally. In contrast, V_{E_W} the within-family environmen-

Table 10. A Model for Twin Data with Polygenic Variance and Two Sources of Environmental Variance

Observed variances	Expected components
$\sigma^2_{B_{MZ}}$	$V_{E_c} + V_{G_A}$
$\sigma^2_{W_{MZ}}$	V_{E_w}
$\sigma^2_{B_{DZ}}$	$V_{E_c} + \frac{1}{2}V_{G_A}$
$\sigma^2_{W_{DZ}}$	$V_{E_w} + \frac{1}{2}V_{G_A}$

tal variance, is assumed to be due to factors that influence the two members of a twin pair differently. Examples of different factors would include such things as dominance of one twin over the other, severe or chronic illness of one twin, or parental favoritism.

As a final step, the observed mean squares can be written according to the model in terms of the expected genetic and environmental components of variance in matrix form as noted in Table 11. This set of simultaneous equations can be solved for the three coefficients of the parameters of the model, either by least squares or by maximum likelihood methods. Fulker, Eysenck, and Zuckerman (1980) have described how to use the computer program LISREL for this purpose. If a sample of unlike-sexed twins is also available, additional parameters representing sex-linked inheritance and/or differential familial influence on males and females could be added to the model.

Similar models can be constructed for other types of family relationships. The more relationships which are included, the more parameters can, in general, be included in the model, at least as long as there are enough individuals represented in each type of relationship. In recent years, there has been a particular interest in MZ and DZ twins, their spouses, and their children. As noted earlier this interest was generated by the realization that the children from two MZ twin members are, genetically speaking, half-sibs: they have a twin parent who is genetically identical to the other twin parent; only the two spouses are genetically different. This situation is equivalent from a genetic viewpoint to a person who married twice, except that in the case of children of MZ twins there is often no age difference between the two sets of children. Besides half-sibs, this design also provides the usual cousins, uncle/aunt–nephew/niece relationships (from the DZ marriages) and similar but closer relations from the MZ pairs. (For details of the method, see Crumpacker et al., 1979.)

Table 11. Twin Data: Expected Genetic and Environmental Components of Variance

Mean squares		Component coefficient		
		V_{G_A}	V_{E_C}	V_{E_W}
MZ	Between	2	2	1
MZ	Within	0	0	1
DZ	Between	1.5	2	1
DZ	Within	0.5	0	1

Another, more generally applicable method of estimating heritability is the calculation of parent–offspring correlations. If calculated
from midparent and midchild values (average scores of both parents
and all children), these correlations give a direct estimate of narrow
heritability if certain assumptions can be made. The major assumption
is that, with regard to the trait in question, there is no evidence that
the trait is under the influence of any common environmental factor
affecting both parents and children. This is a rather strong assumption
for intact families living in the same household but is much easier to
accept in the case of correlations between biological parents and their
children who have been placed in adoptive homes shortly after birth.
How important the assumption is to a valid assessment of genetic
influence also depends on how much common environment is believed to influence the trait under study. For example, because height
is relatively little affected by environmental factors, the assumption
can be made. For infectious diseases, however, it would be obviously
incorrect to assume the absence of a common environmental factor, in
this case, the disease vector.

When the parent–offspring correlation is estimated in this manner
from a sample, it will fluctuate around a hypothetical population value, which itself depends on (i.e., will vary with) the population being
sampled—all white males in England, all students in New York City
high schools, or whatever one chooses to regard as a population. Unfortunately, in most such studies, it has not been possible to define this
population as clearly as one would wish.

Although the value of a correlation is not affected by linear
changes in the units used to measure one or both variables, this is not
true with regard to nonlinear changes in asymmetry (skewness) and in
relative flatness or peakedness (kurtosis) of the distribution of cases.
This means that measures on which the samples under study differ
with respect to either of these characteristics will lead to different
estimates of the parent–offspring correlation. The age distribution,
especially of the children but also of the parents, becomes crucial in
studies of intelligence because it is known that age influences mental
test scores. This can, to some extent, be corrected by using age-
adjusted scores, either as provided by the authors of specific IQ tests or
by directly correcting the data for age effects in a given study. The
latter method is, of course, the more accurate way to insure that the
linear components of variance due to age have been removed.

The methods just discussed for the estimation of heritability are
appropriate for continuous traits, but unfortunately it is not possible to
use the same methods for qualitative traits even with an assumed

underlying continuously distributed liability. Other methods have been developed, however, that allow an estimation of heritability in traits like these. Data on the incidence in relatives of probands, when compared with the incidence in the general population, can be thought of as the response to selection for the disorder in question as if in a genetic experiment. A selection experiment is one in which an attempt is made to "breed" for the increased incidence of a trait. The response to selection can be thought of as the difference in the incidence of the trait under selection in the breeding population, as compared to a control group. How much a character is changed as the result of the selection is a function of, and therefore a measure of, the heritability of the trait: $b = rh^2$ Thus when r is the degree of relationship and b can be calculated from the slope of the line of the various incidence figures for the general population and for relatives with different degrees of relatedness, one can estimate h^2 by the formula $h^2 = b/r$.

Therefore, it is possible to estimate the heritability for any trait, assuming that the underlying genetic mechanism is multifactorial-polygenic, but this does not constitute a test of the hypothesis that the genetic model is polygenic. Methodologies have been developed which allow goodness-of-fit tests for the multifactorial-polygenic (MFP) model. Lange, Westlake, and Spence (1976) and Gladstein, Lange, and Spence (1978) developed methods that utilize actual pedigree structures to estimate parameters and to test the MFP hypothesis. Unfortunately, pedigree data are not always available to test the model. Because this is so, Reich, James, and Morris (1972) and Kidd and Spence (1976) have generalized the original model of Falconer (1965) to include multiple thresholds. The multiple thresholds can correspond to different forms of the disorder (e.g., a mild versus severe form), different frequencies between the sexes, or a combination of the two. This generalization allows the use of family prevalence data for both parameter estimation and a statistical goodness-of-fit test. The only requirement is that it be possible to divide the data on affected individuals into at least two categories (e.g., levels of severity or different frequencies between the sexes) that differ in mean liability to the disorder. This model (with only two thresholds) is completely defined by three parameters: (1) the population prevalence for the more common form of the disorder (or more commonly affected sex); (2) the population prevalence of the less common form of the disorder (or less commonly affected sex); and (3) the correlation between relatives. If the values of these parameters are known, expected values can be calculated, for all prevalences of the one type of the disorder, for relatives of probands of the other type. These expected values are then compared to those observed in the data.

Rice *et al.* (1978) and Cloninger *et al.* (1979a, 1979b) have further extended the model to allow for cultural transmission and nonrandom or assortative mating (correlated behaviors that affect mate selection). The phenotype is now partitioned as $V_P = V_A + V_B + V_E$, where V_A and V_B denote all genetic and cultural factors transmitted from parent to offspring, respectively, and V_E denotes all other random environmental effects, with the covariance $(A,E,)$, and the covariance $(B,E,)$ equal to zero. As with the simpler characterization, all factors are again assumed to be multiple and additive, each having small effect relative to the total phenotypic variance. The phenotypic distribution is again assumed to be normal, and departures from linearity (e.g., dominance, epistasis, and interaction) are neglected. Two additional assumptions are made with regard to the inclusion of a parameter for assortative mating: (1) assortative mating is recurrent and based only on phenotypic preferences; and (2) the phenotypic correlation between mates for a given trait is of constant magnitude through generations. The model is defined by as many as 11 parameters. Using path analysis, correlations between relatives are expressed in terms of these parameters and the system of nonlinear equations generated is used for parameter estimation. Maximum likelihood techniques are used to test various hypotheses about any or all of the parameters. By use of this method, the most likely hypothesis can be determined and the parameters estimated for that hypothesis.

In our opinion, the MFP model has some very real limitations in its application to major behavioral disorders. One serious weakness is the assumption that no epistasis (in its broadest sense) exists. As we learn more about the interactions of genes and environments, the assumption that $P = A + E$ must be considered a rough approximation at best.

Single-Major-Locus Inheritance

The simplest alternative to the multifactorial-polygenic model is one in which the genetic or transmitted component is attributable entirely to a single locus with two alternative alleles, say S_1 and S_2, where one allele, S_1, is considered "normal" and the other, S_2, confers susceptibility to the trait or disorder. This situation gives rise to three possible genotypes: S_1S_1, S_1S_2, and S_2S_2. Development of the general mathematical formulation of this model took place in the early 1970s (Elandt-Johnson, 1971; Elston & Campbell, 1970; James, 1971; Morton, Yee, & Lew, 1971). The model can be conceptualized in two different forms: a graphical representation on a liability scale (Cavalli-Sforza and Kidd, 1971) or an algebraic formulation in which genotypes are assigned penetrances (James, 1971). These two conceptualizations of the model can be mathematically equivalent under certain limiting assumptions. In the simplest algebraic formulation of the model, the population prevalence of the disorder is equal to $q^2f_2 + 2qpf_1 + p^2f_0$. The four parameters are the frequency, q, for one of the alleles (e.g., S_2, the allele associated most strongly with the disorder) and three penetrances, f_0, f_1, f_2, each giving the probability that the respective genotype (with 0, 1, or 2, S_2 alleles) results in the "abnormal" phenotype. The model usually assumes Hardy-Weinberg proportions (i.e., that the genotypic frequencies are stable in the population), but this assumption can be relaxed by adding additional parameters.

General predictions for this model when $0<f_i<1$ for at least one f_i and $f_0<f_1<f_2$ include (1) non-Mendelian patterns and frequencies in families and sets of families; (2) increased risk to subsequent siblings when families are ascertained through more than one affected sibling; (3) increased risk to siblings and offspring of proband when compared with the risk to aunts/uncles or nephews/nieces (the risk will continue to decrease, approaching the population incidence asymptotically as the relationship to the proband becomes more remote); and (4) sex or severity differences may be conceptualized as different penetrance vectors for each type and, when incorporated into the model, usually predict that probands affected with the less common type of the disorder will have a higher frequency of affected relatives than the more common type of proband. These are identical to the general expectations for the MFP model, as discussed by Mendell and Spence (1979).

The SML model is quite general and includes classical Mendelian autosomal dominant and autosomal recessive models as subhypotheses. However, in the general model, the terms *dominant* and *recessive* are not relevant. The SML model is attractive as a working hypothesis because it postulates a single major locus and hence offers the possibility of eventually obtaining a more precise understanding of gene action in the etiology of the disorder. Though many have despaired of ever finding a major locus associated with any behavioral disorder, genetic linkage studies have shown that some disorders long considered to be genetically complex are determined primarily by one locus (Kidd & Matthysse, 1978).

A variety of methods have been proposed for estimating the parameters of the SML model. Using different analytic techniques, it is possible to obtain parameter estimates from average frequencies of affected relatives, from data on segregation patterns in nuclear families, and from more extensive pedigrees. With familial prevalence data on a present/absent trait, the parameters of this model cannot, however, be uniquely specified (James, 1971; Kidd, 1975; Suarez, Reich, & Trost, 1976). Moreover, a goodness-of-fit test cannot be made. Finally, it can be shown that the SML and MFP models are actually only different parameterizations of the same mathematical relationship (Kidd & Gladstein, 1980).

Two-threshold models have been developed for both the MFP and SML models using severity (Reich *et al.*, 1972) or sex differences (Kidd & Spence, 1976) to define the second threshold. These specific models were developed for application to data on pairwise frequency of disease and have the advantage of permitting goodness-of-fit tests. Still, the MFP and SML two-threshold models are closely related (Kidd & Gladstein, 1980); they evince differences only in the inter-relationships of the various frequencies of affected relatives, and discrimination is possible with pairwise frequency data only if several different classes of relationships are studied. In actual applications to data on human disorders, discrimination has been less than perfect: for pyloric stenosis (Kidd & Spence, 1976) and for stuttering (Kidd, 1977) the models only differed appreciably in their predictions for the least frequently observed categories of relationships and therefore the least reliable data set—relatives of female probands.

Analyses based on pairwise prevalences among relatives are not powerful, though it has been shown in simulations (Reich, Rice, Cloninger, Wette, & James 1979) that the parameter estimates are not biased and are approximately correct if the data set is large. Because these methods have the advantage of being reasonably simple to apply to a highly condensed tabulated data set, they are useful as an initial stage in an exploratory data analysis. However, any complete genetic analysis would eventually have to use much more powerful methods. Available methods can be conveniently divided into two general categories: complex segregation analysis and pedigree analysis.

Segregation analysis can give maximum likelihood estimates of the ascertainment probability and other parameters of the genetic model being used (Elandt-Johnson, 1971; Morton *et al.*, 1971). These likelihood ratio tests are then used to compare different hypotheses about the relationships of genotypes to phenotypes. The main drawback of most such analyses is that it must be assumed that all families included have the same genetic disorder and represent a random sample from a homogeneous distribution of environments. For most common diseases, including behavior disorders, both of those assumptions are questionable. Even the less restrictive models can accommodate only a limited amount of genetic heterogeneity.

Pedigree analysis using large multigenerational pedigrees is conceptually similar to segregation analysis of nuclear family data but is generally considered more powerful because each pedigree contains more relationships. Specific hypotheses currently testable by pedigree analysis methods include (1) single-locus inheritance; (2) polygenic inheritance; and (3) multilocus inheritance (influence emanating from two or more major gene loci), among others (Elston & Namboodiri, 1977; Elston & Stewart, 1971; Lange & Elston, 1976; Lange *et al.*, 1976). Parameters in the single-locus and multilocus models include the allele frequencies, the penetrances of all genotypes, and the transmission probabilities. Parameters in the polygenic model can include various components of variance—additive, genetic, environmental, and the like—or more complex conditional transmission functions. A potential difficulty is that analyses of large pedigrees may be biased in favor of one specific hypothesis if only "interesting" pedigrees are analyzed. By establishing rules for the sequential sampling of pedigrees, it is possible to correct for such biases while avoiding unnecessary study of uninformative families (Cannings & Thompson, 1977).

The Mixed Model

Mixed models (Morton & MacLean, 1974) or combined models (Reich, Rice, & Cloninger, 1981) have been developed that, among other things, provide a means of discriminating between SML and MFP models. These can be represented graphically in the same way as the single major-locus model. However, the variation around the genotypic mean is assumed to be in part polygenically inherited with a certain correlation among relatives. Thus, if both parents are heterozygotes, their children will be distributed among the three major-locus genotypes as a result of Mendelian segregation, but each will tend to be in the upper portion of his or her respective distribution because of the additive polygenic contribution to the liability. The model is not a model of heterogeneity because both systems contribute to the same liability.

The mixed model has several statistical advantages over either extreme model separately because both the MFP and SML models are just special cases of the more general mixed model. Allowing the allele frequencies at the major locus to go to 0 and 1 causes the model to become identical to the multifactorial-polygenic model. Allowing the polygenic-multifactorial correlations among relatives to go to zero makes the model identical to the single-major-locus model. The nesting of each of the simple models into a general model allows a likelihood ratio test of either model to the full mixed model. However, because neither of the two extreme models is nested within the other, a direct comparison between them is not interpretable in terms of statistical significance. Lalouel, Rao, Morton, and Elston (1983) have modified the mixed model to allow a specific test of Mendelian transmission. This unified model allows a more complete test of both the mixed model and the SML hypothesis by estimating the transmission probabilities and comparing them to their expected Mendelian values.

LINKAGE ANALYSES

All of the methods reviewed thus far use only the information about affected and unaffected status of family members to attempt to identify mode of inheritance. As noted before, it, unfortunately, is often difficult to differentiate between several different genetic hypotheses using only this information. Hence, the results of many studies conducted to date are inconclusive. Most often the results suggest a genetic component, but the data are not adequate to allow the identification of the mode of inheritance. Genetic linkage relationships are becoming increasingly important because knowledge of this sort can be used as a tool to study the inheritance of complex traits. As we discussed earlier in this chapter, genetic linkage is a normal phenomenon that is a consequence of the way in which the genetic material is organized and transmitted from parent to offspring. It should be clear from that discussion that genetic linkage is useful only when there are only one or two major genetic loci contributing to the variation of the trait being studied. In the future, as more polymorphic marker loci are identified for Homo sapiens the method will probably no longer be limited in this way. However, as currently available, genetic linkage analyses are used primarily in identifying single major loci.

Detection of Heterogeneity. Historically, one of the first uses of genetic linkage studies in humans was the demonstration of genetic heterogeneity. Morton (1956) showed that elliptocytosis, a dominantly inherited disorder of red blood cells, consisted of two distinct genetic types: one that showed linkage to the Rh locus, and one that did not. This was the first indication that what appeared to be a clinically homogeneous disorder was in fact at least two separate disorders. Because many behavioral traits may prove to be heterogeneous, genetic linkage analyses may provide a way to expose various homogeneous subtypes.

Identifying Mode of Inheritance. Another way in which genetic linkage analyses may be useful in studies of behavioral disorders is in the clarification of the mode of inheritance. In fact, it may prove to be a very important aid in resolving mode of inheritance. The best example to date is an analysis of hemochromatosis done by Kravitz *et al.* (1979). They resolved the inheritance of the postulated underlying abnormality in iron concentration by incorporating into their pedigree analysis the information on the HLA system. They were not suggesting that HLA antigens themselves were in any way responsible for the trait but only that the locus affecting serum iron concentrations was sufficiently close to the HLA region that the two would co-segregate in the families being studied. Initial analyses without the information about HLA included were unable to differentiate between a dominant or a recessive mode of inheritance for the serum iron concentration. When the HLA data were included, the researchers were able to rule out the dominant mode of transmission and conclude that the inheritance pattern of the underlying susceptibility to the disease was basically autosomal recessive. With the added HLA information, heterozygotes could also be identified, and the researchers found that heterozygotes had elevated iron concentrations that, however, were usually not sufficiently high for illness to result.

Methods. There are two commonly used methods for linkage analysis: (1) the sib-pair method; and (2) the sequential sampling method.

The sib-pair method was designed to detect the presence of a disease susceptibility locus. First developed by Penrose (1935, 1953) and modified by Suarez, Rice, and Reich (1978) and others, the method examines sibling pairs to see if there are perturbations in the distribution of identity by descent (IBD) scores for sib-pairs at a known marker locus. If there is no population-wide association between a trait and marker locus, but affected sibs share the identical marker locus more often than would be expected by chance, that is taken as evidence for the existence of linkage.

Morton (1955) proposed a method that would utilize data from all individuals in a family pedigree. This method involves calculating likelihoods for specific genetic models and values of the recombination fraction, θ. The likelihood for each $0 < \theta < .5$ is compared to the likelihood when $\theta = .5$ (i.e., the null hypothesis of no linkage). If the ratio of likelihoods (odds) is such that it is 1,000 times more likely for linkage to exist ($\theta < .5$) than not ($\theta = .5$), then by convention that is taken as evidence for linkage. Thus, if the log (odds)>3, then linkage is said to exist between trait and marker. If the ratio is such that the null hypothesis (θ = .5) is 100 times more likely, then, by convention, linkage is rejected. Therefore, if the ratio of the probabilities that the two loci are linked is <1/100, then log (odds)<−2, and the linkage hypothesis would be rejected.

A computer program, LIPED (Ott, 1976), is available to calculate these likelihood or "lod" scores. The program has been modified to incorporate age- and sex-dependent penetrances. LIPED makes the assumption that the genetic model of the trait is known; hence it is not as useful as it could be if it also could estimate the genetic model parameters. Currently available pedigree analysis methodologies allow for the simultaneous estimation of genetic model parameters and θ. This allows for a more precise estimate of all parameters. Recent simulation studies (Goldin, Cox, Pauls, Gershon, & Kidd, 1984) suggest that these estimates are more accurate. However, much work needs to be devoted to the development of more powerful methods for this rapidly developing area of genetic investigation. For a more detailed review of linkage methodologies in general, the reader is referred to Conneally and Rivas (1980).

CHAPTER 5

Hereditary Influences on Epileptic Conditions

INFLUENCES ON EPILEPTIC CONDITIONS

Epileptic attacks are thought to be due to the synchronous discharge of a very large number of brain cells. A seizure occurs when enough cells have been recruited to disrupt the normal, patterned, asynchronous activity in the brain that underlies the organized mental and motor behavior of an intact individual. On the basis of this theory, treatment in some severe cases has been to cut the corpus callosum (the connection between the two hemispheres) to prevent the spreading buildup (or recruitment) from one side of the brain to the other.

The focus of an epileptic attack can now be determined with a technique in which the magnetic field generated by the synchronous currents in a number of adjacent brain cells is picked up outside of the head by superconducting magnetometers (Barth, Sutherling, Engel, & Beatty, 1982; Reite & Zimmerman 1978), but such equipment will remain rare in the near future because it is so expensive.

Because an epileptic attack is such a dramatic phenomenon, one expects epilepsy to be a well-defined entity. On the contrary, convulsive conditions are very heterogeneous, and the meaningfulness of some of the proposed distinctions between epilepsy and other conditions is still uncertain. In addition, increased use of the electroencephalogram (EEG) in making the diagnosis has somewhat blurred the distinction between normal and affected individuals. It is a well-known fact that exposure to flickering lights, hyperventilation, and the use of certain drugs will elicit epileptic symptoms in individuals sensitive to these stimuli. In fact, some medical experts believe that feelings of déjà vu or depersonalization are minor symptoms of epilepsy. If this is so, almost everyone could be diagnosed as epileptic!

CLASSIFICATION OF EPILEPTIC CONDITIONS

The most common distinction is made between secondary or symptomatic epilepsies, due to some known factor affecting the brain, and the primary, essential, or idiopathic ones, without a known cause. The latter are thought to be more likely genetic in origin. In many instances, when a specific focus for the seizure is identified, it is useful in diagnosis. Delgado-Escueta, Wasterlain, Treiman, and Porter (1982) modified a list of such foci compiled by Penfield and Erickson (1941). This modified list is shown in Table 12.

Table 12. Clinical-Anatomical Correlations in Partial Seizures

Initial phenomena	Cerebral origin
Loss of consciousness	Frontal cortex, amygdala-hippocampal complex, or reticular-cortical system
Inability to speak	Broca's area of supplementary motor cortex
Focal clonic movements (contralateral)	Precentral cortex
Tingling sensations (contralateral)	Postcentral cortex
Tingling sensations (bilateral or ipsilateral)	Secondary sensory cortex
Buzzing sound	Heschl's convolution
Vertigo	Heschl's convolution
Unpleasant smell	Uncus
Memories, hallucinations, or illusions	Temporal neocortex or amygdala-hippocampal complex
Epigastric sensation, palpitations	Insula
Black and white geometric patterns	Occipitotemporal cortex
Colored patterns	Occipito cortex
Inability to understand words or meaning of words	Posterior temporal and inferior parietal cortex
Head and eye turning associated with arm movement	Supplementary motor cortex

Note. From "Phenotypic variations of seizures in adolescents and adults" by A. V. Delgado-Escueta, D. M. Treiman and F. Enrile-Bacsal, 1982. In V. E. Anderson (Ed.), *Genetic basis of the epilepsies.* New York: Raven Press. Copyright 1982 by Raven Press. Reprinted by permission.

Volume 34 of the series *Advances in Neurology* is entitled "Status Epilepticus." This name refers to a very severe form of epilepsy in which there are lengthy and/or repeated seizures, up to 100 in 24 hours (Ford, 1973, p. 1332). This can result in lack of oxygen to certain areas of the brain and, hence, brain damage or even death. It can occur at all ages, either spontaneously or as a result of a physical illness. It can also be drug-induced. Within this category further subtypes can be distinguished. Gastaut in his chapter in *Advances in Neurology* distinguishes between convulsive and nonconvulsive types; the latter, an apparent contradiction in terms, refers to such conditions as the so-called "absence status" (also called petit mal or epileptic twilight state). Among the convulsive (grand mal) types, Gastaut distinguishes the tonic, clonic, tonic-clonic and myoclonic subtypes and unilateral and bilateral seizures.

In the same volume, data are reported suggesting that in previously nonaffected children, the consequences of a prolonged seizure episode of the convulsive type were permanent neurological signs in 20%, mental retardation in 33%, and recurring epilepsy in 21%.

More detailed classifications of epilepsy are based on the age of first seizures, severity and type of seizure, and possibly eliciting factors such as photic stimuli or fever, as well as the specific type of EEG abnormality. The World Health Organization and the International League Against Epilepsy each have their own scheme. Delgado-Escueta *et al.* (1982) have provided an especially fine-grained classification shown in Table 13.

Some authors place neonatal seizures in a separate category. Janz and Beck-Mannagetta (1982) believe that neonatal convulsions should be placed in a different category than epilepsy. Febrile convulsions may be another entity, but they may prove to be somewhat related to epilepsy, as Janz and Beck-Mannagetta (1982) found an increased risk for febrile convulsions in offspring of epileptic mothers. Most early convulsions are indeed brought on by fever and Nelson and Ellenberg (1978) reported that only 2% of such affected children become adult epileptics. However, Harrison and Taylor (1976) found somewhat different results when they followed up a group of patients 25 years later. They noted that 22% of children who suffered early seizures were epileptic as adults.

Seizures can be produced by brain lesions and by drugs but also by a large number of Mendelian traits. Anderson (1982) has recently summarized these disorders. He notes that there are 20 autosomal dominant conditions that include seizures among their symptoms as well as 27 autosomal recessive and 7 X-linked recessive conditions. Some of these disorders are not well established and may not be valid single-

Table 13. Classification of Epileptic Seizures Modified by A. V. Delgado-Escueta et al. from the ILAE and WHO Classifications

PARTIAL SEIZURES
- I. Simple partial seizures
- II. Complex partial seizures
  - A. Simple partial onset followed by impairment of consciousness and automatisms
  - B. With impairment of consciousness at onset
    1. Motionless stare with lapse and automatisms
    2. Lapse—automatisms
    3. With drop attack (temporal lobe syncope)
- III. Partial seizures evolving to generalized tonic-clonic seizures

GENERALIZED SEIZURES
- I. Absence seizures
  - A. Classic absence of childhood with 3-Hz spike-wave complexes
  - B. Absence with diffuse 8 to 12-Hz rhythms
  - C. Myoclonic absence with 3-Hz spike-wave complexes
  - D. Myoclonus absence: Staring, fragmentary myoclonus, automatisms, and diffuse 12-Hz rhythms
  - E. Juvenile absence: Staring with 3-Hz spike-wave complexes during adolescence
  - F. Spike-wave stupor or absence status as the only manifestation of epilepsy in adults
- II. Myoclonic seizures
  - A. Infantile spasms (propulsive petit mal: Infantile myoclonic encephalopathy with hypsarrhythmia)
  - B. Myoclonic astatic or atonic seizures (epileptic drop attacks of Lennox and Gastaut in children with mental retardation)
  - C. Myoclonic seizures of early childhood without mental retardation
  - D. Myoclonic seizures of adolescence and late childhood or juvenile myoclonic seizures
- III. Clonic seizures
- IV. Clonic-tonic-clonic seizures
- V. Tonic-clonic seizures
- VI. Tonic seizures

Note. From "Phenotypic variations of seizures in adolescents and adults" by A. V. Delgato-Escueta, D. M. Treiman and F. Enrile-Bacsal, 1982. In V. E. Anderson (Ed.), *Genetic basis of the epilepsies.* New York: Raven Press. Copyright 1982 by Raven Press. Reprinted by permission.

gene entities. In addition, many of these conditions are rare, and some are easily recognized because of obvious physical stigmata or clear medical problems, so that one may be justified in thinking that there is no need to worry about ruling out such convulsive conditions when attempting to do a genetic study of only true, well-defined cases of epilepsy. But if they were by chance improperly included, the fact that these conditions are hereditary could bias a study in the direction of finding a genetic factor and erroneously attributing it to the etiology of epilepsy. Older studies probably included some such cases, as they had not yet been identified as disorders separate from epilepsy. Thus, results of older studies may be in error. Nevertheless, certain general trends should hold true in view of the consistency of findings from study to study. For example, many studies report the incidence of epilepsy at roughly 0.5% (Hauser 1978). A peak onset period occurring between ages 15 and 24 has been reported in Great Britain, and a peak between 20 and 24 years of age was found in a sample gathered in the U.S. The estimate for the incidence of epilepsy varies with age and probably also with the population sampled. Anderson (1982) reported the cumulative incidence rate estimated from data for Rochester, Minnesota, during the years 1935–1974. He noted that although the incidence at any given age fluctuates around 0.5%, the probability of becoming epileptic increases with age, so that the cumulative probability is, for example, 2% at age 55. Ford (1973) mentions an incidence of only three per thousand in the general population in the United States. In the same chapter, Epilepsies and Paroxysmal Disorders of the Nervous System, which also provides much detail about the various subtypes, he cites a paper by Davenport that summarizes the literature on ethnic differences in incidence of epilepsy. The disorder is reported to be low among Maoris, East Indians, natives of the Philippine and Hawaiian islands, Japanese, Finns, Germans, and Scandinavians but high among Koreans, Italians, French Canadians, and English. Ford warns that some of the statistics may have been inaccurate, especially for areas with poor health services or records. Ford also mentions that only 8 to 10% of soldiers with head wounds develop seizures, suggesting that in addition to the injury, there may have to be a genetic predisposition for epilepsy to develop.

Family Studies

As would be expected for a disorder with a genetic component, the incidence in relatives of probands is much higher than the 0.5% reported for the general population. The incidence depends upon the closeness of the genetic relationship. The frequency may be as high as 14% in parents or siblings. Janz and Beck-Mannagetta (1982) reported the results of their own study of offspring of 414 epileptic patients, while also summarizing the results of previous studies of children of epileptics. Taking all the data together, we calculated an incidence of 4.07% for epilepsy in the offspring of patients with idiopathic epilepsy.

When patients with symptomatic epilepsy (associated with some physical trauma) were included, the incidence was reduced to 3.5%.

TWIN STUDIES

The results of the early twin studies summarized by Koch (1967)
are shown in Table 14. For all the studies together, the MZ concordance for epilepsy was .58, and the DZ concordance was .11, which
would result in a (broad) heritability of .94 when using Falconer's formula $H = 2 (r_{MZ} - r_{DZ})$. The rather low MZ concordance in spite of
this suggested high heritability implies reduced penetrance and may be
explained in part by the variability in age of onset of the symptoms.
(*Penetrance* is a term employed to account for the absence of the trait
in the phenotype, even though it is believed to be coded for in the
genotype). Using this explanation, one could hypothesize that some of
the discordant twins might at some later time become concordant.

The ultimate goal of genetic studies is the location of the gene(s)
that have mutated on a specific area of a chromosome. A first step was
taken for epilepsy by Tills, Warlow, Richens, and Laidlau (1981) who

Table 14. Twin Studies of Epilepsy[a]

		MZ Twins		DZ Twins	
Investigators	Year	N	Percentage Concordant	N	Percentage Concordant
Rosanoff et al.	1934	23	.61	84	.24
Schulte	1934	10	.20	12	0
Conrad	1935	30	.67	127	.03
Alstrom	1950	2	.00	14	0
Castellis & Fuster	1952	2	.50	4	0
Ellebjerg	1952	7	.43	12	0
Slater	1953	2	.00	12	0
Schimmelpenning	1955	4	.50	15	0
Bormann	1956	5	.40	15	.13
Lafon et al.	1956	7	.71	—	0
Kamide, Inouye, & Suzuki	1957–60	26	.54	14	.07
Lennox	1960	95	.62	130	.15
Braconi	1962	20	.65	31	.13
Totals		233	.58	470	.11

[a]Heritability, $h^2 = 2(r_{MZ} - r_{DZ}) = .94$ for combined samples.
Note. Adapted from "Epilepsien" by G. Koch, 1967. In H. Becker (Ed.), *Human-genetik: Ein Kurzes Handbuch in Funf Banden.* Stuttgart: Thieme.

tested 30 genetic systems for association with epilepsy and found only one statistically significant difference between patients and controls. This was for a particular typology in the MNSs blood group system. However, until this finding is confirmed by other research, it must be considered to be questionable.

Eeg-Olofsson, Safwenberg, and Wigertz (1982) studied the relationship between HLA (human leucocyte antigen) haplotypes and different types of epilepsy. The HLA system consists of five closely linked loci, each of which has from 8 to 39 alleles. It is located on the chromosome designated as Number 6. *Haplotype* is the term for the particular combination of alleles that an individual has inherited. In the study by Eeg-Olofsson and his colleagues, the only significant difference between epileptic probands and nonepileptic controls and between parents of controls and epileptics was a low incidence of the most common haplotype, A1B8, in families whose members seemed to inherit "benign epilepsy of childhood." Because a number of comparisons were made, however, it is possible that this one difference could have occurred by chance alone.

The Heredity of EEG

A number of twin studies by Davis and Davis (1936), Lennox, Gibbs, and Gibbs (1945), Hanzawa (1957), Vogel (1958, 1965, 1970) Lykken, Tellegen, and Thorkelson (1974), and Lykken, Tellegen, and Iacono (1982) have shown that the EEGs of MZ twins are usually as similar as two records taken from the same person on different occasions, whereas those of DZ twins are quite different. In fact, given paired records of twins, they can be classified as MZ or DZ with few errors. This clearly indicates a high degree of hereditary determination, especially since Juel-Nielsen and Harvald (1958) and Lykken *et al.* (1982) found the EEGs of MZ twins reared apart to be just as similar as the EEGs of MZ twins reared together.

However, a simple comparison of the overall similarity of EEG records is too global a characteristic to lend itself to further analysis. For that reason, later investigators have concentrated on particular EEG features or syndromes such as low-voltage EEGs with few or absent alphawaves (Vogel & Gotze, 1959; Vogel & Helmbold, 1959); 14 to 16 cycles per second positive spikes during sleep in children (Petersen & Akesson, 1968; Vogel, 1965); centrencephalic spike and wave patterns plus petit mal seizure in children (Metrakos & Metrakos, 1960, 1961); abnormal theta wave frequency (Doose, Gerken, Peterson,

& Volzke, 1967); and temporal lobe epilepsy (Barslund & Danielsen, 1963; Bray, Wiser, Wood, & Pusey, 1965; Rodin & Whelan, 1960).

Each of these characteristics is a plausible candidate for a single-gene autosomal "abnormality," and in families of individuals who display one of these syndromes, there is often increased incidence of the same characteristic among several members. When family data for these traits are examined, sex-influenced inheritance seems to be unlikely because in most studies equal proportions of affected parents, sibs, and children of both sexes were found. Sex-influenced genetic systems always result in a preponderance of one sex being affected. The best estimate of the incidence of abnormal EEGs in relatives of epileptics can perhaps be obtained by combining the data from all available studies. This has been done in Table 15.

The average familial estimate of abnormal EEGs is 37%; this much higher value than familial incidence rates for epilepsy implies that what causes an abnormal EEG is not a sufficient explanation for epilepsy. However, abnormal EEG recordings could still prove to be a contributing factor. One could hypothesize that perhaps the one-fifth of the relatives who exhibited the epileptic disorder had either more abnormal genes or life histories more conducive to the expression of epileptic symptoms (i.e., a lower threshold).

As noted before, Lykken et al. (1974) reported extremely high levels of similarity for the EEG spectrum of MZ twins and much lower levels of similarity for DZ twins. Each spectrum consisted of a distribution of the proportion of the total EEG recording that fell in one of

Table 15. Incidence of EEG Abnormality in First-Degree Relatives (Parents, Sibs, Children) of Epileptics

Investigators	Year	Probands	Relatives	Percentage Abnormal EEG	
				Relatives	Controls
Lowenbach	1939	11	37	46	
Strauss et al.	1939	31	93	28	
Lennox et al.	1940	94	183	60	16
Harvald	1954	237	547	36	13
Vercelletto	1955	109	158	45	
Richter	1956	43	87	35	
Total		525	1105	475	

Note. Adapted from "Epilepsien" by G. Koch, 1967. In H. Becker (Ed.), Human-genetik: Ein Kurzes Handbuch in Funf Banden. Stuttgart: Thieme.

the 200 intervals into which the frequency band from 0.1 to 20.0 Hertz was divided. It was then possible to calculate a total similarity score for each pair. The distribution of these similarities could then be compared for MZ and DZ twins. When calculating the similarity for a pair of twins, the difference between the two twins was compared to the variability in recordings noted within each twin and between the spectrum at the beginning and the end of the session. The formula used for what was called the "spectrum difference ratio" is as follows:

$$SDR = \frac{D(A_1 - B_2) + D(A_2 - B_2)}{D(A_1 - A_2) + D(B_1 - B_2)}$$

where A and B are the two twins, the subscripts 1 and 2 refer to the spectra at the beginning and the end, and D is the root-mean-squared difference for the two sets of 200 intervals. When SDR is equal to, or smaller than 1.0, the twins' spectra resemble each other as much or more than the spectra of their own two samples.

The SDR values of 39 MZ pairs tested together had a modal value of 1.0; for 27 DZ pairs, the value was 1.7. In 1982, Lykken et al., reported modes of 1.15 and 1.7 for 50 MZ and 26 DZ pairs. Very similar results were obtained for 25 adult MZ pairs, who had, in every case, been reared apart from one another. Finding that MZ twins reared apart are as similar as MZ twins reared together is, of course, powerful evidence for a genetic influence. In this same paper, the authors also reported concordance rates (intraclass correlations) for the three sets of twins on five parameters of the spectra. These are shown in Table 16.

A major problem with studies of epilepsy is that different studies may have different ascertainment biases—that is, it is generally not known how the particular probands were located. This is especially a problem with epilepsy because most patients are not hospitalized and successful treatment may result in underreporting in family histories. Although in recent years methods have been developed to make statistical corrections for ascertainment biases in a nonrepresentative sample of the population (Elston & Stewart 1971), only a systematic survey of every individual in a well-defined population could circumvent this problem entirely. Earlier studies are probably the most problematic in this regard because it has only been in the last 40 years or so that the ascertainment bias has been recognized as a problem.

The most disconcerting problem, however, is of a different nature. Individuals with epilepsy may have periods of partial or complete remission of symptoms, and, as mentioned earlier, there is in addition a wide range of age of onset of first symptoms. For the centrencephalic

Table 16. Intraclass Correlations of
Five Spectrum Parameters for 25 MZ
Twins Reared Apart (MZA), 89 MZ
Pairs Reared Together (MZT), and 53
DZ Pairs

Parameter	MZA	MZT	DZ
Alpha	.93	.86	.13
Beta	.61	.72	.37
Delta	.90	.84	.26
Theta	.76	.80	.04
Phi[a]	.89	.81	−.15

[a]Phi is the median frequency measured in a 3-Hz
band centered around the peak in the spectrum sec-
tion falling between 7.1 and 13.0 Hz.
Note. From "EEG Spectra in Twins: Evidence for a
Neglected Mechanism of Genetic Determinism" by
D. T. Lykken, A. Tellegen, and W. G. Iacono, 1982,
Physiological Psychology, 10, Copyright 1982 by the
Psychonomic Society. Reprinted by permission.

syndrome, as they denoted a particular epileptic condition, Metrakos
and Metrakos (1960, 1961) calculated the penetrance levels at various
ages. They hypothesized that, overall, if the condition were the result
of a single dominant autosomal gene, parents and sibs of an affected
child should show a 50% incidence of similar EEGs, if penetrance was
complete (i.e., penetrance equal to 1.0).

Departure from this rate was used to calculate the penetrance at
the ages shown in Table 17 to produce Figure 10. If such variability in
expression of the EEG abnormality is the rule in various forms of

Table 17. Calculated Penetrance Levels of Epilepsy at Various Ages
(Based on Rates of Epilepsy Found among Relatives of Probands in
Five Studies)

Age range	Number of sibs/ parents tested	Abnormal EEG	Hypothetical penetrance
2 1/2	16	1	0.13
4 1/2 to 16 1/2	146	65	0.89
16 1/2 to 24 1/2	26	4	0.31
24 1/2 to 40 1/2	147	13	0.18
over 40 1/2	40	1	0.05

Note. From "Genetics of Convulsive disorders" by K. Metrakos & J. D. Metrakos, 1961.
Neurology 11, p. 474–483. Copyright 1961 by Modern Medicine Publications. Reprinted by
permission.

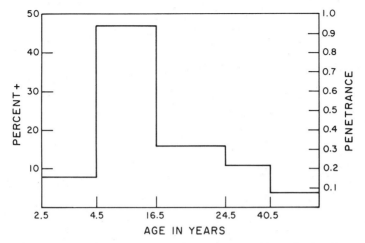

Figure 10. Penetrance levels at various ages for expression of EEG abnormalities. *Note.* From "Genetics of Convulsive Disorders, I, II" by J. D. Metrakos & K. Metrakos, 1960, 1961, *Neurology, 10, 11.* Copyright 1960, 1961 by Modern Medicine Publications. Reprinted by permission.

epilepsy and EEG-designated abnormalities, no high degree of fit to any specific genetic model can be expected. Of course this variability can arise from many possible sources, including such methodological problems as inadequate diagnostic techniques and heterogeneity within the syndrome. Therefore, researchers planning studies in this area would be well advised to utilize the most advanced diagnostic methods, and further, to define specifically the syndrome they wish to study.

THE EFFECT OF EPILEPSY ON INTELLIGENCE

The intelligence of epileptics does not differ from the average, at least when the condition first appears. However, repeated seizures, with their disturbing effects, may lead to lowered performance on IQ tests and in schoolwork and may eventually produce permanent brain damage. Fortunately, this is rather uncommon today because of improved techniques for treating the disorder.

As part of a study of the concordance for epilepsy in twins, Lennox and Jolly (1954) also obtained intelligence test scores on 60 MZ and 67 DZ twin pairs. Their results are shown in Figures 11 and 12. Both figures show that a diagnosis of prior brain damage generally was associated with a lower IQ test score. The 36 MZ pairs without brain

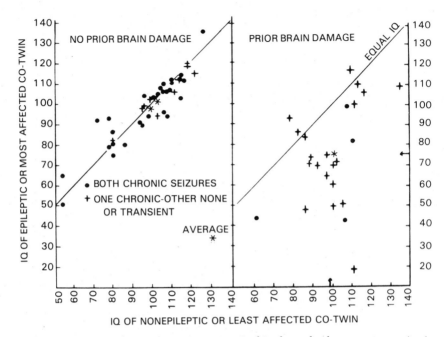

Figure 11. IQ scores of 60 monozygotic twins. In this chart, the dots represent twins in which both have chronic epilepsy. The crosses are for those in which one co-twin either has only transient or no seizures. In the left-hand panel, the stars indicate the average of each of these two groups; the uppermost is for twins when both co-twins have chronic epilepsy. The IQ of the epileptic or the more affected of the co-twins is placed on the ordinate scale. The arrows pointing from the side indicate the average values for the cases in the right panel. *Note.* From "Seizures, Brain Waves and Intelligence Tests of Epileptic Twins" by W. G. Lennox & D. Jolly, 1954. In D. Hooker & C. C. Hare (Eds.), *Genetics and the Inheritance of Integrated Neurological and Psychiatric Patterns.* Copyright 1954 by Williams & Witkins. Reprinted by permission.

damage had an average IQ of 103.5; average IQ scores for the 24 MZ pairs in which one twin had brain damage and the other did not were 75 and 99, respectively, yielding a correlation of only .47. For the 33 DZ pairs without brain damage, the average IQ was 90.5, and the correlation was .65; for the 34 DZ pairs in which one twin had brain damage and the other did not, the averages were 71 and 97, respectively, with a correlation of .39.

    Assuming that the co-twin is a perfect control, the right-hand side of Figure 11 suggests that the effect of the prior brain damage was to lower the average IQ by 24 points, whereas the left side suggests that epilepsy alone does not necessarily lead to a decrease from the mean IQ of 100. This study is an excellent example of how twin studies may be used to investigate the effects of an environmental influence, in this case brain damage, secondary to epilepsy.

COMPARATIVE STUDIES OF EPILEPSY

Mice (Fuller, 1975; Gruneberg, 1952), guinea pigs (Crifo, 1973), rabbits (Nachtsheim, 1939), and cattle and dogs (Collier, 1928) display behavior closely resembling grand mal seizures in humans. This behavior can readily be elicited in certain strains of mice by jingling keys, by ringing an electric bell, or by other sounds. Since mice are easily maintained in laboratories, they are used in many genetic studies. The influence of heredity on such audiogenic seizures in mice is gradually

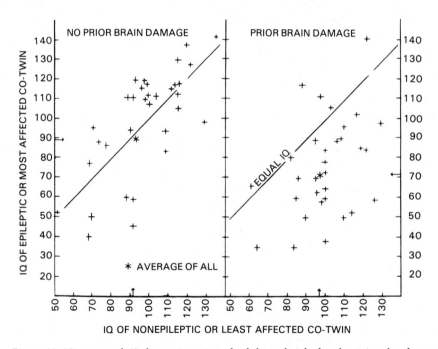

Figure 12. IQ scores of 67 dizygotic twins, the left- and right-hand portion for those respectively without and with prior history of brain damage. The crosses spot the IQ scores of both co-twins. In each case, only one co-twin has chronic seizures. The stars and arrows indicate average values. *Note.* From "Seizures, Brain Waves and Intelligence Tests of Epileptic Twins" by W. G. Lennox & D. Jolly, 1954. In D. Hooker & C. C. Hare (Eds.), *Genetics and the Inheritance of Integrated Neurological and Psychiatric Patterns.* Copyright 1954 by Williams & Witkins. Reprinted by permission.

becoming clear and may provide a model for human epileptic conditions.

Maxson & Cowen (1976) has reported anatomical differences between seizure-prone and other mice. Henry (1967) found that strains of mice not normally seizure prone could be "primed," i.e., made more prone to audiogenic seizures, by exposure to sound stimulation at an earlier age even though no mice of any strains showed any direct effect of the sound at that age. This provides an interesting example of a clear cut effect of early environment interacting with the genotpye to produce the phenotype. Fuller (1975) found that the familial distributions of susceptibility to spontaneous and to primed audiogenic seizures in mice were independent. This evidence suggests that there are at least two independently transmitted forms of seizure-prone behavior in mice. As noted earlier in this chapter, genetic heterogeneity among humans may also be a complicating factor in establishing the mode of inheritance of epileptic conditions.

CHAPTER 6

Hereditary Factors in Schizophrenia

The origin of the most frequently used current classification scheme for schizophrenia can be traced to Emil Kraepelin and Eugene Bleuler. The work by Kraepelin (1856–1926) was the culmination of efforts by the 19th-century psychiatrists to sort out the various types of mental disorders. Although he used the term *dementia praecox*, the disorder he described is very similar to that which is now called *schizophrenia*. His primary concern was to differentiate dementia praecox from manic-depressive psychosis. The major symptoms he described were hallucinations, delusions, negativism, deficient attention, and inappropriate emotional responses. He recognized four types: simple, hebephrenic, catatonic, and paranoid. His general view was that the disease process was organic, perhaps of a hereditary nature.

The term *schizophrenia* was introduced in 1911 by Bleuler (1911/1950). In fact, he referred to the "schizophrenias," suggesting that there are different types that may have different etiologies. Instead of viewing the disease as an organic process, he emphasized the psychogenic aspects. His hypothesis was that the basic defect involved the splitting or disorganization of the personality. Hence the name: split mind. This in turn resulted in inconsistent and inappropriate behavior. He also felt that withdrawal (autism) was central to these patterns of behavior and that this produced the shallowness of affect mentioned by others who had studied the disorder. Although Bleuler's ideas have had much influence in the 20th century, recently researchers have returned to a point of view more in keeping with Kraepelin's physiological theory.

Although the syndrome of schizophrenia may be thought of as being comprised by a set of characteristic symptoms including disturbance of thought processes, of perceptual processes, of affect, of sense of self, and of psychomotor behavior, recent research suggests that there is no single feature that is invariably present in all schizophrenics, nor are any of the previously mentioned symptoms seen exclusively in schizophrenia. The overt behavioral signs that are most strongly associated with this diagnosis are hallucinations and/or delusions, speech that is disorganized and therefore difficult to comprehend, silly, childlike behavior, and "catatonic" posturing of either the stuporous or excited type.

The disorder is considered to be chronic in its overall course. Although some individuals may experience periods after the first onset of symptoms that are relatively symptom-free, most do not. Furthermore, the general course of the disorder does not often include a complete, permanent return to normal, premorbid functioning. Deterioration from a previously higher level of functioning is considered to be an important diagnostic dimension that allows schizophrenia to be distinguished from several other disorders such as mental retardation, manic-depressive illness, and certain personality disorders. This deterioration can be halted or at least slowed down in many individuals through the use of so-called major tranquilizers or antipsychotic drugs. These drugs do not cure the disorder but seem to have an ameliorating effect on disorganized thinking and speech as well as on inappropriate affect and behavior.

There appears to be a higher incidence of schizophrenia in persons of lower socioeconomic status. The reason for this association is unclear. Either lower socioeconomic status puts one at a higher risk for the disorder, or, equally plausible, is the notion that those affected tend to "drift" downward into the lower ranks of society.

Schizophrenia has an early age of onset: the first symptoms can usually be traced to a period beginning in late adolescence and ending early in the third decade of life. It appears to be as prevalent in males as in females, although there is a tendency for the disorder to be diagnosed more frequently in very young males than in young females. However, as the age of onset of first symptoms increases, relatively more females than males are diagnosed, and thus the equal sex ratio is regained.

One of the most precise sets of diagnostic criteria for mental illness was proposed by Spitzer, Endicott, and Robins in 1978. Their RDC

(Research Diagnostic Criteria) manual includes the following specific requirements for the diagnosis of schizophrenia:

A. During an active phase of the illness (may or may not now be present) at least two of the following are required for a definite, and one for a probable diagnosis:

(1) Thought broadcasting, insertion, or thought withdrawal.

(2) Delusions of being controlled (or influenced), other bizarre or multiple delusions.

(3) Delusions having a somatic, grandiose, religious, or nihilistic content, or other delusions without themes of persecution or jealousy lasting at least a week.

(4) Delusions of any type if accompanied by hallucinations of any type for at least one week.

(5) Auditory hallucinations in which either a voice keeps up a running commentary on the subject's behavior or thoughts as they occur, or two or more voices converse with each other.

(6) Non-affective verbal hallucinations spoken to the subject.

(7) Hallucinations of any type throughout the day for several days or intermittently for at least one month.

(8) Definite instances of marked formal thought disorder accompanied by either blunted or inappropriate affect, delusions or hallucinations of any type, or grossly disorganized behavior.

B. Signs of the illness have lasted at least two weeks from the onset of a noticeable change in the subject's usual condition (current signs of the illness may not now meet criterion A and may be residual symptoms only, such as extreme social withdrawal, blunted or inappropriate affect, mild formal thought disorder, or unusual thoughts or perceptual experiences).

C. At no time during the *active* period (delusions, hallucinations, marked formal thought disorder, bizarre behavior, etc.) of illness being considered did the subject meet the full criteria for either probable or definite manic or depressive syndrome to such a degree that it was a *prominent* part of the illness. (Spitzer, Endicott & Robins, 1978, p. 7)

Because the predominant behavior of individual patients seems to differ, four subtypes have been formulated. The *catatonic* type is marked by periods of psycho-motor disturbance and excitement, rigidity, stupor, or posturing. Mutism is particularly common in this type. The *paranoid* subgroup is characterized by systematized delusions, often of persecutory or grandiose type, and frequent hallucinations. Pervasive formal thought disorder may be mild in this particular type, so that the behavior is often relatively normal, until something or someone touches on the subject matter of a particular delusion that the patient holds. Thus a patient may believe that he or she is the focus of a communist plot, or that he or she is working under orders from an otherworldly being, yet be a satisfactory employee, for long periods of time, and may even remain somewhat integrated into the community. The average age of onset of this type is later than that of the other types of schizophrenia, although paranoid schizophrenia is sometimes seen in very young persons. The *hebephrenic,* or *disorganized,* type is characterized by rambling, disorganized thoughts and speech, having a poorly developed delusional aspect to them, which frequently lends an overall absurd or "silly" quality to the behavior of hebephrenics. A final subtype, designated the *simple* or *undifferentiated* type, does not usually exhibit the dramatic behaviors of the other types and may resemble mental retardation in the fact that these patients are generally unable and, seemingly, uninterested in conversing or thinking in a rigorous, logical manner. In fact, because patients in this subgroup are likely to express fewer of the typically schizophrenic symptoms, many diagnosticians feel that simple or undifferentiated schizophrenia should be eliminated from the nomenclature used to classify schizophrenic subtypes (Spitzer *et al.*, 1978).

There is considerable disagreement about whether these subtypes of schizophrenia are really independent disorders with different etiologies and/or outcomes. Some researchers have suggested that a patient can go through various phases during the course of the illness and that the subtypes merely describe these phases. There is also disagreement about whether any or all of the generally recognized types are genetically determined (and to what degree), and finally, whether all four are determined by the same genetic factor(s). Most studies so far have assumed that they are all one genetic entity. However, data have been collected concerning the occurrence of schizophrenia among various relatives of schizophrenic probands that do not suggest any strong concordance for these subtypes (Tsuang, Fowler, Cadoret, & Monnelly, 1974). This evidence notwithstanding, the majority of research on schizophrenia has been done assuming that it is a single disorder. The research to be discussed later reflects this fact.

Kendler, Gruenberg, and Strauss (1981c) reanalyzed the psychiatric records of a large-scale Danish adoption study of schizophrenia (which will be discussed in detail in this chapter) and found no paranoid psychosis in any of the biological relatives of the schizophrenic adoptees in the study, suggesting that paranoia is a distinct genetic entity separate from schizophrenia. Langfeldt (1956) and Schneider (1959) made a distinction between true schizophrenia and schizophreniform psychosis. The latter is characterized by a better premorbid history and a more favorable outcome. This is rather similar to the process-reactive distinction that is better known in the United States, although it has hardly ever been used in genetic research. Yet a division into paranoid, process (or chronic), and reactive (or episodic, periodic, acute) has been suggested by diagnosticians repeatedly (Eisenthal,

Hartford, & Solomon, 1972; Lorr, 1974; Mirsky, 1969; Payne, 1970) Another distinction that is currently being used is that between patients with positive and those with negative symptoms. Positive symptoms (presence of *abnormal* behaviors) are marked by hallucinations and/or delusions, severe formal thought disorders, and bizarre or disorganized behavior. In contrast, the patients with negative symptoms (absence of *normal* behaviors) display affective flattening, anhedonia, apathy, withdrawal, and impaired attention. Sometimes a mixed category is included (Andreasen, 1982). Occasionally, the possibility of a subtype difference existing between sporadic and familial cases is raised. Sporadic cases are those with no known family history of the disorder. A problem with this lack of knowledge of positive family history is that it may not be equated with absence of illness for there may be insufficient data to rule out the latter. In addition, in small families with few or no uncles, aunts, brothers, or sisters, there may not have been a chance for the illness to express itself in any relatives.

HIGH-RISK RESEARCH IN SCHIZOPHRENIA

Although there are far more schizophrenics who seem to be isolated cases in a family with no other known members with a psychiatric history, most researchers have been more interested in the familial type. This is especially true of those interested in studying the genetic aspects. Of particular interest have been children of one or even two schizophrenic parents, because of the environmental and genetic risk factors to which they are exposed. In fact, Pearson and Kley (1957) proposed that children with one or two schizophrenic parents should be followed to determine whether factors could be identified that would distinguish those that became schizophrenic from those that did not. The incidence of risk is said to be between 10 and 15% in the former and almost 40% in the latter. Mednick and Schulsinger (1968) studied children of schizophrenic mothers and reported increased autonomic reactivity that was interpreted as due to overarousal. However, Erlenmeyer-Kimling, Cornblatt, and Fleiss (1979), in a longitudinal study of offspring of schizophrenics, obtained results in the opposite direction from the Mednick and Schulsinger report. Other measures are being investigated by Erlenmeyer-Kimling and her associates, and it is still too early to judge the value of this very difficult, time-consuming, and expensive methodology.

In Europe, the term *schizophrenia* still has about the same meaning as the one proposed by Kraepelin and Bleuler. In the United States, however, until the 1920s a broadening of the definition and a lessening of the distinction between schizophrenia and other severe behavior disorders occurred. This trend was most noticeable with regard to the affective disorders (mania and depression). This approach makes a comparison of results reported by different investigators throughout the years more difficult, and it has often been criticized by British researchers who use a far narrower definition of schizophrenia. Some research has been based on the concept of a spectrum of disorders that runs from mild "schizoid" behavior to definite schizophrenia. Schizoid individuals are thought to be withdrawn, eccentric, or sometimes quarrelsome and suspicious, but not aberrant enough in their behavior to be diagnosed as truly schizophrenic. This spectrum concept actually combines schizophrenia with the currently recognized personality disorders of the schizotypical, schizoid, paranoid, and borderline types. (See, for instance the research by Heston, 1970.) The main differences between these personality disorders and schizophrenia lie in the severity of the symptoms (less severe in the personality disorders) and in premorbid behavior. Unlike schizophrenia, most personality disorders are not characterized by a stage in which marked deterioration in behavior occurs. Rather, the behaviors are reported to have always been a part of that individual's behavioral repertoire (thus the term *personality disorder*). However, in reality, it is often difficult to use this latter dimension in differentiating between schizophrenia and other personality disorders.

Kendler *et al.* (1981b, 1982) in a reanalysis of the Copenhagen sample of the well-known Danish adoption study (Kety, Rosenthal, Wender, & Schulsinger, 1968; Kety, Rosenthal, & Wender, 1978) found an increase in childhood social withdrawal and antisocial traits in biological relatives of adoptees who became schizophrenic. This suggests that these behaviors, which they labeled "schizotypal personality disorder," may be genetically related to schizophrenia, and because such individuals are at high risk for schizophrenia as adults, these behaviors may be predictive of persons at risk. On the other hand, Grove (1982) has reviewed the evidence for the presence of milder forms of abnormalities in unaffected relatives that might be called schizotypic. He found little or no support for either unusual personality traits or cognitive variables such as idiosyncratic thinking presumed to reflect schizotypy. Thus, the evidence regarding a link between schizophrenics and the presence of milder schizotypic behavior in unaffected relatives is mixed.

Can Future Schizophrenia Be Predicted from Childhood Behavior?

Ideally, one would like to know as much as possible about the premorbid personalities of all patients suffering from behavior disorders. Such information would be very useful in determining whether certain personality types are more vulnerable to certain illnesses. Unfortunately, it is very difficult to retrieve accurate information about the personality of a patient before the onset of the illness. Recollections by relatives or acquaintances may exaggerate or minimize prior symptoms, and the investigator has no way of knowing what type of distortion is occurring. Only rarely are there objective data about the premorbid personality.

In one retrospective study (Bowman, 1934), two psychiatrists and four social workers interviewed relatives, employers, and friends of 151 schizophrenics, 74 affective disorder patients, and a group of 96 social workers who served as normal controls. They then used a lengthy checklist to evaluate specific prepsychotic behaviors as well as general personality traits. Bowman summarized the results with respect to schizophrenia as follows:

> The schizophrenic tends to be a model child, to have few friends, to indulge in solitary amusements, to be a follower, to feel superior, to be close mouthed and uncommunicative. As a child, he is not oversensitive and daydreams less than the normal. . . . As he grows up he becomes more seclusive, has fewer friends, becomes more uncommunicative, utilizes humor less, becomes much more sensitive as compared to the normal. (p. 496)

One wonders to what extent factual information about the patients as adolescents would agree with these anecdotal recollections by people who had known them before they became ill. Because the normal controls in this study were social workers, it is possible that they tended more than the actual normative adolescent to be highly sociable, better educated, and to have more friends. Therefore, these results are speculative at best.

In another retrospective study, Bowlby (1942) studied 36 psychotic and 29 neurotic patients at the Maudsley Hospital in London and tabulated the presence or absence of 33 traits for each patient. He suggested that a tendency toward solitariness, having no friends, no interest in the opposite sex, docility, and a lack of a sense of humor were frequent traits in persons who later become schizophrenic. He noted the common occurrence of obsessional traits in the prepsychotic personality of patients with affective illness as well as schizophrenia. Although this study must be considered inconclusive because of the small sample size, it contains many interesting clinical details. An unfortunate weakness of this study is its retrospective nature. Retrospective data may be influenced by knowledge of the present condition. For that reason follow-up (or "follow-back") of children seen in child guidance clinics or of children for whom there exist school records are particularly valuable, because these records could not be influenced by events that have occurred since they were made.

Bower, Shellhammer, and Dailey (1960) compared school records of 44 male schizophrenics and 44 matched controls. While in school, the preschizophrenics were seen as less gifted, less well liked, more submissive and apathetic, and they had poorer grades overall. This tendency toward lack of adequate scholastic achievement was even more marked in high school.

Robins (1966, 1972) used records of 526 children seen at a child guidance clinic in St. Louis who could be followed up to determine their adult status. One hundred controls were also included. Almost 5% of the clinic cases had become schizophrenic, a number considerably higher than the population incidence. When compared to controls, these individuals had shown more and worse antisocial symptoms as children, including running away and poor school attendance. Other frequently noted symptoms were depression and worrying. Although many of these clinic cases were, as adults, diagnosed as antisocial personality types, 95% did not become schizophrenic. Thus, this study does not suggest an association between serious conduct problems in childhood and schizophrenia in adulthood.

Watt, Fryer, Lewine, and Prentky (1979) were able to obtain more objective data on 145 psychiatric patients and 232 controls—all residents of a community in Massachusetts. The subjects ranged in age from 15 to 40. Controls were matched to the patients for sex, age, race, and parental social class; there were three controls for some patients and two for others. Data were obtained from cumulative school records (including teachers' notes, grades, and counseling and guidance files for Grades K through 12). In addition, in Grades 10 and 11, eight 5-point personality rating scales had been completed by each of the students' teachers. The authors were able to construct a number of behavioral scales and clusters from this information. The most striking finding was that the schizophrenics were not significantly more withdrawn as adolescents, but they had been less emotionally stable ($p < .005$) and less agreeable ($p < .05$). Patients with personality disorders also had been less agreeable than controls ($p < .05$). When composite factor scores on these measures were analyzed, schizophrenics were found to score significantly higher than controls on measures of submissiveness. Their scores were significantly lower on measures of security, extraversion, personableness, and considerateness ($p < .05$ for all variables). Patients with personality disorders also were less personable than controls ($p < .05$). The only other significant finding ($p < .05$) was that psychotic depressives were more independent as children and adolescents. A summary of this literature that attempts to elucidate premorbid childhood behavior patterns of adult schizophrenics can be found in Neale and Oltmanns (1980).

INCIDENCE: HOW FREQUENT IS SCHIZOPHRENIA?

Schizophrenia is fairly common. The expected lifetime risk is approximately 1%. This rate seems to be fairly constant among different countries. Because of the chronic nature and early age of onset for this disorder, schizophrenics take up a large number of places in state mental hospitals. Fortunately, new methods of chemical treatment have reduced the average length of stay, particularly for younger patients, although rehospitalization for periods throughout life is still required for many.

The age at first admission is lower for males. However, twice as many females as males are admitted at later ages, so that overall there is no sex difference in incidence. Lewine (1981) has proposed that the sex difference in age of first admission for schizophrenia is not an artifact nor due to a cultural bias resulting from greater tolerance for abnormal behavior in females, but reflects a real age difference in age of onset of the disorder. Men are more likely to be in their 20s and women in their 30s when first admitted. The women show more affective symptoms and are more often diagnosed as atypical schizophrenics.

As one would expect for a hereditary condition, the incidence in relatives of schizophrenics is greatly increased over the population prevalence figures (i.e., 1%). These incidence data are summarized in Table 18. In fact, it is this phenomenon that originally gave rise to the idea of a hereditary factor in schizophrenia. Although the incidence figures among relatives are high, they are generally much too low to fit a simple Mendelian hypothesis. The relatively low incidence of schizophrenia among parents of probands is generally explained by referring to a lowered fertility of potential schizophrenics. This may no longer be true to the same extent now that treatment with antipsychotic

Table 18. Rate of Schizophrenia in Relatives of Schizophrenics

Date	Number of studies	Relationship	N	Number of schizophrenics	%
1928–62	14	Parents	7675	336	4.38
1928–62	12	Sibs	8504	724	8.51
1932–62	10	Sibs (parents free of schizophrenia)	7535	621	8.24
1932–62	6	Sibs (parents not free of schizophrenia)	674	93	13.79
1921–62	5	Children	1226	151	12.31
1930–41	4	Uncles and aunts	3376	68	2.01
1916–46	3	Half-sibs	311	10	3.22
1926–38	5	Nephews and nieces	2315	52	2.25
1928–38	4	Grandchildren	713	20	2.81
1928–41	4	First cousins	2438	71	2.91

Note. Adapted from E. Zerbin-Rudin, "Endogene Psychosen" (p. 446), in *Human-genetik: Ein Kurzes Handbuch in Funf Banden* (Vol. 2), 1967a. Stuttgart: George Theime, Verlag.

drugs permits many patients to remain at home or to return home after a brief hospitalization. However, even recent research has noted that schizophrenics are more likely to remain unmarried than either normal individuals or persons with other severe psychiatric disorders.

TWIN STUDIES

There have been a number of twin studies of schizophrenia. In general, the earlier studies revealed higher MZ concordance rates than those done in recent years. This tendency can be seen by comparing the concordance rates for MZ twins in Tables 19 and 20. This reflects the fact that the earlier studies were somewhat biased in favor of including only twins who were severely schizophrenic and excluding milder cases. Later studies, which started from either a twin register or a register of mentally ill individuals, more frequently included these mild, borderline cases. An example of this trend toward lower concordance rates can be noted in the study by Kringlen (1968; see Table 20). A review of these data reveals that even when the criteria were relaxed to include so-called "borderline" or questionable schizophrenia, the concordance rate for the MZ twins was only 38%. This figure is much lower than any of the earlier studies noted in Table 19, which report concordance rates from 58 to 69%. During the period between 1938 and 1967, several isolated reports of MZ twins reared apart in which at

Table 19. Early Twin Studies of Schizophrenia[a]

Investigator	Date	MZ Pairs			DZ Pairs		
		N	C	%	N	C	%
Luxenburger	1928	19	11	58	13	0	0
Rosanoff	1934	41	25	61	53	7	13
Essen-Möller	1941	11	7	64	27	4	15
Kallmann	1946	174	120	69	296	34	11
Slater	1953	37	24	65	58	8	14
Inouye	1961	55	33	60	11	2	18

[a]N shows the number of pairs investigated, and C the number found concordant, that is, with a schizophrenic co-twin. Monozygotic pairs compared with same-sexed dizygotic pairs.

least one twin was schizophrenic were made. Table 21 summarizes these reports. The fact that 11 out of 17 pairs were concordant is strong evidence for a genetic component. Farber (1981) recently reanalyzed these data and came to a similar conclusion, even though she notes in her book that she started with a bias against heredity as a causal factor in schizophrenia.

One of the most striking findings to come from a twin study of schizophrenia is that of Fischer (1971). She noted that among children of twin participants in her study, schizophrenia was exhibited by the same percentage of offspring of normal MZ co-twins as by offspring of the affected members of the twin pairs. This suggests that the normal co-twin could have carried the gene(s) for schizophrenia and was likely

Table 20. Recent Twin Studies of Schizophrenia: MZ Pairs[a]

	Both strict schizophrenia			Strict schizophrenia + probable schizophrenialike functional psychosis			Including all "Borderline" co-twins		
	N	C	%	N	C	%	N	C	%
Tienari (1968)	10	1	10	14	2	14	16	5	31
Kringlen (1967)	45	12	27	55	17	31	55	21	38
Fischer et al. (1969)	21	5	24	21	10	48	21	10	48
Gottesman & Shields (1972)	20	8	40	22	11	50	22	11	50
Totals	96	26	27	112	40	36	114	47	41

[a]N shows the number of pairs investigated, and C the number found concordant, that is, with a schizophrenic co-twin.

Table 21. Concordance Rates for Schizophrenic MZ
Twins Reared Apart

Investigator	Number of pairs	
	Concordant	Discordant
Kallmann (1938)	1	
Essen-Möller (1941)	1	
Craike & Slater (1945)	1	
Kallmann & Roth (1954)	1	
Shields (1962)	1	
Tienari (1963)		2
Mitsuda (1965)	5	3
Kringlen (1967)	1	1
Total	11	6

to have thus transmitted the tendency to offspring. Her findings further suggest that living with an affected parent did not increase the likelihood that a child would be affected. This is strong evidence indeed for a genetic factor!

An interesting detail reported by Slater and Cowie (1971) is that nobody has yet reported even one case of manic-depressive illness in the MZ co-twin of a schizophrenic. This suggests that these two disorders are indeed different genetic entities. In fact, the same distinction holds in general for family members of schizophrenics and manic-depressive individuals. For instance, in two studies of psychiatric illness in families of schizophrenics, Fowler, Tsuang, Cadoret et al. (1974) reported no cases of manic-depressive illness in relatives. Family members seemed to be at risk in general for schizophrenia and antisocial personality. Further, in an update of the "Iowa 500" investigation (a large-scale interview study of 314 first-degree relatives of 200 schizophrenic probands), Winokur, Tsuang, and Crowe (1982) report that affective disorders, including manic-depressive psychosis, occurred in only 3.7 of these relatives. This rate is actually lower than the risk figure usually reported for affective disorders in the general population (i.e., about 5%).

ADOPTION STUDIES

The first adoption study of schizophrenia was reported by Heston (1966) who located and then interviewed adults born to schizophrenic mothers in the Oregon State Psychiatric Hospital between 1945 and 1951. All of these offspring had been reared in foster homes or in homes of paternal relatives. They were matched with a control group of individuals who had been placed in foster homes by the same agencies. Table 22 reports the major results of this study. Not only were 5 of the 47 children of schizophrenic mothers themselves schizophrenic, but a variety of other mental abnormalities was observed in these individuals. It is noteworthy, however, that there was no case of manic-depressive illness. Within the control group there were no schizophrenics, and there was less mental illness in general than in the offspring of the schizophrenics. A discussion of the Heston research would not be complete without adding a cautionary note, however. Although Heston documented the psychiatric history of the schizophrenic mothers in this study very well, little was known of the mental health status of the fathers of the offspring born to the schizophrenic mothers, except that none of them had been hospitalized for a psychiatric illness. Conclusions made from this study should be drawn with that limitation in mind.

As a side issue, Heston noted that, among those children of schizophrenic mothers who had no psychiatric symptoms ($N = 21$), several had chosen life-styles that were out of the ordinary in that they included creative and/or artistic professions or hobbies. This finding is reminiscent of those anecdotal reports that associate creative genius with eccentric, somewhat nonnormal styles of behavior. Perhaps, Heston concluded, the milder manifestations of the predisposition to

Table 22. Incidence of Some Behavioral Problems in Foster-Home-Reared Children (Mean Age: Approximately 36 Years) of Schizophrenic Mothers Compared to Controls[a]

	Incidence	
	children of schizophrenic mothers ($N = 47$)	Controls ($N = 50$)
Schizophrenia	5	—
Mental deficiency, IQ <70	4	—
Sociopathic personality	9	2
Neurotic personality disorder	13	7
Felons	7	2

[a]The same individual may be represented in more than one category.
Note. Adapted from "Psychiatric Disorders in Foster Home Reared Children of Schizophrenic Mothers" by L. L. Heston, 1966, British Journal of Psychiatry, 112.

schizophrenia result in positive rather than negative deviations from normative behavior.

In addition to Heston's study, a large-scale adoption study of schizophrenia was conducted in Denmark (Mednick & Schulsinger, 1968; Wender et al., 1968). This study was more systematic because it was based on complete state registries of adoptions and of the mentally ill. In one report from this study, individuals who had a history of mental illness (in all but one case, schizophrenia) and whose children were adopted away at an early age were matched to a group of controls whose children were also given up for adoption. The authors then arranged for psychiatric evaluations to be made of these adopted individuals by interviewers who were blind to the mental health status of the biological parents. This resulted in 13% of the offspring of a schizophrenic parent being diagnosed as having symptoms within the spectrum of schizophrenia-like disorders whereas only 7% of the children of the control parents were so diagnosed. A follow-up study, in which a larger group of subjects was utilized, revealed that of the children of the mentally ill biological parents, 31.6% had a diagnosis within the schizophrenia spectrum, whereas this was true of only 17.8% of the control offspring. This difference was statistically significant. However, 17.8% is a much higher rate than one would expect in a control sample. An interesting fact that may be relevant to this high rate of schizophrenia among the controls comes from work by Horn, Green, Carney, and Erickson (1975). These researchers collected personality test data on 363 women who had given up their children for adoption. The test used was the Minnesota Multiphasic Personality Inventory (MMPI) that includes a measure of tendencies toward schizophrenic attitudes (the so-called Schizophrenia scale or Sc scale). When these women were compared to matched controls (mothers who had not relinquished a child for adoption), there was a significant difference on this particular scale, with the scores of the mothers of adopted-away children being more deviant. None of these mothers were frankly schizophrenic, yet their elevated Sc scores did suggest that they had schizophrenic-like tendencies that, to the extent that they are heritable, might place adopted children, in general, at a higher risk for schizophrenia.

Another utilization of the adoption design is that of Kety et al. (1968, 1978), also done in Denmark. In this case, the researchers attempted to locate all individuals adopted between 1924 and 1947, who had, as adults, been diagnosed schizophrenic. These probands were then matched by age, sex, age at adoption, and socioeconomic status of adopting families to nonschizophrenic adoptees. Finally, a concentrated effort was made to ascertain the mental-health status of all the adoptive and biological relatives of both the probands and the controls. The authors reported that, among the 173 identified biological relatives of schizophrenic probands, 37 (or 21%) had been diagnosed schizophrenic. Among the biological relatives of controls, 19 of 174 were schizophrenic (approximately 11%). This difference was statistically significant ($p < .006$). Adoptive relatives of the proband and control groups were also compared for frequency of schizophrenia. The rate of schizophrenic to normal in these groups of relatives was 4/74 (5%) and 7/91 (8%), respectively. This difference was not significant. Further, the percentage of schizophrenics in both of these latter groups was somewhat less than the 11% found among the biological relatives of controls. When Kendler et al. (1981b) reanalyzed the psychiatric records of this adoption study, they also found significantly more schizotypal personality disorder in the biological relatives of the schizophrenic adoptees than in those of the control adoptees.

Wender, Rosenthal, and Kety (1968), also using the same core sample of Danish adoptees described before, published data suggesting that although the biological parent–offspring relationship was most critical in the transmission of schizophrenia, there is some evidence that adoptive parents of schizophrenics are more frequently mentally ill than are the adoptive parents of nonschizophrenics. In this case, however, the direction of transmission is not clear, and we will have to wait for future studies to clarify the issue. Although parent-to-child transmission seems the most logical direction, one could argue that having a schizophrenic child might be very damaging to the psychological well-being of an adoptive parent. However, a small U.S. adoption study reported by Wender et al., (1977) made this later premise somewhat questionable. In this study, the adoptive parents of 19 schizophrenic adoptees were compared with a group of biological parents who had reared their own offspring, all of whom had, as adults, been diagnosed as schizophrenic. In addition, a third group of individuals was included, consisting of mentally retarded children and their biological parents who had reared them. In this study, elevated rates of schizophrenia were noted only among the biological parents of schizophrenics, and in neither of the other two groups. This sugests that the general stress of rearing a behaviorally abnormal child is not sufficient in itself to bring about schizophrenic symptomatology in parents.

A review of adoption studies of schizophrenia would not be complete without mention of the studies by Karlsson (1966, 1973, 1981) that were made in Iceland. When the results of these small studies are combined, they yield an overall significant difference in the comparison of the amount of schizophrenia in biological relatives of schizophrenic, adopted probands and the amount of schizophrenia found in adoptive relatives of those affected probands.

GENETIC MODELS OF THE INHERITANCE OF SCHIZOPHRENIA: SINGLE GENE VERSUS POLYGENIC

Kallmann (1946) was one of the first to suggest a single autosomal gene model. He proposed a recessive mode of inheritance. He suggested that deviations from the model could be explained by lack of penetrance, in which case an individual could possess the genes for schizophrenia, but because of mitigating factors, still be phenotypically normal.

Slater (1958) proposed something similar to a theory of incomplete penetrance—namely a partially dominant gene that manifests itself in all homozygotes but not in all heterozygotes. This idea came from Böök's (1953) detailed study of a small population living in the far north of Sweden, where the incidence of schizophrenia was extremely high (around 3%). Slater worked out the consequences of this interesting model in considerable detail. Given a frequency, p, of the schizophrenic gene, there will be p^2 homozygous schizophrenics; $2p(1-p)$ heterozygous individuals, of whom a percentage, m, are also schizophrenic; and $(1-p)^2$ normal homozygotes. Thus s, the incidence of schizophrenia in the general population is

$$s = 2mp(1-p) + p^2,$$

where m must lie between 0 and 1 (for complete recessivity or complete dominance, respectively). Finally, defining h as the proportion of schizophrenics who are homozygotes, Slater used Kallman's data shown in Table 23 to construct the graph shown in Figure 13. The

Table 23. Schizophrenia among Relatives of Schizophrenics

Type of familial relationship	Percentage expected	Percentage observed	Study
Children of one schizophrenic	14%	16%	Kallmann
Children of two schizophrenics	40%	39%	Elsasser
Sibs of schizophrenics	14%	14%	Kallmann

Note. Adapted from "The Monogenic theory of Schizophrenia" by E. Slater, 1958, *Acta Genetica, 8* p. 50.

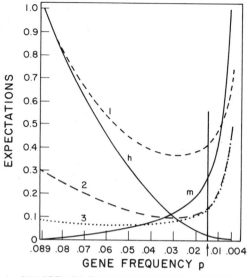

I = CHILDREN OF TWO SCHIZOPHRENIC PARENTS
2 = CHILDREN OF ONE SCHIZOPHRENIC PARENT
3 = SIBS OF SCHIZOPHRENICS

Figure 13. Expectations for schizophrenia as a function of gene frequency and biological relationship: 1 = children of two schizophrenic parents; 2 = children of one schizophrenic parent; and 3 = sibs of schizophrenics. *Note.* From *The Genetics of Mental Disorders* by E. Slater & V. Cowie, 1971, p. 59. London, Oxford University. Copyright 1971 by Oxford Press. Reprinted by permission.

various values of m (and of h) are shown for $s = .008$ at different values of p. In addition, the expected incidence ("expectations") for schizophrenia in children of two schizophrenic parents, in children of one schizophrenic parent, and in siblings of schizophrenics was calculated for each value of m. Using the assumption that people mate randomly with respect to schizophrenia, these risks were calculated as shown in Table 24. Because the observed risks were very close to the expected ones at that point, Slater suggested that p is 1.5% and m is 26%. Using new values, Slater and Cowie (1971) further tested the fit of the model as shown in Table 25.

What can perhaps be thought of as a final version of this model has been proposed by Karlsson (1966), who suggested that two pairs of allelic genes are involved—one that predisposes toward schizophrenia and one that determines whether a particular person will actually become ill or not.

Heston (1966), using a modification of the hypothesis that in-

Table 24. Expectations in Terms of p and m in Offspring by Type of Parental Mating

Mating	Frequency	Weighting	Offspring Schizophrenic	Not schizophrenic
Independently of psychiatric status of parents				
AA × AA	p^4	1	1	0
AA × Aa	$4p^3(1-p)$	$1/2(1+m)$	$1/2(1+m)$	$1/2(1-m)$
AA × aa	$2p^2(1-p)^2$	m	m	$1-m$
Aa × Aa	$4p^2(1-p)^2$	$(1+2m)/4$	$(1+2m)/4$	$(3-2m)/4$
Aa × aa	$4p(1-p)^3$	$1/2m$	$1/2m$	$1/2(2-m)$
One parent schizophrenic				
AA × Aa	$4(1-m)p^3(1-p)$	$1/2(1+m)$	$1/2(1+m)$	$1/2(1-m)$
AA × aa	$2p^2(1-p)^2$	m	m	$1-m$
Aa × Aa	$8m(1-m)p^2(1-p)^2$	$(1+2m)/4$	$(1+2m)/4$	$(3-2m)/4$
Aa × aa	$4mp(1-p)^3$	$1/2m$	$1/2m$	$1/2(2-m)$
Neither parent schizophrenic				
Aa × Aa	$4(1-m)^2p^2(1-p)^2$	$(1+2m)/4$	$(1+2m)/4$	$(3-2m)/4$
Aa × aa	$4(1-m)p(1-p)^3$	$1/2m$	$1/2m$	$1/2(2-m)$

Note. From *The Genetics of Mental Disorders* (p. 61) by E. Slater & V. Cowie, 1971, London: Oxford University Press. Copyright 1971 by Oxford University Press. Reprinted by permission.

vokes a single gene, proposed that what is inherited is "schizoidia." This is a broader concept of the disorder that includes schizophrenia but also the frequently milder personality problems such as social isolation, suspiciousness, eccentricity, or quarrelsomeness that are associated with certain types of personality disorders. According to Heston, environmental factors determine whether a person becomes schizophrenic or schizoid. In support of his theory, he cites the fact that the MZ co-twin of a schizophrenic has a 46.4% chance of being schizophrenic and a 41.1% chance of being schizoid but only a 12.6% chance of being in good mental health. Heston also compared expected and observed incidences in other relatives of schizophrenics (see Table 26) and found a good fit to his model as shown in Figure 14. However, in a study by Mosher, Pollin, and Stabenau (1971), no evidence of these schizoid personality problems were found among nonpsychotic MZ co-twins of schizophrenics.

Rao, Morton, Gottesman, and Lew (1981) reanalyzed reported data on the incidence of schizophrenia in a wide variety of relatives of schizophrenia patients. These relatives included spouses and children,

Table 25. Expectancies for Schizophrenia in Relatives of Index Cases

Relationship	N	No. a	No. b	% a	% b	Theoretical expectation %
Sibs (all)	8805	724	865	8.5	10.2	10.2
Sibs (neither parent schizophrenic)	7535	621	731	8.2	9.7	9.4
Sibs (one parent schizophrenic)	675	93	116	13.8	17.2	13.5
Children	1227	151	170	12.3	13.9	8.8
Children of mating schiz. × schiz.	134	49	62	36.6	46.3	37.1
Second-degree relatives						
Half-sibs	311	10	11	3.2	3.5	4.7
Uncles and aunts	3376	68	123	2.0	3.6	4.7
Nephews and nieces	2315	52	61	2.2	2.6	4.7
Grandchildren	713	20	25	2.8	3.5	4.7

Note. From *The Genetics of Mental Disorders* (p. 62) by E. Slater and W. Cowie, 1971, London: Oxford University Press. Copyright 1971 by Oxford University Press. Reprinted by permission.
[a] Diagnostically certain cases only.
[b] Also including probable schizophrenics. The theoretical expectations are calculated on the values for best fit: general population risk of schizophrenia $s = 0.0085$; frequency of schizophrenic gene $p = 0.03$; manifestation rate of gene in heterozygote $m = 0.13058$. For these values, the proportion of schizophrenics who will be homozygotes is about 10%.

first cousins, and grandchildren. They used a path analytic model that considered cultural inheritance and biological transmission as well as assortative mating and a familial environment unique to twins. The fit of the data to this model is remarkably good. They report approximately 70% of the phenotypic variability is due to polygenic factors and 20% to environmental factors common to the family. O'Rourke,

Table 26. Percentages of First-Degree Relatives Found to be Schizophrenic or Schizoid

Relationship	Number of individuals	Schizophrenia[a] %	Schizoid %	Total: Schizoid plus schizophrenic %
Children	1,000	16.4	32.6	49.0
Siblings	1,191	14.3	31.5	45.8
Parents	2,741	9.2	34.8	44.0
Children of two schizophrenics	171	33.9	32.2	66.1

Note. From "The Genetics of Schizophrenia and Schizoid Disease," by L. L. Heston, 1970, *Science*, 167. p. 253. Copyright 1970 by The American Association for the Advancement of Science. Reprinted by permission.
[a] Age-corrected rates.

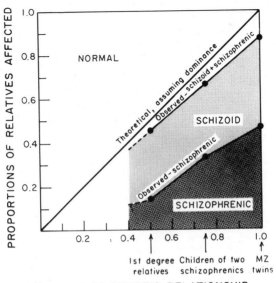

Figure 14. Observed and expected proportion of schizoids and schizophrenics. *Note.*
From "The Genetics of Schizophrenia and Schizoid Disease," by L. L. Heston, 1970,
Science, 167. p. 253. Copyright 1970 by the American Association for the Advancement
of Science. Reprinted by permission.

Gottesman, Suarez, Rice, and Reich (1982) attempted to fit published
data on familial incidence of schizophrenia to a simple major gene
model with two alleles, and obtained such a poor fit that they confidently rejected that model. Thus, the evidence for a simple single-gene
model of schizophrenia is tenuous at best. For a thorough review of the
evidence for a genetic basis for schizophrenia, see Gottesman and
Shields (1982).

The results of a number of studies have led to various etiological
hypotheses, including the possibility that (a) there could be several
heterogeneous genetically determined forms of schizophrenia; (b) there
is only one homogeneous genetically determined type with several
different manifestations; and (c) there is one predominantly hereditary
form of the disease (the nonparanoid group) and one predominantly
nonhereditary form (mainly the paranoid type). Such a diversity of
theories is a result of the difficulty of taking into account the varying
forms and degrees of schizophrenia. Of course, many nongenetic
etiological theories of schizophrenia have been suggested over the
years. In particular, various environmental ("life-experience") theories

have been proposed (see Neale and Oltmanns, 1980, for an account of these).

As might be expected, there are many problems with the genetic studies. Nearly every study has been criticized either because of the statistical procedures, the method of data collection, or the diagnostic criteria. Many critics claim that the familial concentration of the disease could as easily be due to environmental as to genetic factors. The environment certainly plays an important part in the expression of schizophrenia. But even if one took a strong hereditarian stand and argued that the environment is only eliciting a genetic predisposition, those environmental factors are still important, indeed critical, in determining who becomes schizophrenic. For that reason, all possible environmental correlates of the disorder should be explored. In keeping with this concept is a theory that Rosenthal has termed the "diathesis–stress" model. He postulates a genetic predisposition that interacts with the psychological trauma a person may encounter in his or her life to produce the illness.

Rabkin (1980), after reviewing the evidence for a relationship between stressful life events and schizophrenia, concluded as follows:

> Comparing schizophrenic and normal respondents, available evidence is inconclusive. For independent events no differences have been observed, although for all events, [i.e., the chain of events following a primary psychological trauma] schizophrenics did report more than normal respondents. The few studies of life events and of the probability of relapse among schizophrenics suggest that relapsing patients report more events than do those who continue in remission. (p. 424)

Critics of research on schizophrenia often make the legitimate complaint that the criteria for a diagnosis differ from one study to another. For this reason, it is quite likely that different investigators have been dealing with different phenotypes. In addition, many of the diagnoses have been conducted by investigators who, because they had a strong theoretical bias and "knew" exactly what they were looking for, might have made subjective observations. For instance, various critics of the twin studies have claimed that the determination of zygosity has been inaccurate or carelessly conducted. It must also be remembered that modern serological methods of determining zygosity are new so that older studies, which relied mostly on subjective judgment about physical similarity, could have been influenced by preknowledge of concordance (or lack of it) for the disease.

A final complication that could affect attempts to define a genetic mechanism associated with schizophrenia involves the differential diagnosis of schizophrenia from other disorders. Mention has already been made earlier in this volume of physical illnesses that can produce symptoms that mimic psychopathology. In addition, several conditions believed to be separate etiological entities from schizophrenia share symptomatology with this disorder. These "phenocopies" of schizophrenia are often misdiagnosed as being the true schizophrenic condition. Included in this group of disorders often misidentified are certain temporal lobe epileptic manifestations, acute amphetamine psychosis, several personality disorders, and schizoaffective conditions. As noted already in this chapter, the differential diagnostic status of these last two types of mental disorders is currently under debate. Some researchers believe that schizoaffective disorders, the so-called "schizoid" personality type, and perhaps the antisocial personality type are more accurately perceived as being milder manifestations of schizophrenia and thus are a part of the spectrum of schizophrenic disorders. Others feel that they are truly independent entities. It is easy to see, however, that any successful identification of a particular mode of inheritance for schizophrenia probably will not be accomplished until these diagnostic uncertainties are resolved and a specific unitary disorder is identified. The diagnostic procedure would be much more clear-cut if distinctive biochemical differences could be found for "pure" schizophrenia, or if selective improvement of symptoms with specific drugs proved to be diagnostic. Literally hundreds of attempts have been made along these lines, but in spite of many promising reports, nothing has stood the test of time.

There is a growing body of evidence that some schizophrenics have enlarged cerebral ventricles, as demonstrated by computerized axial tomography (CAT scan). This and other evidence that schizophrenia may be due to brain dysfunction has been reviewed by Seidman (1983). Among laboratory-type neuropsychological tests, a deficit in attention seems to be one of the most consistent findings among schizophrenics. However, in determining the value of these neurophysiological findings as they relate to the etiology of schizophrenia, one must consider the possibility that the physiological abnormalities are *effects*, not *causes* of the disorder.

BIOCHEMICAL THEORIES

Any genetic hypothesis presupposes underlying biochemical events. For several decades, researchers have tried to identify a biochemical factor in schizophrenia.

After the accidental discovery that a miniscule amount of lysergic acid diethylamide (LSD) produces a condition resembling a psychotic episode in normal individuals, a period resulted in which induced abnormality was seen as a model of mental illness that might produce insights in the biochemical pathways responsible. That idea has lost most of its attractiveness because the drug-induced behavior is not very similar to the symptoms of schizophrenia. At about the same time (around 1950), drugs such as reserpine and chlorpromazine (thorazine) were found to have a beneficial effect on most schizophrenics: these drugs quieted down aggressive symptoms, made patients accessible to therapists, and seemed to eliminate or reduce the number of episodes of delusions and hallucinations. There are now a number of these "antipsychotic" drugs. Because there are considerable individual differences in the side effects of each particular drug, it is generally possible to find one that will be best for a given patient. Among the variety of drugs that ameliorate symptoms of certain behavior disorders, five types are often distinguished: the antipsychotics described previously (sometimes called "neuroleptics" or major tranquilizers), antianxiety drugs (also called "ataractics" or minor tranquilizers), antidepressants, central nervous system stimulants, and a type consisting mainly of those sedatives used as sleeping aids ("hypnotics"). Following are some examples of each of these five types of drugs: *antipsychotic*—phenothiazines, rauwolfia alkaloids, indoleamines, butyrophenones, thiozanthines; *antianxiety*—diphenylmethanes, tri- and tetracyclics, benzodiazepines; *antidepressants*—monoamine oxidase (MAO) inhibitors, tricyclics; *hypnotics*—barbiturates, bromides, aldehydes and alcohols, opiates; and *stimulants*—amphetamines, piperidines.

It would take too lengthy an excursion into neuropharmacology to summarize in detail the emerging theories about the actions of the various psychotropic drugs. Briefly, they seem to affect synaptic action in the nervous system by affecting neurotransmitter substances. Neurotransmitters, of course, are the biochemicals that facilitate or inhibit neural activity. Of the ever-growing number of possible neurotransmitters that are presently being discovered, there are at least three that affect monoamine metabolism in the central nervous system; two are catecholamines and one is an indoleamine. The two catecholamines are dopamine and noradrenaline (also called norepinephrine). The indoleamine is serotonin. Yet another neurotransmitter is acetylcholine (ACh). Atropine and scopolamine are two drugs that lower the ACh level in the brain. They have an amnesic effect. Various other anticholinergic drugs are known, but most are not used in treatment of psychiatric patients, because their effects include anxiety, disorientation, and hallucinations.

There is no simple one-to-one relationship between the five types of psychotropic drugs and the various types of neurotransmitters. In many cases there are no "geographic" or brain site differences (i.e., various areas in the brain, such as the cortex, hypothalamus or cerebellum, produce more than one type of neurotransmitter). Some pathways, however, such as the limbic system, do display some degree of preference for one neurotransmitter. Norepinephrine, which is the primary neurotransmitter in the peripheral sympathetic nervous system, is another example of site specificity. With regard to neurotransmitters and schizophrenia, there is some evidence that the monoamine oxidase (MAO) level is altered, at least in some schizophrenics, but no clear correlation has been established. This could be due to heterogeneity within the patients studied.

A recent research finding has been reported that suggests the central nervous system metabolic activity is altered in some individuals suffering from schizophrenia. This evidence comes from positron emission tomography (PET) scans of the brain. Specifically, carbohydrate metabolism seems to be affected. However, this evidence is still contested by many as being just an artifact of the PET scan technology. It may be that someday most mental illnesses will be shown to be due to abnormal alleles of genes controlling brain chemistry, so that if individuals homozygous for the abnormal alleles can be identified, they may be treated by biochemical means or by being placed in environments that will minimize the consequences of the biochemical defects. However, despite all the efforts that have been made to establish such a link between abnormalities in brain biochemistry and schizophrenia, there is no strong evidence, to date, of any atypical neurochemical activity that is specific to, and characteristic of, most schizophrenia.

Is There a Selective Advantage for Relatives of Schizophrenics?

Heston (1966, 1970) and Karlsson (1981), both of whom advocate simple genetic models, are among those who have suggested that individuals who are likely to be heterozygous for "schizophrenia genes" (i.e., relatives of patients) may be more "creative" and more frequently be artists, musicians, inventors, and the like. This is an interesting hypothesis but one that is difficult to test rigorously. The main problem lies in the difficulty of establishing criteria that clearly define "creativity." Should creativity be regarded primarily as high achievement in one of the arts or sciences, or can it be equated with high intelligence? An additional problem is that a strict test of this theory would require counting the creative relatives of patients, and comparing this figure to the proportion of creative individuals in the general population.

This particular hypothesis regarding a selective balance for genes associated with mental illness is a modern version of the old idea that genius and mental illness are expressions of the same trait and that many geniuses eventually end up insane. The prototypical "mad scientist" of novels and films would fit this theory. Lange-Eichbaum has (1967) collected many such instances from biographies of famous persons and from historical accounts. Kurth (1967) added further cases in a revised edition of Lange-Eichbaum's book. Unfortunately, the information on most of the individuals included in these summaries came from biographies written by authors with no medical training, some of whom did not even know their subjects personally. Even in those rare instances when personalities of the individuals were described by psychiatrists, the diagnosis of mental illness was often not certain. For example, many biographical accounts of Adolf Hitler express doubts about his sanity. However, there is very little agreement about what disorder he suffered from and very little clinical evidence that could be used to establish a diagnosis. Nevertheless, the summaries by Kurth leave one with several impressions: the main one is that great artists, poets, philosophers, and other famous people seem to have become mentally ill rather often. One can only guess, of course, whether the frequency of mental illness in this group exceeded the rate of the general population because, of course, the total number of nonaffected famous persons is also high. Also, the significance of the tentative conclusion that there is a relationship between genius and mental illness is weakened by the fact that much of the illness was obviously due to the effects of syphilis.

A much simpler hypothesis than those of the studies described before merely states that relatives of schizophrenics produce offspring at a higher rate than the general population. To date, two studies have been reported that provide evidence for a selective advantage. Erlenmeyer-Kimling and Paradowski (1966) and Carter and Watts (1971) reported a small increase in the number of children of unaffected relatives compared to the average number of offspring in the general population. These studies certainly should be replicated, if for no other reason than the fact that if a true selective advantage can be substantiated, the reason for the advantage will likely hold an important key to understanding the etiology of schizophrenia.

CHAPTER 7

Hereditary Factors in Affective Disorders

For some time, Freudian theories postulating that disorders of the emotions (or affect) have a psychodynamic origin were held in higher esteem than was the thesis of Emil Kraepelin—that affective disorders have a constitutional basis. However, Kraepelin's concept is now being substantiated by a large body of more recent research findings. Both the Freudian theories and the biological hypotheses for the etiology of mania and depression will be discussed in this chapter.

The Kraepelinian notion of depression was influenced by a set of theories originating with the physician Hippocrates, of ancient Greece. He suggested that disposition is determined by the ratio of various body fluids, or "humors." Melancholia (depression) was the result of a humoral imbalance, specifically, a surfeit of black bile and phlegm.

In the 2nd century A.D., Aretaeus of Cappadocia noted an association between depression and mania. He described several cases in which both conditions were expressed at different times in the same individual. (This combination is referred to as "bipolar affective disorder"). He also noted the cyclical, episodic nature that is even today considered to be a hallmark of these emotional abnormalities (Woodruff, Goodwin, & Guze, 1974).

Slight variations on these early ideas about affective disorders appeared in updated forms throughout the centuries. However, Freud's psychoanalytic explanations deviated markedly from the earlier "constitutional theories." For Freudians, depression is always caused by the loss of a love object, and is specifically brought about when feelings of hostility and ambivalence to the love object become turned inward. This, it is postulated, results in despair, loss of self-esteem, and suicidal feelings. Mania, according to the same theory, is nothing more than a reaction formation to the original feelings of depression. (Reaction formation is a psychoanalytic defense mechanism. As Freud defined them, defense mechanisms are techniques that the mind utilizes to reduce anxiety. In the case of reaction formation, this is accomplished by transforming a set of behavioral symptoms into second-order behaviors that are the polar opposite of the originals. Thus, depression becomes mania.)

This psychoanalytic interpretation was very influential until the middle of the 20th century, despite little confirmatory evidence. However, in the last several decades, the Kraepelinian view has again become more popular. It should be noted that, even though the Freudian ideas about the etiology of depression and mania were in ascendency throughout the first part of this century, several researchers still held to the constitutional explanations. One in particular, Kretschmer, speculated that emotional disorders are merely an accentuation of a basic premorbid personality type. He suggested that depression is more likely to occur in people who are introverted and passive. Since the 1930s when Kretschmer first presented these ideas, both positive and negative evidence for them have been published. The issue has never been adequately resolved, and there is still much research being done in this area. (For a recent review of research regarding premorbid personality factors associated with affective disorders, see Akiskal, 1983). The return to constitutional theories of affective disorders has come about in part because of interest in research such as this and also because of mounting evidence for a strong underlying hereditary component in many cases of depression and mania.

INCIDENCE OF AFFECTIVE DISORDERS

Robins *et al.* (1984) reported lifetime rates for 15 DSM-III psychiatric diagnostic categories obtained from three large epidemiological surveys. Their data on affective disorders suggest that the overall frequency is approximately 5% for major depressive disorder and that about 1% of the population has experienced both a manic and a depressive episode (i.e., meet criteria for bipolar illness). When broken down by sex, there was a preponderance of females with major depression. Approximately twice as many females as males have experienced a major depressive episode during their lifetime. This sex difference did not occur for bipolar illness, where the sex ratio was not significantly different from 1:1.

A particularly interesting finding in the Robins *et al.* study was a significant age effect. A significantly higher frequency of affected individuals occurred in the group aged 25 to 44 years of age, when compared to the older groups. One would expect that because the rates reported were lifetime rates, the frequency of affective disorders should increase with age. That is, the longer you live the more likely it is that you will experience a depressive episode. Hence the lifetime rate should increase with age. Thus, the results obtained are in direct contradiction to the expected outcome. The authors offer several possible explanations for their findings. They suggest that the decrease in rates could be the result of death, immigration, or institutionalization of many older people. Alternatively, they suggest that older people have forgotten earlier depressions or mislabeled depression as some other type of illness. It is also possible that there has been a true increase in affective disorder in the last few generations and that these results are an accurate reflection of that increase. Considerable work is now in progress attempting to discover the cause of this age effect.

BIPOLAR AND UNIPOLAR DISTINCTION

In the late 1950s, there was growing support for the idea that there were at least two distinct subtypes of affective disorders: one in which there is only severe depression (unipolar), and one that is typified by periodic behavior having a manic or euphoric quality, most frequently alternating with phases of depression (bipolar). The major symptoms of depression include feelings of worthlessness, sadness, guilt, insomnia, loss of appetite, anorexia, loss of energy, inability to focus one's thoughts, and suicidal ideation. The manic episodes that occur in bipolar affective disorder are characterized by hyperactivity, push of speech (need to keep talking), reduced need for sleep, euphoria, grandiosity, and, occasionally, hallucinations.

In some bipolar patients, the episodes of euphoria and depression are separated by a rather lengthy period of normal behavior. Other patients seem more likely to "cycle" directly from mania into depression. Woodruff *et al* (1974) describe a type of bipolar manifestation in which symptoms of depression and mania are expressed simultaneously (e.g., patients who, while speaking in a euphoric manner, are also weeping). Finally, there are certain individuals diagnosed as bipolar-affective type whose pathology includes no evidence of depressive episodes. However, this latter type accounts for only a small proportion of bipolar illness.

As noted before, incidence rates differ markedly for the two subtypes (see table 27). Bipolar affective disorder occurs in approximately 1% of the population (no sex difference), whereas major depressive disorder is diagnosed in about 5% of the population with females outnumbering males by approximately 2:1. Bipolar affective disorder has a much narrower range of average age of onset than does unipolar disorder. The first manic episode usually occurs before age 30. An initial episode of depression can occur with almost equal frequency from late adolescence throughout adulthood.

Leonard (1957) was the first to suggest that bipolar and unipolar disorders were etiologically and genetically distinct. Much of the evidence that has been used to substantiate the difference between unipolar and bipolar affective disorder has come from family studies. Two monographs, by Angst (1966) in Switzerland and by Perris (1966) in Sweden, reported a higher incidence of illness among parents and siblings of patients with unipolar symptoms (see Table 28). The incidence of bipolar symptoms was low in relatives of unipolar probands, whereas unipolar symptoms occurred very frequently. Both Angst and Perris also reported a higher incidence of affected females than males among the relatives of unipolar probands. Similar findings were reported by Winokur and Pitts (1965) and Winokur and Clayton (1967b). An overall greater risk for affective disease in relatives of bipolar than unipolar probands has been reported in Japan (Asano, 1967) and in Germany (von Trostorff, 1968). Since 1966, a series of independent investigations have consistently shown that the relatives of bipolar probands have higher rates of bipolar illness than do relatives of unipolar probands (Angst, Frey, Lohmeyer, & Zerbin-Rudin, 1980; Cadoret & Tanna, 1977; Gershon, Mark, Cohen et al., 1975; Gershon et al., 1982a; Helzer & Winokur, 1974; James & Chapman, 1975; Mendlewicz & Ranier,

Table 27. Population Incidence of Affective Disorders in Both Sexes

Diagnosis	Males	Females	Total	F/M Ratio
Mania	.009	.009	.009	1.00
Major Depression	.031	.071	.052	2.29

Note. Adapted from "Lifetime Prevalence of Specific Psychiatric Disorders in Three Sites," by L. N. Robins et al., 1984, Archives of General Psychiatry, 41.

Table 28. Percentage of Affective Disorders in Relatives of Bipolar and Unipolar Probands

	Relatives	
Proband	Bipolar	Unipolar
Bipolar		
Angst, 1966	3.7	11.2
Perris, 1966	10.8	0.56
Winokur & Clayton, 1967b	10.2	20.4
Helzer & Winokur, 1974	4.6	10.6
Mendlewicz and Ranier, 1974	17.7	22.4
James & Chapman, 1975	6.4	13.2
Gershon, Mark, Cohen et al., 1975	3.8	8.7
Smeraldi, Negri, & Melica, 1977	5.8	7.1
Gershon et al., 1982a	4.5	14.0
Unipolar		
Angst, 1966	0.3	5.1
Perris, 1966	0.3	6.4
Gershon, Mark, Cohen et al., 1975	2.1	14.2
Smeraldi, Negri, & Melica, 1977	0.6	8.0
Gershon et al., 1982a	1.5	16.6
Weissman et al., 1984a	1.0[a]	17.2[a]
	0.8[b]	18.4[b]

[a]Nonhospitalized probands.
[b]Hospitalized probands.

1974; Shields, 1975; Smeraldi, Negri, & Melica, 1977; Suslak, Shopsin, Silbey, Mendlewicz, & Gershon, 1976; Winokur, Clayton, & Reich, 1969; Winokur, Cadoret, Dorzab, & Baker, 1971; Weissman, 1984a; Zvolsky 1973).

Bertelson, Harvald, and Hauge (1977) reported an interesting finding from a twin study of affective disorders. In addition to noting a higher concordance rate among MZ twins than DZ twins for affective disorders in general, they found that MZ twins as a class are much more frequently concordant for bipolar affective illness than for the unipolar type (74% vs. 43%). This phenomenon was not apparent in the DZ twins. The increase in concordance for the bipolar subtype in MZ twins suggests that the expression of bipolar affective disorder is either influenced to a greater degree by genetic factors, or alternatively, by some cultural influence(s) peculiar to the shared environments of MZ twins.

Not all family studies suggest that the unipolar and bipolar affective illnesses are genetically distinct entities. Taylor and Abrams

(1980) summarize the findings of several studies that suggest that the recurrence risk for unipolar and bipolar affective disorder is not different in relatives of both unipolar and bipolar probands. In addition, in their review of the "Iowa 500" patients, Winokur et al. (1982) found approximately the same frequencies of unipolar depression among first-degree relatives of bipolar and unipolar index cases: 9.4% compared to 8.2%. Nevertheless, the majority of studies have shown a difference in recurrence rates for relatives of bipolar probands when compared to relatives of unipolar probands. This does not necessarily imply that the two are genetically separate disorders. As Gershon et al. (1982a) point out, the patterns observed in these families are consistent with the hypothesis that bipolar and unipolar illness are part of a continuum, with bipolar representing the more severe form of the disorder. Results of their analysis using multiple thresholds and assuming a common underlying liability are consistent with this hypothesis, if the mode of transmission is assumed to be multifactorial-polygenic (Gershon et al., 1982a). However, Price et al. (1986) were unable to replicate these results with a group of families that partially overlapped the sample used by Gershon et al.

Using a larger sample of unipolar families, Price et al. were unable to fit a multiple threshold model that assumed bipolar and unipolar to be part of a continuum. Their results suggest that the two disorders are genetically distinct. As the authors point out, the assumption that bipolar and unipolar illness are part of a continuum was only one of several assumptions of the model being tested, and rejection of the model may have resulted from the violation of any one of these additional assumptions. Yet, given what is known about the affective disorders, it is imperative to consider the possibility that the forms may be etiologically heterogeneous. It is clear from studies on course of illness and treatment that they are clinically heterogeneous. Patients vary with regard to symptoms, onset and course, response to pharmacological and psychological treatments, and biological findings. Certainly, the effectiveness of lithium in the treatment of bipolar illness suggests some underlying differences between the two classes of affective disorder. Within unipolar disorder there is some evidence for heterogeneity as well. As early as 1970, Rosenthal suggested that major depression was comprised of several phenotypically similar but etiologically distinct disorders. Efforts to define these disorders have led to the formulation of several possible subtypes of major depression (Leckman 1984a, 1984b; Merikangas, Leckman, Prusoff, Pauls, & Weissman, 1985; Nelson & Charney, 1980; Weissman et al., 1984a; Weisman, Prusoff, & Merikangas, 1984b).

Interest has also focused on subtypes of nonbipolar depression that seem to be biologically mediated. A number of categories have been proposed. These categories include endogenous, melancholic, autonomous, agitated, retarded, psychotic, and delusional among others. Evidence in support of these subtype distinctions is mainly differential response to therapy (Avery & Lubrano, 1979; Bielski & Friedel, 1976; Glassman & Paykel, 1979; Reisby et al., 1979).

There is also suggestive evidence that bipolar affective disorders may be genetically heterogeneous (Kidd et al., 1984). If affective disorders are etiologically heterogeneous, it follows that analyses done on data sets comprised of heterogeneous disorders would give inconclusive and possibly conflicting results. It is true that all genetic analyses reported to date have assumed etiologic homogeneity. Therefore, if affective disorders are heterogeneous, the results from these analyses could be totally invalid. Subsequent work should, of course, be done using samples that are as clinically homogeneous as possible.

ALCOHOLISM AND DEPRESSION

In addition to identifying possible subtypes for study, it is important to determine whether etiologically homogeneous subtypes of the disorder may be expressed in different forms. Winokur, Clayton, and Reich (1969) found a greatly increased incidence of heavy drinking among relatives of depressed patients and have suggested that alcoholism may mask a depressed state.

This hypothesis could be used to explain the different incidence of depression in the two sexes, as well as in alcoholism (where male alcoholics are far more prevalent than female). The idea has not yet been tested adequately. However, in an Amish population where alcohol abuse is not tolerated, there seems to be no strong sex difference in the incidence of affective disorders (Egeland & Hostetter, 1983).

In other work along these same lines, Winokur (1975) has suggested that a diagnostic distinction, and possibly an etiological one as well, could be made between pure unipolar depression and what he terms "depression spectrum disorder." In this latter type, one sees unipolar depression occurring in some female family members and alcoholism and sociopathy in male members of the same family. Based on these observations, Winokur and co-workers (Van Valkenberg, Lowry, Winokur, & Cadoret, 1977) have operationally defined pure depressive disorder as that which occurs in an individual whose first-degree relatives are neither alcoholic nor sociopathic. An additional difference is that symptoms of depression occur earlier in women with the spectrum-type disorder. If several features are found that distinguish between these two proposed types of unipolar depression, one could then assume with some amount of certainty that they are indeed separable entities. Successful refinement of diagnostic categories within the mental illnesses will certainly result in more accurate information about etiology and treatment of disorders. Therefore, this type of research is extremely valuable. It is difficult, however, to test for possible genetic differences between these two possible subtypes because family information is used to make the diagnosis. Thus, for example, because pure unipolar depression is that type where alcoholism does not appear in the relatives, it is not possible to test hypotheses about the etiological relationship between alcohol and depression using family data of pure unipolar depressive probands. Different sorts of data are needed. Merikangas *et al.* (1985) analyzed family data of depressed probands with and without alcoholism. Their results suggest that there may be some etiological difference between individuals with depression only when compared with individuals expressing depression and alcoholism. It is clear that much additional work is needed before this diagnostic issue is settled.

OTHER POSSIBLE SUBTYPES OF DEPRESSION

Besides the pure/spectrum distinction, there may be another dichotomy. As we noted previously in this chapter, some researchers have proposed that of the several possible types of unipolar depression, a distinction is often made between reactive and endogenous depression. Such theorists frequently express the notion that most reactive depressions are in response to environmental conditions and that endogenous depression is more likely to have a genetic component. This distinction between reactive and endogenous depression has rarely been used in studies related to psychiatric genetics. One exception is a report by Kiloh and Garside (1963) who studied various symptoms in 143 depressed patients and found that they were able to form two groups that resembled this kind of subtyping. They noted that the two types could be distinguished to some degree on the basis of two different sets of symptoms. The reactive depressed often showed obsessive symptoms, whereas the endogenous depressed exhibited sleep problems, weight loss, and affective retardation. The researchers pointed out, however, that some patients had both types of symptoms. They also could not rule out the possibility that the difference in symptoms was merely indicative of a time trend associated with the course of depressive illness. Perhaps obsessive symptoms occur soon after onset of the disorder and are replaced by other symptoms as the disorder becomes more severe.

Leckman *et al.* (1984a) used family data to address the validity of subtype distinctions. They separated families on the basis of whether the proband met criteria for endogeneous, melancholic, autonomous, and/or delusional depression. Rates of depression were then compared among relatives in the various categories. They found that the rate of depression was highest among relatives of delusional depressives, with the other rates being somewhat lower but still significantly greater than rates in a control group. They also found that the affected relatives tended to exhibit the same kind of depression as the proband. That is, there was some evidence that the subtypes *bred true.*

In the DSM-III an older term, *neurotic depression,* has been replaced by *dysthymic disorder.* Akiskal (1983) has reviewed this new concept and proposed methods of distinguishing several types of milder chronic depressions, in part on the basis of age of onset. These particular distinctions have not yet been used extensively in psychiatric genetic studies.

REVIEW OF TWIN AND ADOPTION STUDIES

Other data that suggest a genetic component come from twin and adoption studies. Bertelsen *et al.* (1977) have summarized the results of a number of studies comparing MZ and DZ twin-pair concordance rates. Table 29 illustrates the findings from major twin studies done over the years. An interesting aspect of these studies in general is that so many more DZ pairs (322) than MZ pairs (166) seem to have been included. One frequently sees a selection bias in the opposite direction, especially in early twin studies (i.e., identical pairs, whether or not concordant for the disease, would often come to the attention of the investigators more frequently than fraternal pairs). However, these numbers accord well with the incidence in the population of both types of twins, as DZ twinning is a more frequent phenomenon. The fact that early studies did not attempt to collect a representative sample of both MZ and DZ twins may account for some of the variability in reported concordance rate.

By combining the results of all the studies reported in Table 29, even acknowledging probable differences between studies in diag-

Table 29. Twin Concordance for Affective Disorder

Author	MZ concordance rates	N	DZ concordance rates	N
Luxenburger, 1930 (Germany)	0.67	3	0.00	13[a]
Rosanoff et al., 1935 (U.S.A.)	0.70	23	0.16	67[a]
Essen-Möller, 1941 (Sweden)	0.25	8	0.00	3
Slater, 1953 (U.K)	0.50	8	0.24	30*
Kallmann, 1954 (U.S.A.)	0.93	27	0.24	55
Da Fonseca, 1959 (U.K.)	0.71	21	0.38	39
Kringlen, 1967 (Norway)	0.33	6	0.00	20*
Allen et al., 1967 (U.S.A.)	0.33	15	0.00	34
Bertelsen, Harvald, & Hauge, 1977 (Denmark)	0.58	55	0.17	52
Average Concordance Rate (Combined Studies)	0.62	166	0.17	313

Note. From "A Danish twin study of manic-depressive disorder" by A. Bertelsen, B. Harvald & M. Hauge, 1977, *British Journal of Psychiatry, 130.* Copyright 1977 by Headley Brothers, Ltd. Reprinted by permission.
[a]Concordance based on both like-sex and unlike-sex pairs.

nostic and ascertainment criteria, one can obtain a rough estimate of the importance of genetic factors. The overall concordance rates of 62% for MZ twins versus 17% of DZ twins suggests a strong genetic component to this class of disorder ($H = .90$).

Mendlewicz and Rainer (1977) have reported the results of a Belgian adoption study of the manic-depressive condition (bipolar affective disorder). Admissions for 5 years to psychiatric services in and around Brussels were searched for adopted patients who had both manic and depressive episodes. Only if they had been sent to their adoptive home before the age of 1 year and had remained with those parents until adulthood were they included in the study. The biological parents were located through the cooperation of the adoption agencies. Biological and adoptive parents of 29 manic-depressive adoptees and 22 normal adoptees were interviewed blindly. Also included in the study were the biological parents of a group of nonadopted bipolar index cases and parents of children who had been disabled by polio. The results indicated that biological parents of the bipolar patients (both those who relinquished their children and those who kept their children) more often showed signs of psychopathology than did the adoptive parents or any other group. On the average, 28% of the biological parents of patients with bipolar disorder were diagnosed as having affective disorder. The incidence in the other parental groups ranged from 2 to 10%. A small study by Cadoret (1976) reported that among eight biological mothers who were ascertained to have a depressive disorder, three of their adopted-away offspring (37.5%) subsequently developed symptoms of depression. In this study, the incidence of psychological disorder other than affective disorder was no higher in the biological parents of the affected adoptees than in the parents of normal adoptees.

Are Some Affective Disorders X-Linked?

Given our discussion and current understanding of the mode of transmission in affective disorders, it may seem somewhat premature to begin looking for linkage of these disorders with known genetic markers. Nevertheless, several investigators have reported results suggesting that in some families such a linkage relationship can be observed. Winokur and Tanna (1969) have suggested that the pattern of familial incidence is frequently compatible with sex-linked dominant inheritance of the bipolar condition as it is expressed in many families. Table 30 shows incidence figures for male and female first-degree relatives that suggest a reduction of father-to-son transmission. Helzer and Winokur (1974) presented further support for the absence of father–son transmission in bipolar patients.

The sex-linkage hypothesis led to a search for affected families with other known sex-linked traits. Winokur et al. (1969) reported on two families in which the transmission of color blindness was consistently associated with affective disorder in 12 persons, whereas Mendlewicz, Linkowski, Guroff, and Van Praag (1979) found another eight families in which color blindness and affective disorder were

Table 30. Incidence in Male and Female Relatives of Bipolar and Unipolar Probands

	Bipolar proband		Unipolar proband	
	Male	Female	Male	Female
Brother	29%	7%	16%	7%
Son	15%	23%	5%	9%
Father	7%	17%	12%	10%
Sister	18%	23%	12%	13%
Daughter	15%	24%	7%	26%
Mother	27%	23%	11%	12%

Note. Adapted from "Possible role of X-linked dominant factor in manic-depressive disease," by G. Winokur and V. Tanna, 1969, *Diseases of the Nervous System, 30,* 89.

associated. This does not mean that color blindness is necessarily more frequent in individuals with affective disorders. Rather, it suggests that the genes for both are closely linked on the X-chromosome. Therefore, if one of the maternal Xs can be shown to contain both abnormalities, any one of the offspring is likely to get both or neither but rarely only one or the other. Winokur and Tanna (1969) also reported possible linkage to the genetic site Xg, a blood group locus located on the X-chromosome. This was further confirmed by Mendlewicz, Fleiss, and Fieve (1975).

However, there have been several reports of negative evidence for sex-linked inheritance of bipolar affective disorder. Gershon, Targum, & Matthysse *et al.* (1979), Leckman, Gershon, McGuiness, Targum, and Dibble (1979), and Kidd *et al.* (1984) present evidence refuting close linkage to either red-green color blindness or the Xg blood group. Incidentally, these two markers are too far apart on the X chromosome for a gene to be linked to both. In addition, Von Grieff, McHugh, and Stokes (1975) reported pedigrees in which patterns of inheritance for bipolar disorder were frequently in contradiction to a theory of sex-linked inheritance. However, in 1980, Mendlewicz, Linkowski, and Wilmotte reported linkage between glucose-6-phosphate dehydrogenase (G6PD) deficiency and manic-depressive psychosis. G6PD is closely linked to color blindness.

Glucose-6-phosphate dehydrogenase is an enzyme, lack of which causes a hemolytic reaction after treatment with primaquine, an antimalaria drug. The hemolytic reaction can also occur after eating fava beans and is therefore sometimes called "favism." G6PD deficiency occurs mainly among people living in Mediterranean areas where malaria is prevalent, as well as in Africa and India. This trait seems to confer resistance to malaria.

One possible way of resolving these inconsistent data is to assume that bipolar affective disorder is transmitted as an X-linked genetic factor in only certain subpopulations, whereas in other cases the mode of transmission is quite different.

SEARCH FOR AUTOSOMAL LINKAGE

Weitkamp, Purdue, and Huntzinger (1980) investigated 29 autosomal marker genes in a family with 19 members having affective disorder to see whether there was any indication of linkage of these marker genes with a hypothesized "susceptibility" gene for depression. Not only was no linkage suggested, but the data ruled out linkage for most markers in this family. It is, of course, always possible to suppose that there are several types of depressive illness and that in other families linkage relationships may be found. But, until this is actually demonstrated, the more conservative approach is to accept this as negative evidence for linkage to autosomal markers in general.

HLA (human lymphocyte antigen) is an autosomal system that is part of the major histocompatibility complex in man. It is perhaps the most complicated human genetic system elucidated at the present time. It is characterized as having a number of closely linked loci, each with a larger number of alleles. HLA plays an important role in immune reaction and self-recognition by cells and may play a role in the development of at least certain types of cancers. Although in the single-family study mentioned no evidence for HLA linkage was found, Weitkamp, Stancer, Persad, Flood, and Guttormsen (1981) have described an increase in identical HLA haplotypes for pairs of depressed and nondepressed siblings in families with one or two affected siblings but not in families with more than two affected members.

Other studies of HLA linkage (Kidd et al., 1984; Shapiro, Ryder, Svejgaard, & Rafaelson, 1977; Smeraldi, Negri, Melica, & Scorze-Smeraldi, 1978; Targum, Gershon, Van Eerdewegh & Rogentine, 1979) have not been consistent in their findings. The absence of increased HLA linkage identity when more than two siblings are affected is explained in the report by Weitkamp et al. by suggesting that liability to depression in such families is affected by more than one HLA haplotype in either parent. Thus, different predisposing haplotypes can be transmitted to affected offspring. On the basis of this hypothesis, the authors have predicted that "affected pairs of siblings would have the greatest probability of being HLA-haplotype-identical if neither parent was affected, a lower probability if one was affected, and an even lower probability if both were affected" (p. 1302). This somewhat complicated hypothesis clearly must be tested, but it is an interesting explanation for some of the ambiguity that has arisen from results of studies in this area.

Johnson, Hunt, Robertson, and Doran (1981), in Australia, have reported it unlikely that a gene for affective disorder is closely linked with the ABO blood groups, the Rh factor, haptoglobins, or HLA alleles. Further, no significant associations were found for the MN blood system. Other blood groups (Kell, Duffy) were also uninformative in this particular study. Nurnburger (1981) found no linkage with color blindness or the following known genetic markers: Xg blood group, HLA, platelet monoamine oxidase (MAO), plasma dopamine-beta-hydroxylase (DBH), or catechol-o-methyl-transferase (COMT).

In an attempt to identify autosomal markers for affective illness, Goldin *et al.* (1982) studied the inheritance of markers DBH, COMT, and MAO in different subsets of 162 patients with affective disorders and in 1,125 relatives. The results for both DBH and COMT were consistent with a single major gene hypothesis displaying no dominance relationships. The MAO data did not fit a single major locus hypothesis. There was some weak evidence for linkage with the ABO blood group and for the DBH locus, but no other linkage was even likely. However, in a later report, Goldin *et al.* (1983) noted the absence of any linkage in 21 autosomal markers, including those noted before, to the hypothesized major gene for affective disorder. In the same paper, they reported the failure of segregation analysis to support the hypothesis of a single major gene model of affective disorder. Thus, the overall evidence for linkage of affective disorder with known genetic markers is quite sparse.

A possible explanation for the somewhat discouraging results of attempts to find a specific genetic mechanism for affective disorder is that affective disorder may not be a unitary disorder at all. It is quite likely that there exists a group of phenotypically similar illnesses with different modes of transmission that have historically been conceived of as a single phenomenon. In light of the various ways in which affective symptoms are expressed in different patients, heterogeneity within the disorder is very plausible. For example, Dunner, Fleiss, Addonizio, and Fieve (1976) have suggested two subtypes of patients, one of which is characterized by far more frequent suicide attempts.

Other support for this idea of heterogeneity comes from a study by Turner and King (1983). They provide evidence that there may be two distinctly different forms of bipolar disorder. They selected seven large extended families with father-to-son transmission of the disorder and showed that these pedigrees were consistent with a model of autosomal dominant transmission. They also reported linkage with HLA. Linkage analysis of these families, using a very narrow criterion, yielded a highly significant likelihood of linkage (specifically, a lod score of 8.02 and a recombination value of 0.15). This suggests there is a strong likelihood that the two genes are segregating together. In these families, affected siblings had high concordance for HLA haplotypes. The authors proposed the designation BPD-2 (Bipolar Disorder 2) for this hypothesized HLA-linked condition and BPD-1 (Bipolar Disorder 1) for the non-HLA-linked types which they suggest may be a sex-linked form. They also argue for a spectrum of expressivity because using broader criteria for defining affective disorder, including schizotypic behaviors with a depressive component, anorexia nervosa, and hypochondria led to very similar linkage patterns.

Laboratory Tests for Depression

A specific biochemical test for clarifying the diagnosis of "melancholia" or depression was reported by Carroll et al. (1981). The idea for this specific test dates back to the early part of this century when it was first noted that individuals suffering from an overactive adrenal gland (or Cushing's syndrome) were often depressed. This led to a theory that high levels of the adrenal hormone, cortisol, can affect emotional tone. Attempts to test this theory were implemented, and evidence was presented that high doses of cortisol could cause mood disturbance in control subjects. Later, it was noted that dexamethasone acts as a cortisol suppressor in normal subjects but is not effective in individuals with Cushing's syndrome or many other depressed individuals. Therefore, the implication is that depression may be related to the neuroendocrine system that is referred to as the *hypothalamic-pituitary-adrenalin axis.*

The so-called "dexamethasone suppression test" (DST) for depression, developed at the University of Michigan, consists of the administration of dexamethasone, which normally suppresses cortisol production, and an assay 24 hours later. Abnormally high levels of plasma cortisol testing have been found to be associated with depression. The authors report a diagnostic accuracy of 83 to 95%, depending on the dosage level considered critical and the time when the blood sample is taken. Although a positive test result is strong evidence for endogenous depression, a negative test cannot, however, be used to rule out such a diagnosis. In addition, a number of other organic conditions that can lead to high cortisol levels need to be excluded, such as Cushing's syndrome, pregnancy, diabetes, significant weight loss, acute withdrawal from alcohol, and others. Although the dexamethasone suppression test is close to becoming a routine procedure (Greden 1982; Schatzberg et al. 1983), its clinical use has been criticized. At a 1983 meeting of the American Psychiatric Association, for example, data were presented suggesting that certain schizophrenics, manics, and normal controls also tested positively. Thus, the suppression test may not be sufficiently specific to be used for differential diagnosis.

Extein, Pottash, Gold, and Cowdry (1982) have proposed using protirelin (synthetic thyrotropin-releasing hormone) as a test of thyroid-stimulating hormone (TSH) secretion to distinguish specifically between mania and schizophrenia. Patients with a history of affective disorder had less of a response than did schizophrenics or normals. However, alcoholism, hyperthyroidism, and various drugs (including central nervous system depressants such as barbiturates and opiates) will produce the same decrease in response. Despite this obvious problem with the method, Extein, Pottash, and Gold (1982) report that combining this assay with the dexamethasone suppression test resulted in the correct identification of psychiatric condition in 85% of patients tested.

TREATMENT

Although electroconvulsive therapy is still used in some cases that prove resistant to other treatment, the treatment of choice for unipolar affective disorder is now pharmacological in nature. Management of depressive symptoms is most frequently achieved by using tricyclic antidepressants and monoamine oxidase (MAO) inhibitor substances. Some individuals seem to respond better to one class than the other, but to date these individual differences have not been associated with any systematic differences in expression of the disorder. Thus, although the drug response variability held out the hope of a differential diagnosis dimension, one has not yet been developed.

Mania in general can be treated effectively by using lithium medications and/or a major tranquilizer such as one of the phenothiazines. When lithium has been used for the relief and prevention of mania, there is frequently also amelioration of depressive symptomatology in the treated individual. Many manic patients respond to lithium, but a minority respond less favorably. It remains to be determined whether the heterogeneity in drug response noted among patients with affective disorder is in general the result of separate etiological entities having been classified together as one affective illness. If this were to be the case, trial administration of the various forms of antidepressants or antimania agents could become a powerful diagnostic tool.

LIFE EVENTS AND ENVIRONMENTALLY INDUCED DEPRESSION

The idea that depression can be brought on by events in one's life is an old one and figured prominently in the classic treatise *The Anatomy of Melancholy*, by Burton (1621). In recent years, there have been efforts to develop measures of such events, so that their impact can be systematically evaluated. Lloyd (1980a, 1980b) has reviewed some of this work and concludes that the childhood loss of a parent by death appears to increase the risk of depression by a factor of 2 or 3. Yet most depressives have not experienced such an event. He also concluded that, later in life, the risk of a depression after a loss or severe threat to one's well-being may be significantly increased (by as much as a factor of 5 or 6). Lloyd warns that this association between depression and life events is based on retrospective studies that may overemphasize the seriousness of events linked to depressive symptoms and that would tend to make causal connections between experiences and later behavioral aberrations when none are really warranted. Nevertheless, it seems promising to try to combine genetic studies with an investigation of life events preceding the onset of depressive episodes. We may find, for example, that prolonged stress leads to an imbalance in the hypothalamic-pituitary-adrenalin axis more frequently or more easily in some families than in others.

There are some facts that raise serious questions about the contribution of stress to mental disorders. These are the absence of an increase in mental illness during natural disasters and wars. Even cases of shell shock, after repeated prolonged exposure to wholesale slaughter during World War I, often recovered completely in a surprisingly short time. Rachman (1978) has summarized some of the reports on the effects of air raids and combat on civilians and military men. The consensus derived from various sources is that there was a notable absence of both short-term and long-term harm to those exposed.

It is an amazing fact that even in concentration camps, amid the brutality, starvation, and constant threat of death, there was not much of the kind of mental illness that would have stood out from the general deterioration of personality in most prisoners. Further, among the survivors, there were special psychiatric problems, but not a marked increase in the number of major psychiatric syndromes—affective disorders, for example.

Distinctions have been made between stressful events in terms of their predictability and one's ability to feel in control of the events. For instance, doing something useful during an air raid was reported by air raid wardens or firemen to help them remain calm. There have also been several animal studies which report that the condition of being helpless to control or escape from stressful events is far more deleterious than exposure to the same events for the same amount of time while maintaining the ability to alter the situation. This factor may explain how certain appalling experiences seem to leave few serious psychological side effects, whereas others, of a milder nature, result in more disturbance.

Sociologist Jessie Barnard (1972) suggested that one could make the following interpretation of the statistics of depression: on the whole, marriage is a good thing for men and bad for women. For example, the incidence of depression is higher for married women than for unmarried ones, whereas the reverse is true for men. This pattern seems more likely to be related to a cultural factor rather than a genetic one. However, before we can even conclude that marriage has important implications for the expression of depression in males and females, the statistics would have to be carefully corrected for such things as age, socioeconomic status, educational level, length of marriage, and the like. If the basic concept is correct, one should be able to find an increased incidence of affective disorder in women that would relate to length of marriage independently of their age. Perhaps the opposite effect would be noted for men. This particular concept can be thought of as a special case of the more general theory that seeks a relationship between depression and stress. If one looks at it from that perspective, it is probably not realistic to think that the institution of marriage is always related to depression in females. It is far more likely to assume that marriage in *certain* cultures and in *certain* periods in history will prove to be a common stressor for many females. For example, in a recent study of women living in Camberwell, England (Brown & Harris, 1978), evidence somewhat contrary to the marriage-as-stressor premise was noted. The study included 114 psychiatric patients and 2 random samples of normal women ($N = 458$).

The researchers examined the role of environmental stresses in the origin of depression. They concluded that "a woman who has a confiding relationship, particularly with a husband, has much less chance of developing depression once a provoking agent occurs" (p. 271). Thus, it may be that in cultures and times that do not encourage confiding relationships within marriage, the marital status of individuals may be related to the development of depressive disorder. In other situations, the correlation between marriage and affective disorder could be expected to vary quite markedly.

CONCLUSION

In summary, depression is one of the most prevalent forms of mental illness. Although much of the time it is mild enough to allow those affected to maintain jobs and family responsibilities, one only need talk to persons so affected to comprehend the tremendous anguish that is associated with this form of mental disorder. In considering the high prevalence rate of the combined forms of affective disorder, it becomes obvious that research leading to better treatment and a better understanding of the etiology of this type of behavioral disorder would increase the quality of life for a substantial segment of the general population. Therefore, it seems incumbent upon researchers, and even more importantly, those government agencies that provide the principal source of funds for mental health research, to set research on affective disorders at a high level of priority.

CHAPTER 8

Hereditary Factors in Neurotic Conditions

Although the clinical utility of the term *neurosis* has been questioned (see DSM-III, 1980, for a discussion of this issue), an extensive body of psychiatric data has been collected regarding neurotic conditions. Before summarizing the genetic studies in this field, we need to review the terms used in that body of research. A *neurosis* has usually been defined as a mental abnormality in which there is no serious loss of contact with reality (i.e., there are no hallucinations or delusions), no serious disorganization of personality, and no pervasive change in mood. Rather, the central symptom is thought to be anxiety, which is expressed in a variety of ways, frequently manifested in compulsive or obsessive behavior, difficulty in making decisions, panic attacks, phobias, or conditions characterized by temporary loss of memory. Some neurotics can be difficult to live with because of extremely rigid behavior patterns. They may also be quarrelsome or appear withdrawn, and when this latter symptom is present the condition may be confused with schizoid personality.

Freud and most of his followers believed that neuroses are caused by environmental influences in childhood. Others believe that neuroses result directly from the reinforcement of inappropriate behaviors. Could there also be a hereditary contribution? As we shall see, more evidence is needed before that can be definitely established.

One of the first researchers to look for hereditary factors in neuroses was Slater (1943). He studied the relatives of World War II soldiers diagnosed as neurotic and reported that over half had parents, siblings, or children with some psychiatric problem. Brown (1942) had also reported the incidence of psychopathology in first- and second-degree relatives of 63 probands with anxiety neurosis, 21 with hysteric neurosis, and 20 with obsessional neurosis. He found a significant increase among relatives of neurotics when compared to that in relatives of a control group. Similar findings were reported by McInnes (1937) and Cohen, Badal, Kilpatrick, Reed, and White (1951). None of these studies dealt adequately with the possibility that the neurosis might be due to exposure to a familial environment that was predisposing to the acquisition of neurotic behavior. This problem can be circumvented to a degree by the twin study method because it may be assumed in many circumstances that family influences are similar for both members of identical and fraternal twin pairs.

Slater (1953) reported having studied 8 MZ and 43 DZ twin pairs in which the twin index case had been judged psychopathic or neurotic. Among the MZ twins, 2 pairs were concordant. For the DZ pairs, this number was 8. Although based on a very small sample, these results do not suggest an important hereditary effect. In a later paper, Shields and Slater (1971) reported the results of a rediagnosis by Slater of 192 index cases, known to have a twin, admitted to the Maudsley Hospital in London. Their findings are summarized in Table 31. Combining the incidence of anxiety state, other neuroses, and personality disorders, it may be noted from the data in the columns labeled 1 that 18 out of 62 MZ pairs and 3 out of 84 DZ pairs were concordant. This is somewhat

Table 31. Concordant Pairs of Twins by Psychiatric Diagnosis and Zygosity

	MZ Pairs			DZ Pairs		
	No. of Pairs	1[a]	2[b]	No. of Pairs	1[a]	2[b]
Anxiety state	17	7 (41%)	8 (47%)	28	1 (4%)	5 (18%)
Other neuroses	12	0	3 (25%)	21	0	5 (24%)
Personality disorders	33	11 (33%)	18 (55%)	35	2 (6%)	10 (29%)
Schizophrenia	6	2 (33%)	4 (67%)	7	0	2 (29%)
Endogenous depression	11	3 (27%)	7 (64%)	14	1 (7%)	8 (57%)
Other (organic)	1	0	0	7	0	3 (43%)
Total	80	23 (29%)	40 (50%)	112	4 (4%)	33 (30%)

Note. Adapted from "Diagnostic Similarity in Twins with Neuroses and Personality Disorders" by J. Shields and E. Slater. In J. Shields & L. I. Gottesman (Eds.), Man, Mind and Heredity: Selected Papers of Eliot Slater on Psychiatry and Genetics, 1971, Baltimore: The Johns Hopkins Press.
[a]Concordance based on both twins displaying symptoms of the same psychiatric dosorder.
[b]Concordance based on both twins displaying a psychiatric syndrome of any sort.

more indicative of a genetic effect than Slater's earlier study. In this second study, Shields and Slater raised an interesting possibility, namely that the co-twin might also be suffering from a psychiatric disorder, albeit a different one. The columns labeled 2 contain these results. When that possibility is considered, the concordance figures become 29 out of 62 MZ pairs and 20 out of 84 DZ twins, which is stronger evidence for a genetic factor.

The table results seem to suggest that co-twins of a schizophrenic or depressed parent may present with a different mental disorder such as neurosis or character disorder. It will be remembered that Heston (1966) also found some sociopathic and neurotic personalities among the adopted-away children of schizophrenic mothers. These two reports taken together suggest that there may be a general vulnerability to a variety of mental illnesses that might be due to hereditary factors. This idea resembles the distasteful 19th century notion of an hereditary "taint." It is as likely, however, that such results merely reflect the inadequacy of the present state of psychiatric diagnosis or at least the fact that diagnoses may not be made as carefully as they should. For example, when Kendler, Gruenberg, and Strauss (1981a) reexamined the recorded interviews from the Danish adoption study of schizophrenia (Kety et al., 1968, 1978) for the presence of relatives with anxiety neurosis, they found neither a genetic nor a familial-environmental relationship between the two illnesses. This finding is contrary to the results of three earlier studies in which relatives of probands with anxiety neurosis were examined (Brown, 1942; McInnes, 1937; Mitsuda, Sakai, & Kobayashi, 1967), and schizophrenics were found. The difference between the Kendler et al. study and the others may be in the quality of the diagnostic process.

The bulk of the other twin studies of neuroses that have been made are each based on very small numbers of twins. Summing across these studies revealed the following results: out of a total of 655 MZ pairs, 117 or 26.4% were concordant, and out of 824 DZ, there were 124 or 12.4% concordant (Braconi, 1961; Essen-Moller, 1941; Ihda, 1961; Inouye, 1961; Juel-Nielsen, 1964; Legras, 1933; Parker, 1966; Pollin, 1976; Schepank, 1971, 1974; Shapiro, 1970; Shields, 1954; Slater, 1953, 1961; Stumpfl, 1937; Tienari, 1963).

It should be noted that among these studies there was much diversity in methods used to ascertain probands, in diagnostic procedures, and in symptomatology. If these overall figures are taken at face value, however, they would lead to two conclusions: first, there must be strong environmental factors affecting the expression of neurosis because the concordance for the MZ twins was only 26.4%. Second, there is a considerable genetic component as reflected by the MZ-DZ difference in the concordance rates.

From results of seven family studies summarized by Pollin (1976), the familial nature of general neurosis seems to be reinforced. For example, in those studies he reviewed, he noted an overall sizable increase of neuroticism in relatives of probands, when compared to the incidence in the general population (although the incidence varied widely between studies). Studies of "normal" individuals who were administered a neuroticism questionnaire also fit into this body of research findings. Neuroticism has been variously defined in these studies by the specific questions asked, which usually deal with anxiety, worry, being tense, and the like. It is generally thought that neuroticism is a milder form of neurosis, so that evidence for a genetic contribution to neuroticism is deemed to be relevant evidence for a genetic factor in neurosis. These studies generally show higher concordance for MZ than DZ twins, even when the twins were reared apart (see Shields, 1962). A review by Miner (1973) presents thorough coverage of these genetic studies of neuroses and neuroticism.

In conjunction with studies of neurotic personality traits noted in normal individuals through the use of questionnaires, two interesting questions may be raised. First, do persons who later become mentally ill show signs before that time that could be interpreted as early warning signals? At least part of the rationale of the child guidance clinics consists of the belief that appropriate treatment can prevent later problems. The fact that relatively few children treated by such programs later develop mental illness might attest to the success of the programs and may validate the need for early treatment (Robins, 1966). However, that fact may also be interpreted as a negative answer to the question posed. Perhaps childhood problems are not as prognostic of later problems as is usually assumed. Of course, this would not diminish the value of child guidance clinics, but it does render questionable the concept of premorbid signs of mental illness.

The second question is perhaps even more basic. Can various mental illnesses be viewed as extremes of normal variation in personality? Some questionnaires developed for the measurement of personality traits are certainly used in that manner, whether their authors intended such use or not. Eysenck's personality scales were constructed from responses of psychiatric patients but proved useful with normals, as does the Minnesota Multiphasic Personality Inventory and the California Psychological Inventory. Whether scales developed on normal persons, sometimes even restricted to college students, can be of value in describing psychiatric patients is yet another question. These questions might be answered to some extent by studies that examine mentally ill and normal persons to see if test scores reflecting a trait thought to be affected by the illness form a continuum, with the clinical patients being represented at a different site than normals. On the other hand, the patients should show no marked difference from the normals if the trait is not one that is affected.

Also needed are personality test scores on persons before and after the onset of illness, preferably free of the effects of treatment with drugs, electric shock, and other therapeutic techniques. However, it may well be that psychological disorders do not form a continuum with normal personality. There are several reasons for thinking that this is so. Beyond the often bizarre nature of certain symptoms, there is the argument from behavioral genetic studies. These studies support the notion that although there is substantial agreement about a considerable genetic component in most types of mental illness, evidence from studies of normal personality traits is much weaker. Would one not expect the same degree of heritability, if normal personality traits and mental disorders are on the same continua? But perhaps we have been too concerned with the refining of our personality tests. Maybe we are attributing too much stability to personality.

Mischell, for example (1968, 1971), has argued that there is insufficient stability in human behavior to allow precise prediction—that trait theories of personality are unrealistic. Although this extreme position is fast being abandoned, as more and more evidence for continuity of personality traits across the life span emerges, there is some merit to acknowledging that under certain conditions personality can be drastically altered. The need for attention to present and past environmental conditions may be particularly important for psychiatric disorders. Whether or not mentally ill persons have been subjected to greater environmental stress than have others is uncertain. Although this is widely assumed, it is only recently being investigated systematically. To do so, we need to assess life histories in a more comprehensive and standardized way than is usually done. Ideally, one would want to quantify stressful events. Holmes and Rahe (1967) developed a checklist of stressful events, which was somewhat predictive of physical illness. Dohrenwend and Dohrenwend (1974) continued this work, focusing more specifically on psychological consequences. Although cultures may differ in their interpretation of certain events, work by Hough, Fairbank, and Garcia (1976), Wainer, Fairbank, and Hough (1978), and Mirowsky and Wheaton (1970) show that many life changes produce similar stresses in various ethnic groups. However, life event questionnaires may not allow prediction of *individual* illness, even when showing promise for comparing groups, as Horowitz, Schaefer, Hiroto, Wilner, and Levine (1977) warn. Lewinsohn and Talkington (1979) divided stressful life events into the following categories: (1) health; (2) achievement; (3) daily inconvenience; (4) close personal relationships; (5) legal; and (6) financial. They report substantial relations with daily mood and clinical depression. Related to this concept of life stress, Kobasa (1979) suggested that persons differ in "hardiness," so that some persons can withstand more stress than others, without developing illness. This may provide another way to conceptualize and operationalize the term *liability* to mental illness. For the reader who would like to know more about this area, Hurst, Jenkins, and Rose (1976) have written a thorough general review of life events research.

Over the years, psychiatric genetics research has moved away from studying global, undifferentiated "neurosis." For example, the most recent research has been directed toward investigating specific, clearly defined, clinical syndromes that have been classified as particular types of neurotic conditions. Anxiety neurosis, phobic neuroses, and obsessional neurosis have all been the focus of genetic studies of this kind. The study findings for specific conditions will now be discussed.

ANXIETY NEUROSIS (PANIC DISORDER)

In the early 1950s a paper was published in the *American Journal of Human Genetics* (Cohen *et al.*, 1951) presenting data suggesting that anxiety neurosis is familial in nature. Anxiety neurosis over the years has also been referred to as neurocirculatory asthenia, effort syndrome, soldier's heart, panic disorder, or DaCosta's syndrome. The prevalence in the general population was reported between 1 and 5.6%. In contrast, when the families of probands suffering from anxiety neurosis were examined by Cohen and co-workers, it was noted that among relatives of these probands ($N = 67$) the proportion of affected fathers was 17.5%, of mothers, 54.8%, of brothers, 13.3%, and of sisters, 12.1%. The much higher risk for mothers was explained by the fact that anxiety neurosis traditionally affects twice as many females as males. Although this paper was the first specific attempt to fit genetic models to familial data regarding anxiety neurosis, the fact that the disorder "runs in families" has been noted as early as the 19th century. A review of the studies of anxiety neurosis made between 1869 and 1948, which mention the familial aspects of the disorder, was included in the Cohen *et al.* report. An updated version adapted from this material appears in Table 32. In concluding their report, Cohen *et al.* state that anxiety neurosis, of the chronic type, seems to be inherited as a single dominant gene disorder.

In most diagnostic systems, one requisite for the diagnosis of anxiety neurosis is a positive history of anxiety attacks. These attacks typically take place in a short period of time. During that time, however, the experience is usually reported to be one of sheer terror. It may begin quite unexpectedly, at home, at work, even while sleeping. Deep apprehension usually marks the beginning of an attack and is followed quickly by several somatic symptoms, including rapid heart beat (tachycardia), hyperventilation, sweating, dilated pupils, nausea, and often loss of consciousness. Within a few minutes, the anxiety attack usually subsides completely, although between attacks, the affected individual often reports continued low levels of anxiety. Anxiety attacks are experienced quite frequently by some persons (as often as daily) whereas, for others, a full-blown anxiety attack will occur only once or twice a year. The age of risk is from the mid-teens into the mid-30s. Anxiety neurosis rarely requires hospitalization. In fact, it is probably underdiagnosed as many affected individuals with mild manifestations do not seek psychiatric assistance. The symptoms seem to become exacerbated during times of stress and often spontaneously remit during nonstressful periods. There is no evidence that any type of existing therapy can effectively eliminate these attacks in the majority of people.

In addition to the earlier work of Cohen *et al.* (1951), several other studies have been reported that relate to the familial aspects of anxiety neurosis (Crowe, Pauls, Slymen, & Noyes, 1980, 1983 and Noyes, Clancy, & Crowe, 1978). Noyes *et al.* report a prevalence rate of 18% (out of 919 cases) among first-degree relatives of 129 anxiety neurosis patients, as compared to 3% found among the relatives of 140 controls. In keeping with earlier reports, female relatives were at greater risk than males (24% vs. 13%).

The studies by Crowe *et al.* are unusual in several respects, including the fact that the risk rate in first-degree relatives of probands was calculated at about 30%, a figure much higher than those reported by Noyes *et al.* (1978) and Cohen *et al.* (1951). Crowe and his co-authors attribute the difference to the fact that theirs are the first studies of anxiety neurosis in which direct diagnoses of relatives were made based on psychiatric interviews administered personally or by telephone to the relatives participating in the studies. They believe that this approach is much more sensitive than relying on secondhand re-

Table 32. Literature Concerning the Familial Aspects of Anxiety Neurosis

Date	Author	Terminology	Total number of cases reported	Were cases studied from familial standpoint?	Are conclusions based on data presented?
1869	Beard	Nervous exhaustion (neurasthenia)	0	No	No
"Hereditary descent terribly predisposes to neurasthenia."					
1871	Da Costa	Irritable heart	200	No	No
No comments on familial appearances.					
1895	Freud	Angstneurose	0	No	No
"In some cases no etiology can be readily ascertained . . . in such cases it is seldom difficult to demonstrate a marked hereditary taint."					
1899	Savill	Neurasthenia	0	No	No
"General hereditary taint"					
1902	Hartenburgh	Nevrose d' Angoisse	58	No	No
One family had nervousness in mother and father.					
1907	Savill	Neurasthenia	205	No	No
"Heredity as a predisposing cause of neurasthenia may and does sometimes act."					
1911	Ballet	Neurasthenia	0	No	No
"The proportion of neurasthenics in whose antecedents one finds hereditary taints more or less marked may be estimated at 40%."					
1917	Heckel	Nevrose d' Angoisse	0	No	No
"There is not the least doubt of familial predisposition."					
1918	Lewis	Effort syndrome	558	No	No
"One of the largest groups is that of constitutional weakness, nervous, or physical or both."					
1918	Oppenheimer, Levine,	Neurocirculatory	558	No	No

Year	Author	Condition	No.		
	Morrison, Rothchild St. Lawrence, & Wilson	asthenia		Yes	Yes

"Must lay stress on the importance of a complete anamnesis even at times including family history."

| 1918 | Oppenheimer & Rothschild | Irritable heart | 100 | Yes | Yes |

Family history shows that there is more nervousness, alcoholism, irritability insanity, tuberculosis, epilepsy and stigmata in parents than there is in family history of Wolfsohn's controls.

| 1918 | Robey & Boas | Neurocirculatory Asthenia | 89 | No | No |

"The vast majority of the patients give a family history of nervous disorder."

| 1925 | Myerson | Neurasthenia | 0 | No | No |

"... that 'some' people 'are' predisposed to neurasthenia in that from the first days of their lives they showed lowered energy and endurance, irritability, emotional unrest, etc."

| 1940 | Lewis | Effort syndrome | 860 | No | No |

"One of the largest groups is that of constitutional weakness, nervous or physical or both ..." "Many show defective physical development.... The defects are certainly derived from both hereditary and acquired sources."

| 1941 | Wood | Da Costa's syndrome | 265 | Yes | Yes |

41.9% of patients have family history of "neuroses" or "nerves" as compared with 9.6% in controls.

| 1942 | Brown | Anxiety state | 63 | Yes | Partly |

Anxiety state appeared in 21.4% of parents and 12.3% of siblings as compared with 0% and 0% respectively in controls. Concludes that three types of neurosis, i.e., "anxiety state," "hysteria," and "obsessional state" are "genetically related," although his published data do not support this.

| 1943 | Slater | Anxiety neurosis | 647 | Yes | Yes |

56.7% of patients had "general positive family history" i.e., there was definite neurotic illness, psychosis, epilepsy, psychopathy (drunkenness, shiftlessness, violent or brutal habits). No data on control subjects. Concludes: "The neurotic constitution is then a useful hypothesis."

| 1946 | Cohen, Badal, Johnson, | Neurocirculatory | 70 | Yes | Yes |

(continued)

Table 32. (*Cont.*)

Date	Author	Terminology	Total number of cases reported	Were cases studied from familial standpoint?	Are conclusions based on data presented?
	Chapman, & White	asthenia, effort syndrome, anxiety neurosis			

The disorder occurred in 47% of mothers, 40% of fathers, and 13.2% of brothers and sisters of patients as compared with 0%, 4.9%, and 0% in normal controls.

Date	Author	Terminology	Total number of cases reported	Were cases studied from familial standpoint?	Are conclusions based on data presented?
1948	Wheeler, White, Reed, & Cohen	Neurocirculatory asthenia, effort syndrome, anxiety neurosis	50	Yes	Yes

Prevalence in sons and daughters of patients is 48.6% as compared with prevalence of 5.6% in general population of 234 healthy controls.

Date	Author	Terminology	Total number of cases reported	Were cases studied from familial standpoint?	Are conclusions based on data presented?
1948	Cohen, White, & Johnson	Neurocirculatory asthenia, anxiety neurosis; chronic and acute types	67	Yes	Yes

Neurocirculatory asthenia (anxiety neurosis, effort syndrome) occurs in 18.5% of fathers, 58.0% of mothers, and 12.6% of brothers

Year	Authors	Disorder	N			Findings
1951	Cohen, Badal, Kilpatrick, Reed, & White	Neurocirculatory asthenia, anxiety neurosis, effort syndrome	139	Yes	Yes	Manifestation of the disorder occurs in a high proportion of family members of affected probands diagnosed as having the *chronic* form of the disorder. There is little familial involvement in patients who were diagnosed as acute cases. and sisters of patients with chronic neurocirculatory asthenia in contrast to no cases in fathers, mothers, brothers, and sisters of 54 control subjects.
1978	Noyes, Clancy, & Crowe	Anxiety neurosis	129	Yes	Yes	Morbidity risk in first-degree relatives of anxiety neurosis probands calculated at 18% as compared to 3% in controls.
1980	Crowe, Pauls, Slymen, & Noyes	Anxiety neurosis	21	Yes	Yes	Psychiatric interviews of 121 relatives of anxiety neurosis probands reveal a morbidity risk of 31% as compared to 4% in 90 relatives of controls.
1983	Crowe, Noyes, Pauls, & Slymen	Panic disorder	41	Yes	Yes	Structured psychiatric interviews of 540 relatives of panic disorder probands and controls gave estimates of morbidity risks of 27.4% in relatives of patients as compared to 2.3% in relatives of controls.

Note. Adapted and updated from "The High Familial Prevalence of Neurocirculatory Asthenia (Anxiety Neurosis, Effort Syndrome) by M. E. Cohen, D. W. Badal, A. Kilpatrick, A. Reed, & P. White, 1951, *American Journal of Human Genetics*, 3, p. 126.

porting of relatives' conditions. In fact, if only interviewed relatives were included in the calculations, the morbid risk approached 50%, or that expected if the trait was due to an autosomal dominant gene.

Another unique aspect of this study is its suggestion that some patients who display symptoms of anxiety neurosis may in fact be suffering primarily from the cardiac disorder, mitral valve prolapse syndrome. This differential diagnosis problem was first noted by Wooley (1976). Mitral valve prolapse syndrome is characterized by a faulty mitral valve in the heart itself. It can be detected by using the sonar detection method of echocardiography. Wooley suggests that, because many of the somatic symptoms of anxiety neurosis are similar in nature to those experienced by mitral valve prolapse patients, a heart defect might underlie the symptoms of what is commonly thought to be a functional, or psychologically induced disorder. To some extent, Crowe et al. (1980) have corroborated this. Among 21 patients ascertained to have a definite diagnosis of anxiety neurosis, 8 (38%) were found to have mitral valve prolapse as detected by echocardiography.

One hundred twenty-one first-degree relatives of 19 of the anxiety neurosis proband group were interviewed. These data were compared to interviews from 90 first-degree relatives of 19 normal controls. At least 1 first-degree relative with definite anxiety neurosis was found in 14 of the 19 family groups of patients afflicted with the disorder. Only 4 of the 19 control family groups contained an individual with anxiety neurosis, and in each family, just one instance of the disorder was noted. A significant difference in rate of alcoholism was also found between the proband and control relatives. The morbidity risk for relatives was calculated at 15% and 4%, respectively ($p < .05$). This was the only evidence that families of anxiety neurosis probands were more heavily loaded for other psychiatric disorders.

The authors of this study also compared relatives of anxiety neurosis probands with mitral valve prolapse to relatives of probands who did not screen positively for prolapse. There were no differences between the two groups in the number of relatives at risk for anxiety neurosis. Further, there were no differences noted in risk for the two groups by class of relative or by sex of relative. On the basis of this admittedly small study of anxiety neurosis with or without mitral valve prolapse, the authors conclude that "the two sets of families were indistinguishable" (Crowe et al., 1980, p. 79; see also Pauls, Noyes, & Crowe, 1979; Pauls, Bucher, Crowe, & Noyes, 1980).

The preceding review of studies investigating the heritable nature of anxiety neurosis reveals a strong familial component to a disorder that is sometimes accompanied by an underlying structural heart defect. The reports of MZ twins reared apart (see Slater & Shields, 1969) and other small studies suggest at least a portion of this familial component is likely to be of genetic origin. Further, the earlier studies of anxiety neurosis concur by and large with the latest study by Crowe *et al.* (1983) in suggesting that a single dominant-gene mode of transmission is likely.

FEARS AND PHOBIAS

Another type of neurosis, somewhat less common than anxiety disorder, consists of unreasonable fears and worries that the patient often realizes should not cause the reaction they do but that cannot be controlled. These phobias can be so strong that they interfere markedly with a normal life. The patient may be unable to leave the house (agoraphobia) or to enter an elevator or a revolving door. The fear of flying is one particularly well-known example. It is not known how frequently phobias occur in the general population. However, Agras, Sylvester, and Oliveau (1969) interviewed a representative sample of adults in Burlington, Vermont. From their data, they estimated that 7.7% of the population have some strong, unreasonable fears, but only .2% have a disabling phobic condition. Other recent estimates suggest that 1.0% of women and 0.5% of men seen in outpatient clinics are diagnosed as having a phobia. Although some fears are rather common, the incidence of truly disabling phobias does seem to be low. There may, however, be under-reporting of this condition because patients often are ashamed of their phobia and do not seek help. Refusal to leave the house, as is often the case in agoraphobia, poses a special problem. Occasionally, elderly persons may die of malnutrition or from extremes in temperature rather than attempt to overcome their fear of leaving their house.

The most dramatic phobia is definitely agoraphobia (Matthews, Gelder, & Johnston, 1981). Although there are some indications of familial tendencies toward neurosis, there have been only a few studies of the familial aspects of phobias. Solyom, Beck, Solyom, and Hugel (1974) reported that 55% of mothers and 24% of fathers of agoraphobic patients were neurotics, whereas Burns and Thorpe (1977) reported that several relatives of 35 agoraphobics were neurotics. Buglas, Clarke, Henderson, Kreitman, and Presley (1977) found 28% of mothers and 17% of fathers neurotic. There were very few cases of concordance for a specific fear or phobia. In contrast, a study by Harris, Noyes,

Crowe, and Chandhry (1983) revealed that among the relatives of agoraphobic probands, there was an increased rate of agoraphobia when compared to families of panic disorder probands and controls. However, there was also an increased rate of other phobias and anxiety. These results are somewhat consistent with a recent study of phobias in twins that yielded evidence suggesting that MZ twins are more concordant for specific fears than are DZ twins. Togerson (1980) studied phobic fears in 50 MZ and 49 DZ twin pairs, about equally divided between male and female pairs. They ranged in age from 20 to 70 years. Fifty-one questions were used to assess fears.

The types of fears reported were found to define five independent factors in a factor analysis with a Varimax rotation (which results in uncorrelated factors). These five factors were interpreted by the researchers as (1) agoraphobia or fear of separation; (2) fear of animals; (3) castration anxiety, or fear of mutilation; (4) social fears, that is, of embarrassment; and (5) a mixture of agoraphobia and claustrophobia plus fears of fires, heights, the ocean, and other natural phenomena. Togerson computed heritability estimates from scores derived from each of the five factors. The results of this analysis are summarized in Table 33 in which it can be noted that phobias about animals (snakes, spiders, etc.) seem to be very concordant in MZ twins, along with separation anxiety and mutilation fears.

Carey (1978) administered the MMPI to twins from the Maudsley Hospital Twin Registry in England. At least one member of each pair had been diagnosed as suffering from obsessional or phobic disorder. Of the MZ co-twins, 85% also displayed evidence of obsessive or phobic symptoms, whereas 50% of DZ co-twins did. There was a trend toward

Table 33. Five Phobia Factors. Intraclass Correlations and
Heritability Estimates

	Intraclass correlations		Falconer's estimate of heritability[a]
	MZ Twins	DZ Twins	
Separation factor	.69	.39	.60
Animals factor	.48	.05	.86
Mutilation factor	.35	−.20	.70
Social factor	.88	.65	.26
Mixed fears factor	.55	.35	.40

Note. Adapted from "Hereditary-Environmental Differentiation of General Neurotic, Obsessive, and Impulsive Hysterical Personality Traits" by S. Torgerson, 1980, Acta Genetica Medica Gemellologiae, 29.
[a] $2(r_{MZ} - r_{DZ})$

Table 34. Twin Analysis of Fear Survey Data (MZ Pairs =
222; DZ Pairs = 132)

Fear factor	r_{MZ}	r_{DZ}	$2(r_{MZ} - r_{DZ})$
Negative Social Interaction	.50	.28	.44
Social Responsibility	.54	.24	.60
Dangerous Places	.43	.14	.58
Small Organisms	.53	.20	.66
Deep Water	.52	.36	.32
Loved One's Misfortunes	.52	.38	.28
Personal Death	.52	.16	.72

Note. From "A Developmental-Genetic Analysis of Common Fears from Early
Adolescence to Early Adulthood" by R. Rose & W. B. Ditto, 1983, Child Development 54, p. 365. Copyright 1983 by Society for Research in Child Development. Reprinted by permission.

symptom specificity, although details of the content of the phobia or
obsession frequently differed. The author reports that familial-environmental factors also seemed to play a role in producing phobic personalities as revealed by the fact that the DZ concordance rate was quite
high (50%).

Rose and Ditto (1983) studied the concordance for common fears
in MZ and DZ twins pairs ranging in age from 14 to 35 years. A 51-item
fear survey was administered to 354 pairs of like-sex twins along with
over 1,800 nontwin individuals. The fear survey was factor analyzed,
and the seven factors noted in Table 34 were reported by the authors.
MZ and DZ concordance rates for the seven factors are also shown in
Table 34. As in the Torgerson (1980) data reported before, fear of small
organisms (snakes, spiders, rats) yielded a high heritability estimate.
The authors note that when the concordances were analyzed separately for younger (19 years of age and less) and older (20 to 34 years of
age) twin pairs, the DZ concordance for certain factors was noticeably
reduced in older twins, when compared to the overall DZ data. No
such phenomenon was noted for MZ concordance rates. This resulted
in higher heritability estimates for the older twins than for the younger. The authors speculate that the difference is a result of the fact that
the older twins rarely shared a household, and therefore, common living experiences were more rare among this group. This in turn resulted
in an increased emphasis on genetic differences.

In her reanalysis of MZ twins reared apart, Farber (1981) mentioned several pairs with similar phobias. Although she was able to
find only a few cases of such shared phobias, her attempt provides

Table 35. *Percentages of Males and*
Females in the U.S. Reporting Specific
Fears

	Percentage having a specific fear	
	Men	Women
Speaking before a group	36	48
Heights	26	38
Deep water	13	30
Loneliness	11	16
Dogs	9	14
Lifts	4	11
Escalators	2	8

Note. From *Twins, An Uncanny Relationship* by P.
Watson, 1981, New York: Viking Press. Copyright 1981
by Viking Press. Reprinted by permission.

further evidence for the possibility of a genetic component in phobic
disorder.

Peter Watson (1981), in his popular book on twins, makes the
useful comment that certain mild or moderate fears are common
enough in the general population to make resemblances even between
strangers fairly probable just by chance alone (see Table 35). If one adds
to that the common living conditions and shared experiences that
influence family members, similar fears would certainly be expected to
occur quite often and yet not be related to any genetic influence. The
same argument can be made even more forcefully for twins. This may,
in fact, account for the high concordance rates one often finds for both
MZ and DZ twins with regard to phobias.

OBSESSIONS AND COMPULSIONS

Obsessions and compulsions are, respectively, thoughts and actions that are seemingly irrational but that keep reoccurring despite
the obvious discomfort they cause in the individual experiencing
them. The age of onset for this kind of neurotic condition is usually in
late adolescence or early adulthood, with onset of symptoms rarely
occurring after the age of 40. Attempts to prevent or inhibit compulsions are generally anxiety-producing and are often unsuccessful. Behavior modification techniques seem to be the most effective type of
therapeutic intervention.

That obsessions in particular are related to general neuroticism is suggested by an analysis reported by Clifford, Fulker, and Murray (1981). The responses of 404 pairs of MZ and DZ twins, aged 16 to 70 years, to the Brief Leyton Obsessional Inventory and the Neuroticism scale of the Eysenck Personality Questionnaire (Eysenck & Eysenck, 1977) were analyzed into their genetic and environmental components. The Leyton scale measures four types of obsessions: a need for perfection that cannot be met, excessive cleanliness and tidiness, intrusion of gloomy thoughts, and constant repetitive checking, such as "Is the gas off?"—"Is the door locked?" and the like. The heritability estimates for these four components and for the Neuroticism scale were .31—need for perfection; .43—excessive cleanliness; .41-intrusion of gloomy thoughts; .39—constant checking; and .42—score on the Neuroticism scale. All of these values are surprisingly similar. Genetic correlations among these five variables are shown in Table 36 above the diagonal, with the environmental correlations below the diagonal. It should be noted that the genetic values are generally larger. The standard errors of the genetic correlations were .10 or less, and for the environmental components, .05 or less.

Hare, Price, and Slater (1971) estimated that obsessive-compulsive neuroses comprised 0.5% of first admissions to psychiatric hospitals and 3% of all neuroses. Black (1974) summarized 11 studies reported up to 1964 and estimated that among psychiatric outpatients between 0.3 and 0.6% had obsessive-compulsive neuroses.

Rachman and Hodgson (1980) reviewed the relevant studies and concluded that a genetic factor exists not so much for a specific obsessive-compulsive disorder as for general neuroticism or emotional oversensitivity. These same authors also conclude that there is no firm basis for the idea that there is an obsessional personality type that is more likely to develop an obsessive-compulsive disorder. They, however, posit a relationship between neurotic depression and obsessive-

Table 36. Genetic and Environmental Correlations between Leyton Scale Scores and Eysenck's Neuroticism Scale for 404 Twin Pairs[a]

Need for perfection	1.00	.57	.43	.80	.50
Cleanliness and tidiness	.26	1.00	.23	.30	.38
Gloomy thoughts	.28	.09	1.00	.24	.64
Checking and counting	.18	.22	.50	1.00	.48
Neuroticism scale	.09	.04	.19	.05	1.00

Note. Adapted from "A Genetic and Environmental Analysis of Obsessionality in Normal Twins" by C. A. Clifford, D. W. Fulker, R. M. Murray, in L. Gedda, P. Parisi & N. E. Nance (Eds.), *Twin Research 3, Part B. Intelligence, Personality, and Development*, 1981, New York: Alan R. Liss.
[a]Genetic correlations appear above diagonal and environmental correlations appear below.

compulsive disorder. Earlier we mentioned the proposed distinction between neurotic depression and endogenous or psychotic depression, in which the latter is seen as more likely to be genetically determined and neurotic depression as more due to experiential factors. There have been no specific studies of the relationship of life stresses to obsessive-compulsive behavior, but it could well be that certain individuals are predisposed to this disorder because of inherited factors, whereas others might become obsessional or compulsive because of certain learning experiences to which they have been exposed. Probably before one could take this notion further, a more refined diagnosis of the disorder is necessary. Particular attention would have to be paid to evidence of individual differences that could suggest the possibility of there being more than one form of the disorder (a mild and severe subtype, for example).

In a study that relates to the preceding issue, Pollak (1978) reviewed the literature on the obsessive-compulsive personality. This personality type is thought to be characterized by orderliness, cleanliness, thrift, carefulness, rigidity, and conservatism. This personality type is to be distinguished from the psychiatric entity called obsessive-compulsive neurosis and should not be regarded as a precursor of the psychiatric condition. People who are characterized by these traits are most frequently not clinically neurotic. Further, there is no evidence that the obsessive-compulsive personality is more frequent in normal relatives of patients with the psychiatric condition. This suggests that there is no genetic relationship between the so-called obsessive-compulsive personality type and obsessive-compulsive neurosis. The review by Pollak also discusses several personality tests that measure this personality constellation.

CONVERSION DISORDER (OR HYSTERICAL NEUROSIS)

The description of conversion disorder as noted in DSM-III is an alteration of physical state *not* caused by an obvious extraneous factor such as a physical trauma or a toxic agent. Conversion disorder can include a twilight state in which the patient's judgment is weakened, as well as more dramatic symptomatology. Frequently, there are fits, paralysis of parts of the body, anesthesia in areas of the body, and muteness. Hallucinations are not an essential criterion for the diagnosis and tend to be minor if they do occur. "Hysterical conversion neurosis," as it was traditionally referred to in early psychiatric literature, can include blindness or deafness. A hysterical personality is often characterized as a person who has a pressing need for variety and enjoys being the center of attention; his or her enthusiasm is easily aroused, but his or her endurance tends to be limited. The hysteric often complains in a dramatic manner about many physical symptoms that cause pain and discomfort. Upon medical examination, however, most frequently no evidence of conditions that could explain the pain is found. Early Freudians believed that suggestibility and distractibility were two of the most characteristic traits.

The concept of hysteria has had a curious history (Veith, 1965). Although it was a common diagnosis in the 19th century and played a crucial role in the development of psychoanalysis, Freud himself used the term relatively little (Krohn, 1978). Even though hysteria is still included in several psychiatric diagnostic systems, it is diagnosed less and less frequently today. It thus appears to have become much less prevalent, but it is also probable that this diagnosis is really just no longer fashionable. In other words, not only the patients have changed but also the physicians. Conversion symptoms are still diagnosed but are usually attributed to psychosomatic illness, malingering, or hypochondriasis.

The DSM-III includes a new diagnostic entity, somatization disorder, that was previously referred to as Briquet's syndrome of hysteria. It is characterized by multiple and chronic physical complaints without a known physiological origin. As was hysteria in earlier times, this is predominantly a female disorder. The specific diagnostic criteria in the DSM-III (p. 243) require at least 14 symptoms in females and 12 in males from the list of 37 noted next.

- Conversion or pseudoneurological symptoms: difficulty swallowing, loss of voice, deafness, double vision, blurred vision, blindness, fainting or loss of consciousness, memory loss, seizures or convulsions, trouble walking, paralysis or muscle weakness, urinary retention or difficulty urinating.
- Gastrointestinal symptoms: abdominal pain, nausea, vomiting spells (other than during pregnancy), bloating (gassy), intolerance (e.g., gets sick) to a variety of foods, diarrhea.
- Female reproductive symptoms: judged by the individual as occurring more frequently or severely than in most women: painful menstruation, menstrual irregularity, excessive bleeding, severe vomiting throughout pregnancy or causing hospitalization during pregnancy.
- Psychosexual symptoms: for the major part of the individual's

life after opportunities for sexual activity: sexual indifference, lack of pleasure during intercourse, pain during intercourse.
- Pain: pain in back, joints, extremities, genital area (other than during intercourse); pain on urination; other pain (other than headaches).
- Cardiopulmonary symptoms: shortness of breath, palpitations, chest pain, dizziness.

Throughout the period of time in which the terms *hysteria, hysterical conversion,* or *conversion disorder* have been in use, many researchers have deplored the fact that there were few clear-cut distinctions one could make among these psychiatric labels. Indeed, there was enough overlap to create a diagnostic confusion in the minds of many diagnosticians. Chodoff and Lyons (1958) attempted to clarify the use of "hysteria," "hysterical personality," and "hysterical conversion." In 1962, Perley and Guze suggested the symptoms for hysteria shown in Table 37 but noted various other criteria that must be met before hysteria is diagnosed (see table footnote).

Many textbooks written before 1951 emphasized the hereditary nature of hysteria. Göring (1910) found hysterical reactions in relatives of a proband with hysterical dizziness. Other early studies were by Kraulis (1931), McInnes (1937), and Brown (1942). Kraulis studied only paroxysmal cases and patients who exhibited twilight states. Among 212 parents of 105 probands, $9.4 \pm 2.0\%$ exhibited a hysterical mode of reaction, and $2.4 \pm 1.0\%$ had been hospitalized. For siblings over the age of 5, these figures were $12.5 \pm 1.7\%$ and $6.3 \pm 1.2\%$, respectively. McInnes found that 6.0% of the parents and 3.3% of the siblings of 30 probands with conversion hysteria had similar symptoms, whereas only 1.1% of 75 control cases showed symptoms of conversion hysteria. Of 104 neurotics studied by Brown, 21 were classified as conversion hysterics. The frequency of hysteria was 19% in the parents of these probands and 6% in their siblings over the age of 15; for a control group, the frequency was 0.8%.

In 1957, Ljungberg reported on a genetic study of 233 males and 453 females who exhibited one or more of the symptoms of conversion hysteria as listed in Table 38. One patient was briefly described as having suffered from a fall that caused amnesia; in fact, in this report, Ljungberg noted 61 cases with head injuries. Such cases do not seem to fit the diagnosis of conversion hysteria because cases resulting from physical injury are usually excluded. Nonetheless, within his sample of 686 cases, Ljungberg probably did have quite a few accurately diagnosed cases. He found widely varying ages of onset, with a peak at

Table 37. Symptoms for Hysteria[a]

Group 1	Group 6
Headaches	Abdominal pain
Sickly most of life	Vomiting
Group 2	**Group 7**
Blindness	Dysmenorrhea
Paralysis	Menstrual irregularity
Anesthesia	Amenorrhea
Aphonia	Excessive bleeding
Fits or convulsions	**Group 8**
Unconsciousness	Sexual indifference
Amnesia	Frigidity
Deafness	Dyspareunia
Hallucinations	Other sexual difficulties
Urinary retention	Vomiting 9 months pregnancy or
Ataxia	hospitalized for *hyperemesis*
Other conversion symptoms	*gravidarium*
Group 3	**Group 9**
Fatigue	Back pain
Lump in throat	Joint pain
Fainting spells	Extremity pain
Visual blurring	Burning pains of the sexual organs, mouth,
Weakness	or rectum
Dysuria	Other bodily pains
Group 4	**Group 10**
Breathing difficulty	Nervousness
Palpitation	Fears
Anxiety attacks	Depressed feelings
Chest pain	Need to quit working or inability to carry on
Dizziness	regular duties because of feeling sick
Group 5	Crying easily
Anorexia	Feeling life was hopeless
Weight loss	Thinking a good deal about dying
Marked fluctuations in weight	Wanting to die
Nausea	Thinking of suicide
Abdominal bloating	Suicide attempts
Food intolerances	
Diarrhea	
Constipation	

Note. Adapted from "Hysteria—the Stability and Usefulness of Clinical Criteria" by M. G. Perley & S. Guze, 1962. *New England Journal of Medicine, 266.*
[a]Twenty-five symptoms or more for 9 of 10 groups are required, with onset before age 35. To qualify, symptoms (1) must interfere with patient's life and/or (2) patient should have taken medication for symptoms and/or (3) patient must have consulted a doctor for symptoms.

Table 38. Conversion Symptoms
Noted among Hysterics

Astasia-abasia	Amnesia
Fits	Visual field defects
Tremor	Aphonia
Twilight state	Speech defects
Anaesthesia	Mutism
Paralysis	

Note. Adapted from "Hysteria—A Clinical, prognostic and genetic study" by L. Ljungberg, 1957, *Acta Psychiatrica et Neurologica Scandinavica, 32* (Suppl. 112).

about 22 years of age. Many patients improved spontaneously and were reportedly unaffected thereafter. Among the relatives of the probands, 3 fathers, 18 mothers, 12 brothers, 27 sisters, 1 son, and 3 daughters had been or were subsequently diagnosed as conversion hysterics. When uncertain cases were included, the figures became 6, 27, 14, 35, 3, and 5. These figures are higher than the risk in the general population, which Ljungberg estimated at about 0.5%. But because it appears that head injury cases were included in the family study, the specific results are not to be taken uncritically. This study is, however, another that reports a higher risk factor in families of affected individuals.

Cloninger, Reich, and Guze (1975) have suggested an association between Briquet's syndrome and antisocial behavior by noting that in many families one finds a high rate of hysteria in females and a corresponding high rate of antisocial behavior in male family members. Flor-Henry, Fromm-Auch, and Tapper (1981) have also suggested that hysteria in females may be equivalent to psychopathy in males. This particular suggestion did not rest on a genetic analysis but on the results of an extensive neuropsychological test battery, which indicated that both hysteria and psychopathy are due to a dysfunction of the dominant (left) hemisphere. Attempts to relate various types of mental illness to patterns of neuropsychological test results, including evoked potentials, are too new to have led to a consensus of opinion, so we shall not discuss them further here. It is possible that they may eventually provide another means of grouping psychiatric patients more objectively.

CHAPTER 9

Heredity and Alcoholism

Hereditary Factors in Alcoholism

The temperance movement (and Prohibition) was based on a 19th century realization that drunkenness was a vice, not only of the wastrel rich and the improvident poor, but also of the middle classes. Alcohol itself was seen as the culprit. However, modern views of alcoholism emphasize that many individuals enjoy drinking without experiencing any alcohol-related difficulties and that one therefore should focus on problem drinkers rather than on alcohol use. In fact, alcoholism is now thought by many to be a disease or a psychiatric disorder rather than a moral weakness. This is reflected in the inclusion of alcohol abuse and of alcohol dependence in the DSM-III. Tables 39 and 40 describe the diagnostic criteria for these two conditions.

Although the existing literature on alcoholism perhaps justifiably places predominant emphasis on environmental influences, there are strong indications that hereditary factors also play a role. One line of evidence is the often-noted remarkable racial difference in response to a small amount of alcohol. Orientals frequently experience a nearly instantaneous, unpleasant flushing reaction of the face and skin in general, and many of them have a lower tolerance than Caucasians to the inebriating effects of alcohol (Lieber, 1972). Similarly, in animals, there are well-documented differences among strains of mice in preference for alcohol (McClearn, 1973), and these differences can be enhanced by selective breeding.

Most convincing, however, are three related studies of adopted-

Table 39. Diagnostic Criteria for Alcohol Abuse

A. Pattern of pathological alcohol use: need for daily use of alcohol for adequate
    functioning; inability to cut down or stop drinking; repeated efforts to control or
    reduce excess drinking by "going on the wagon" (periods of temporary
    abstinence) or restricting drinking to certain times of the day; binges (remaining
    intoxicated throughout the day for at least 2 days); occasional consumption of a
    fifth of spirits (or its equivalent in wine or beer); amnesic periods for events
    occurring while intoxicated (blackouts); continuation of drinking despite a
    serious physical disorder that the individual knows is exacerbated by alcohol use;
    drinking of nonbeverage alcohol.
B. Impairment in social or occupational functioning due to alcohol use: e.g.,
    violence while intoxicated, absence from work, loss of job, legal difficulties (e.g.,
    arrest for intoxicated behavior, traffic accidents while intoxicated), arguments or
    difficulties with family or friends because of excessive alcohol use.
C. Duration of disturbance of at least 1 month.

Note. From *Diagnostic and Statistical Manual of Mental Disorders* (3rd ed.), pp. 169–170, by the
American Psychiatric Association, 1980. Copyright 1980 by the American Psychiatric Association.
Reprinted by permission.

Table 40. Diagnostic Criteria for Alcohol Dependence

A. Either a pattern of pathological alcohol use or impairment in social or
    occupational functioning due to alcohol use:
    Pattern of pathological alcohol use: need for daily use of alcohol for adequate
    functioning; inability to cut down or stop drinking; repeated efforts to control or
    reduce excess drinking by "going on the wagon" (periods of temporary
    abstinence) or restricting drinking to certain times of the day; binges (remaining
    intoxicated throughout the day for at least 2 days); occasional consumption of a
    fifth of spirits (or its equivalent in wine or beer); amnesic periods for events
    occurring while intoxicated (blackouts); continuation of drinking despite a
    serious physical disorder that the individual knows is exacerbated by alcohol use;
    drinking of nonbeverage alcohol.
    Impairment in social or occupational functioning due to alcohol use: e.g.,
    violence while intoxicated, absence from work, loss of job, legal difficulties (e.g.,
    arrest for intoxicated behavior, traffic accidents while intoxicated), arguments or
    difficulties with family or friends because of excessive alcohol use.
B. Either tolerance or withdrawal:
    Tolerance: need for markedly increased amounts of alcohol to achieve the desired
    effect, or markedly diminished effect with regular use of the same amount.
    Withdrawal: development of alcohol withdrawal (e.g., morning "shakes" and
    malaise relieved by drinking) after cessation of or reduction in drinking.

Note. From *Diagnostic and Statistical Manual of Mental Disorders* (3rd ed.) p. 170, by the American
Psychiatric Association, 1980. Copyright 1980 by the American Psychiatric Association. Reprinted
by permission.

away children of alcoholic parents. Goodwin, Schulsinger, Hermansen, Guze, and Winokur (1973) used information in the Danish adoption registry to compare 78 male controls to 55 men separated early in life from their biological parents, after one of the parents had received a hospital diagnosis of alcoholism. The outcomes shown in Table 41 suggested a hereditary component to alcoholism. For example, even though the control group reportedly engaged in frequent drinking, only 5 of them were ever diagnosed as alcoholic as compared to 18 of the children of alcoholic biological parents.

In the second study, Goodwin *et al.* (1974) compared 30 sons of 19 alcoholics reared by the alcoholic biological parent with 20 of their brothers who had been adopted away from the family before the age of 6. Five men in each group were alcoholic, which means that the percentage was higher in the adopted group. In addition, if one of the brothers was alcoholic, there was a tendency for the other also to be alcoholic, and this was related to the seriousness of their biological father's condition.

The third study (Bohman, 1978) utilized the Swedish adoption registry to make comparisons in a manner similar to the studies just described. Again, an association was found between alcohol abuse in biological parents and their adopted-away offspring. In a further analysis, new light was thrown on these data. Bohman, Sigvardsson, and Cloninger (1981) studied the maternal inheritance of abuse in 913 Swedish adopted women. Adopted-away daughters of alcoholic mothers were three times as likely to be alcohol abusers. Alcoholic fathers fell into two groups. Biological fathers with mild alcoholic abuse not associated with criminality often had daughters who abused alcohol, but fathers with serious alcoholism and crime problems had no excess

Table 41. Incidence of Drinking in Adopted Children Born to Alcoholic or Control Parent

Classification	Children of alcoholic parents $N = 55$	Children of control parents $N = 78$	p
Moderate drinker	51	45	ns
Heavy drinker, ever	22	36	ns
Alcoholic, ever	18	5	.02

Note. From "Alcohol Problems in Adoptees Raised Apart from Alcoholic Biological Parents" by D. W. Goodwin, F. Schulsinger, Hermansen, & Guze, 1973, *Archives of General Psychiatry, 28.* Copyright 1973 by the American Medical Association. Reprinted by permission.

of alcohol-abusing daughters. Alcohol abuse by adoptive parents did not increase later alcohol abuse by the adopted women. Thus, the authors propose that there are two distinct types of alcoholism. The first is expressed only in certain environments and affects men and women. Here, alcoholism is generally not connected with criminality. Both the inherited factor and environmental provocation are necessary for a person to become an abuser. If either the inherited factor or the provocative environment alone is present, the risk of alcohol abuse is lower than in the general population. If both are present, the risk is twice as great.

In the second type of families, the biological fathers have an earlier onset of alcoholism (often in adolescence) and serious criminality. The risk for the adopted-away sons of this type is nine times as great and not dependent on the environment. Daughters do not seem to be affected, however. In these latter families, the mothers do not differ from mothers of nonalcoholics. Similar results were obtained in Copenhagen by Goodwin *et al.* (1973) and Goodwin, Schulsinger, and Knop (1977) who studied 55 adopted sons and 49 adopted daughters of severely alcoholic biological parents. Alcoholism was not increased in the daughters but increased four times in the sons.

Schuckit, Goodwin, and Winokur (1972) studied half-sibs of 60 male and 9 female alcoholic probands. When 32 alcoholic half-sibs were compared with 32 nonalcoholic half-sibs, the results in Table 42 were obtained. At the very least, this study suggests that the effect of having an alcoholic progenitor is much more important then the effect of being reared by an alcoholic.

A further analysis of these data brought out this contrast even more clearly. Half-sibs were categorized in two ways—as having a

Table 42. Incidence of Precipitating Factors in Alcoholic and Nonalcoholic Half-Sibs of Alcoholic Probands

Precipitating factors	Alcoholic $N = 32$	Nonalcoholic $N = 32$
At least one alcoholic biological parent	62%	19%
Living with any alcoholic parent figure (for 6 or more childhood years)	28%	22%
Broken home	81%	71%

Note. Adapted from "The Half-sibling Approach in a Genetic Study of Alcoholism" by M. Schuckit, D. W. Goodwin, & G. Winokur, 1972, in M. Roff, L. N. Rolins, & M. Pollack (Eds.), *Life History Research in Psychopathology* (Vol. 2), Minneapolis: University of Minneapolis Press.

Table 43. Incidence of Alcoholism in Persons Born to Alcoholic or
Nonalcoholic Parent and Raised by Alcoholic or Nonalcoholic Foster
Parent

| | | Foster Parent | | |
		Alcoholic	Nonalcoholic	Total
Biological parent	Alcoholic	11/24 (46%)	11/22 (50%)	22/46 (47.8%)
	Nonalcoholic	2/14 (14%)	8/104 (8%)	10/118 (8.5%)

Note. Adapted from "The Half-Sibling Approach in a Genetic Study of Alcoholism" by M. Schuckit, D. W. Goodwin, & G. Winokur, 1972, in M. Roff, L. N. Rolins, & M. Pollack (Eds.), *Life History Research in Psychopathology* (Vol. 2). Minneapolis: University of Minneapolis Press.

biological parent who was alcoholic or not and as having a foster parent who was alcoholic or not. The results are shown in Table 43, where the entries are the proportions of half-sibs who were themselves alcoholic. It may be seen that having an alcoholic foster parent only doubled the proportion, whereas the proportion increased by a factor of almost 8 in those cases in which the biological parent was an alcoholic, even though the offspring had no contact with that parent. In appraising this last study, it should be kept in mind that the subjects were half-sibs of probands who were alcoholics, so that they were not a random sample of individuals with alcoholic or nonalcoholic parents. Thus, they must be considered as a subset that was particularly predisposed to alcoholism.

Earlier twin studies by Jonsson & Nilsson (1968), Kaij (1960), and Partanen, Brunn, and Markanen (1966) found higher MZ than DZ concordance for alcoholism, for amount of drinking, and for drinking large amounts of alcohol, respectively. However, the fact that all the twin pairs were reared together makes the interpretation somewhat less clear-cut.

ARE ALCOHOLISM AND DEPRESSIVE STATES RELATED?

We mentioned earlier the suggestion that some alcoholics are attempting to fight depression by self-medicating with alcohol. Are these alcoholics possibly hidden cases of affective disorder? Could their presence "spoil" behavior genetic analyses of the latter condition? This question has been raised by Winokur and his associates (Winokur & Clayton, 1967a), by Reich, Winokur, and Mullaney (1975), and by Woodruff, Guze, Clayton, and Carr (1973). In the latter report, the incidence of a number of problems in the family or the personal history of alcoholics with (N = 39) or without (N = 29) depression and of depressive patients (N = 136) was examined. The results were somewhat different for men and women. Table 44 summarizes the data (after excluding items known to be directly related to alcoholism, such as number of arrests due to drinking because inclusion of these items would result in circular reasoning.) The patients with depression alone differed more from the group with the combined symptoms than did the patients who were alcoholics without depression. In fact, most of the distinguishing items occurred at an age before drinking had developed; yet they were almost never found in the group with depression only. This finding strengthens the impression that alcoholics are a distinct group. For both sexes, the items distinguishing alcoholics included outbursts of rage, fights, and number of arrests (without counting those due to drinking). These antisociallike behaviors are suggestive of a personality disorder quite different from the symptoms of psychotic depression. For men only, there was also often a family history of alcoholism noted, frequently including a father who drank heavily.

Merikangas, Leckman, Prusoff, Pauls, and Weissman (1985) also found evidence suggesting that depression and alcoholism are distinct disorders. They found that the relatives of depressed probands did not have increased rates of alcoholism, whereas rates were increased in relatives of probands who had both symptoms of depression and alcoholism. The rates of depression were the same in both types of families. They conclude from these results that depression and alcoholism are independent. Interestingly they found an elevated rate of anxiety disorders in the relatives of probands with combined symptoms. This suggests that instead of self-medicating for depression, these relatives may be self-medicating for anxiety.

The incidence of alcoholism is always lower in females than in males (lifetime expectancy rates range from 0.1 to 1% and 3 to 5%, respectively). Reich et al. (1975) used the "inheritance of liability" model of Falconer (1965) to compare male and female incidence of alcoholism in white and black populations. The model uses a comparison of the incidence in first-degree relations of affected individuals with the incidence in the population at large to estimate the correlation (r) of liability between relatives. When the correlation is between first-degree relatives, given that their environments are uncorrelated, the degree of genetic determination, or heritability (h^2), is: $h^2 = 2r$. Using this method, they obtained the results in Table 45. It can be seen that the value of r for relatives is always lower for female probands. To

Table 44. Comparison of Three Diagnostic Groups on History Items after Removal of Variables Directly Due to Alcohol

Men	Alcoholism without depression (N = 19)	p	Alcoholism with depression (N = 22)	p	Depression alone (N = 33)
Family history of alcoholism	58%	NS	73%	0.01	33%
Father drank heavily	37%	NS	55%	0.01	15%
Mean socioeconomic index	26	NS	25	0.05	38
No history of serious injury	58%	0.05	18%	0.02	55%
Mean number of injuries	0.5	0.05	1.5	NS	0.8
Fighting before age 18	21%	NS	45%	0.001	3%
History of outbursts of rage	37%	NS	59%	0.05	27%
Demoted in service	11%	NS	23%	0.05	0%
School difficulty, fights	16%	NS	45%	0.01	6%
Mean number of arrests	1.6	NS	1.9	0.05	0.7

Women	Alcoholism without depression (N = 10)	p	Alcoholism with depression (N = 17)	p	Depression alone (N = 103)
History of outbursts of rage	50%	NS	59%	0.01	20%
Mean number of jobs last 10 years	2.6	NS	3.4	0.01	1.8
School difficulty, fights	20%	NS	24%	0.05	5%
Traffic violations	0%	NS	24%	0.05	6%
Ever arrested	20%	NS	35%	0.05	12%
Ever jailed	0%	NS	24%	0.001	1%
Mean number of arrests	0.2	NS	0.9	0.001	0.1

Note. "Alcoholism and Depression" by R. A. Woodruff, S. B. Guze, P. J. Clayton, & D. Carr, 1973, Archives of General Psychiatry, 28. Copyright 1973 by the American Medical Association. Reprinted by permission.

Table 45. Correlations in Liability between Male and Female Probands and Their Like-Sexed and Opposite-Sexed Relatives in White and Black Populations

		Whites First-degree relatives		Blacks First-degree relatives	
		Male	Female	Male	Female
Probands	Male	0.53 ± 0.05	0.24 ± 0.07	0.76 ± 0.06	0.40 ± 0.09
	Female	0.33 ± 0.09	0.18 ± 0.10	0.36 ± 0.10	0.29 ± 0.13

Note. Adapted from "The Transmission of Alcoholism" by T. Reich, G. Winokur, & J. Mullaney, 1975, in R. Fieve, D. Rosenthal & H. Brill (Eds.), *Genetic Research in Psychiatry*, Baltimore: The Johns Hopkins University Press.

try to explain these differences, a model was employed in which sex difference in the expression of alcoholism was attributed !o a higher threshold for females, but with the same proportions of genetic and environmental variance operating for both sexes as shown in Figure 15. This particular model did not fit well in either ethnic group. An attempt was then made to fit the data to a model basing the sex differences on cultural effects (i.e., the social proscriptions against heavy drinking in females are much stronger in most cultures). The fit to this model was more satisfactory. This suggests that the sex difference in prevalence of alcoholism may be a result of strong social pressure against women's drinking, especially to excess.

SOCIETAL FACTORS IN ALCOHOLISM

Not all researchers are impressed with the findings of genetic factors in alcoholism. In fact, some authors question the validity of current concepts in research on alcohol abuse that focus on personal differences between problem drinkers and the rest of the population.

The moderate or social drinker is often seen as someone who has "control" over his or her intake, in contrast to the problem drinker who has no control. These critics point out that this control is only in part a personal characteristic and is also a function of the social situation in which the drinking takes place. Both the personal and the social factors are, in turn, influenced by the prevailing cultural attitudes toward drinking, intoxication, and alcoholism. An example of this critical attitude is provided by Beauchamp (1980) who believes that the personal characteristics will not account for much of the variation in drinking behavior and that, therefore, the search "for the 'stuff' that alcoholics and social drinkers are made of" (p. 93) will be fruitless. In fact, he argues that personal control only becomes a meaningful concept when the individual is "at risk," that is, finds himself or herself in a situation when he or she is tempted to drink more than a "safe" amount. But studies of the distribution of alcohol consumption show that only a small proportion of Americans drink as much as two drinks or one ounce of absolute alcohol per day. It is only for those persons that the concept of personal control would be meaningful, according to Beauchamp (1980). He notes that

> the myth of social drinking functions as a powerful and pervasive ideology that legitimates and alibis the new situation for alcohol consumption that emerged with the collapse of Prohibition and the decline of traditional or fundamentalist perspectives. This ideology located the source of society's alcohol problems solely within the skin of the alcoholic, forcing the moral

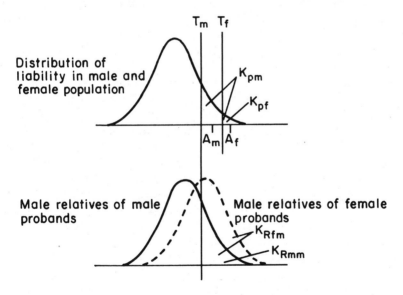

Figure 15. The two-threshold model illustrates the distribution of liability in the male and female population (top) and in male relatives of male and female probands (bottom). T_m: male threshold; T_f: female threshold; K_{pm}, K_{pf}: proportion of affected males and females in the general population; A_m, A_f: mean liability of affected males and females; K_{Rfm}, K_{Rmm}: proportion of affected male relatives of male and female probands. *Note.* "The Transmission of Alcoholism" by T. Reich, G. Winokur, & J. Mullaney, 1975, in R. R. Fieve, D. Rosenthal & H. Brill (Eds.), *Genetic Research in Psychiatry*, Baltimore: The Johns Hopkins University Press. Reprinted by permission.

gaze of society away from the larger issues surrounding alcohol and the conditions of its availability in society. (p. 95)

In his contribution to a 1980 conference on alcoholism and clinical psychiatry, Klerman (1982) took a rather similar position. Without denying the individual differences and the possible genetic factors, he emphasized the public health aspects of alcoholism. He estimated the economic costs of alcohol misuse to be well over $40 billion a year and discussed ways in which general consumption of alcoholic beverages might be reduced.

Kissin and Hanson (1982) sketched an even more complicated model in which a number of feedback loops between various social supports and pressures and the psychological and physiological aspects in the individual drinker's progression from social to heavy drinker to problem drinker and alcoholic are considered.

A recent study of demographic variables related to alcohol use by Overall (1982) provides some support for such a complex view. Two dimensions were found: one of frequency separated abstainers, moderate drinkers, and frequent drinkers, whereas the second dimension separated problem drinkers from the other groups. The variables presented on this second dimension were low social class and family responsibilities.

If one accepts the evidence that some persons are genetically predisposed to alcoholism and are more apt to lose control over their drinking, the question can be asked whether this is due to their psychological makeup or to a biochemical anomaly that produces a different reaction to alcohol. The possibility that alcoholism masks depression, at least in some men, supports in general the psychological explanation, but the differences in flushing mentioned in the early part of this chapter and the alcohol-related research in mice suggest a biochemical factor. Of course, it is very likely that both explanations are correct, and in fact there may be more than two critical factors. This chapter must end with a cautionary note. There has been so little research done on alcoholism in women that it is impossible to determine if alcoholism in females is etiologically similar to alcoholism in males. Both sexes seem, however, to respond to similar forms of treatment.

CHAPTER 10

Hereditary Factors in Antisocial Personality Disorder

The phenotypes to be discussed in this chapter form a rather complicated set of behaviors that display certain common characteristics.
However, a distinction should be made between criminality and antisocial personality disorder (until recently, more frequently referred to
as "psychopathy"). Criminality, in general, is not considered to be a
psychiatric disorder. Antisocial personality disorder, however, is a
well-established psychiatric syndrome, one symptom of which is often
criminal behavior.

An essential dimension in making the diagnosis of antisocial personality disorder is a history of behavior in which the rights of others
are violated. This can be manifested by acts of aggression either against
another's person or property. In addition, many diagnosticians feel that
the symptoms of the disorder must be present by age 15 and that the
antisocial life-style be chronic in nature. In adults, specific symptoms
associated with the disorder include criminality, fighting, vagrancy,
sexual promiscuity, excessive drinking or drug use, failure to accept
the behavioral norms of society, failure to maintain good job performance, and failure to be a responsible parent.

The course of this disorder is often marked by encounters with law
enforcement agencies, lack of career success, and general ostracism
from society. The disorder has been estimated to occur in 3% of American males and less than 1% of American females. Both antisocial
personality and criminality occur with a much higher frequency in

some families than one would expect from the incidence rate in the general population. The disorder is quite common among biological fathers of both males and females who manifest criminal or antisocial behavior. This clustering of cases in single families has influenced a number of etiological theories, some dating back to the 19th century. Many of these theories invoke a hereditary influence. As many more theories point to the execrable environmental conditions in which many criminals and antisocial personality types were reared, as the most likely critical element. To date, most studies of the influence of heredity have focused on criminality, rather than antisocial personality disorder. The following discussion reflects this fact.

Hereditary Factors

The idea that there may be a hereditary predisposition toward crime has never been widely accepted by criminologists, psychiatrists, or other social scientists, even though it has been advocated for many years (Lombroso 1887; Lange 1929; Mednick, Pollock, Volavka, & Gabrielli, 1982).

Lombroso proposed that there exists a born criminal, who is an "atavism," that is, a reversion to an almost prehuman type. He included in his studies pictures of individuals illustrating features that Lombroso believed to be typical of such persons. These included, among other things, more pronounced eyebrows that were continuous across the brow ridge, as well as coarser and heavier facial characteristics. Such ideas have, by and large, been discredited today. However, during the early part of this century this theory was well regarded, and its influence was felt in the practice of social work, psychiatry, and law enforcement.

In one of the first twin studies of criminality, Lange (1929) reported results in which 10 of 13 identical pairs, but only 12 of 17 fraternal pairs were concordant for criminal behavior. He concluded that some individuals are "fated" to become criminals. There is no indication of how the twins were selected. Results of this study along with a number of other twin studies are summarized in Table 46. Observation of these results reveals quite a bit of variability among studies. In some cases, there is a much higher degree of concordance among identical than fraternal twins; in others, there is very little difference in rate of concordance.

An early family study by Sheldon and Eleanor Glueck (1939) investigated 510 young delinquents in the Massachusetts Reformatory and

Table 46. Twin Studies of Criminal Behaviors

	MZ		DZ	
	Pairs (N)	Concordant (N)	Pairs (N)	Concordant (N)
Lange, 1929, Germany	13	10	17	2
LeGras, 1933, Holland	4	4	5	0
Rosanoff, 1934, USA	37	25	28	5
Kranz, 1936, Germany	31	20	43	23
Stumpfl, 1936, Germany	18	12	19	7
Borgstrom, 1939, Finland	4	3	5	2
Slater, 1953, England	2	1	10	3
Yoshimasu, 1961, Japan	28	17	18	2
Tienari, 1963, Finland	5	3	—	—
Christiansen, 1968, Denmark	81	27	137	15
Dalgaard & Kringlen, 1976, Norway	31	8	54	8
Totals	254	130 (51%)	336	67 (20%)

found that the records in 302 cases showed some criminal offense by other members of the family. However, they pointed out that this did not necessarily indicate biological inheritance and that social learning might indeed play a major role. For example, they note that

> familiarity with a certain type of antisocial experience may gradually elimi-
> nate any deterrent influence, even if it does not go so far as to breed con-
> tempt for it. Within families with a tradition of vice and criminality it is a
> difficult task to instill in any member the enduring desire to abide by the
> laws. (pp. 112–113)

The concept of a hereditary factor predisposing toward crime was recently given a temporary boost by the report by Jacobs, Brunton, Melville, Brittain, and McClemont (1965) of a high incidence of males with XYY syndrome among criminals in a maximum security prison. There have since been a number of concurring reports, as well as some negative ones. The incidence of this type of chromosome aberration at birth has been estimated by Kessler (1975) to be slightly over 1 per 1000. However, it is certainly not the case that all these individuals will grow up to be criminals; so it is clear that having two Y chromo-somes is not a sufficient condition for criminality. Such individuals tend to be quite tall and frequently suffer from mild mental retarda-tion. It has been suggested that these factors may contribute to both a lack of psychological adjustment and higher arrest rates by law enforc-ers. Alternatively, a supernormal level of androgens has been hypothesized as the explanatory factor for both the increased height and aggressive behavior of XYY individuals. To date, there is little evidence for this latter theory. One of the better designed studies of XYY syndrome is reported by Witkin *et al.* (1977). Four thousand one hundred and thirty-seven men 184 cm (6 feet) or taller of all 31,436 men born in Copenhagen in 1944 to 1947 were karyotyped. Twelve XYY men were found, and the Danish criminal records searched. No violent crime was recorded for any of these men, but significantly more criminality was noted among this group than for normal (XY) men of the same age, height, intelligence, and social class. The EEGs of these XYY men also revealed slower alpha waves and more theta waves than did the normals (Volavka, Mednick, Sargeant, & Rasmussen, 1977). Summarizing, we can say that most XYY men seem not to be criminals, and most criminals are not XYY. Further, violence does not seem to be associated in any obvious way with the XYY disorder in the Witkin et al. study.

Recently, there has been a revival of the idea of a genetic predisposition toward misbehavior, possibly due to lack of control or excess aggressiveness. Marvin Zuckerman (1979) suggests that the amount of sensation sought by an individual is genetically determined and that this physiological factor determines in part, four, somewhat unrelated behavioral tendencies, which he calls (1) thrill or adventure seeking; (2) experience seeking in nondangerous situations; (3) disinhibition (i.e., not being restrained by social conventions); and (4) susceptibility to boredom. To date, there has been one twin study supporting the idea of a genetic component to this factor (Fulker, Eysenck, & Zuckerman, 1980).

All of the aforementioned traits could be described as forms of impulsivity, a trait that forms a major component of the personality dimension commonly referred to as "extraversion" by Eysenck and others. Eysenck has written a book entitled *Crime and Personality* (1977), in which he states that criminals and juvenile delinquents score high on personality scales designed to measure extraversion, neuroticism, and psychoticism. These first two traits are well-established dimensions of his personality theory. The third is a somewhat more recent addition to the theory.

Extreme extraverts are thought by Eysenck (1977) to condition less well and, therefore, to be less likely to become as quickly or as thoroughly socialized as others. It could be the impulsivity component of Eysenck's measure of extraversion that is responsible for this. Eysenck also reasons that neurotics are highly anxious and the need to alleviate anxiety could drive them toward antisocial behaviors. Finally, high scores on the psychoticism scale are related to callous, uncaring, and insensitive behavior to others. Eysenck believes that these tendencies are inherited and thus, indirectly, are in part responsible for genetic factors in crime. Some support for Eysenck's ideas was provided by a series of studies reported by Rushton and Chrisjohn (1981). They found substantial correlations between self-reported delinquency and extraversion as well as psychoticism. However, no relationship was noted between delinquency and neuroticism.

Twin Studies

Table 46, as noted earlier, summarizes 10 twin studies of criminality. There is a tendency for the percentage of MZ twins that are concordant to be lower in more recent studies. This is especially true of the last two studies noted in the table, which were based on complete registries of twins. Even in those two studies, however, there is still a significant difference between MZ and DZ concordance rates, suggesting an appreciable role for genetic factors in crime. For more details of the studies included in Table 46, see Dalgaard and Kringlen (1976).

An earlier review of twin studies, and an important research document in its own right, was contributed by Christiansen (1968). His sample was based on a complete registry listing of all twin pairs born in Denmark between 1880 and 1910 in which both members of the pair survived until age 15. Of these, 900 pairs were entered into the central or local police register. Data from the study are included in Table 46. Christiansen's concordance rates were considerably lower than those previously reported. When only actual criminal offenses were considered, the MZ and DZ concordances were .53 and .22, respectively.

In 1977, Christiansen broadened his study to include 3,506 twin pairs from the Danish twin registry. The results based upon this larger group are shown in Table 47. The pairwise concordance rates for male and female MZ twins were .35 and .21, respectively; for male and female DZ twins, the rates were .13 and .08.

It is clear that concordance rates were lower in this unselected sample. Christiansen believed that this was due not only to the completeness of his sample but also to changing social conditions. He held that strong social norms require more of a deviant personality in the law breaker, whereas urbanization and industrialization lead to weakening of norms. This explains, he believes, his somewhat paradoxical findings that genetic factors influencing unlawful behavior appear to

Table 47. Data from Danish Twin Study of Criminality by Christiansen
(1977)

	Male-Male Pair		Female-Female Pair	
	MZ	DZ	MZ	DZ
Number of Twin Pairs	325	611	328	593
Pairs in which criminality was found	71	120	14	27
Concordant Pairs	25	15	3	2
Pairwise concordance rates	35%	13%	21%	8%

Note. Adapted from "A Preliminary Study of Criminality among Twins" by A. L. Christiansen, 1977, in S. A. Mednick & K. O. Christiansen (Eds.), *Biosocial Bases of Criminal Behavior*, New York: Gardner Press.

play a stronger role in upper-class than in lower-class persons and in rural rather than urban areas. When he divided his data by chronological periods, he also found greater concordance in MZ twins and, therefore, evidence for a stronger genetic component in the earlier, less industrialized period than in the later.

In a presentation of his data, Christiansen (1968) mentioned that in doing this study it was brought to his attention that one MZ twin occasionally was mistaken by the police for his brother and, whether falsely accused or not, this experience often seemed to produce a negative attitude on the part of the misidentified twin toward the law and its officers. This in turn could lead to actual delinquent or criminal behavior.

Christiansen also mentioned cases where one MZ twin was waiting somewhere for his brother who was committing a crime, and when arrested claimed to have been ignorant of the crime, and in some cases probably was totally innocent. Christiansen noted that such occurrences were less frequent with DZ twins. Other researchers have described how behavior of the police toward misbehaving youngsters can sometimes lead toward more, rather than the intended less, delinquency. In this case, it might prove to have been a factor that on certain occasions influenced MZ concordance rates for criminal behavior.

Christiansen also introduced an interesting technique for calculating the expected rate of occurrence of the crime in a particular population of twins. By comparing the observed concordance to this number, he obtained what he called a "twin coefficient." He believed that this index expressed how much the probability of crime increases for a twin (as compared to the general crime rate for all twins) when the other member of the twin pair is criminal. He attributed this increase not only to genetic factors but also to the twins' shared social background, and he thought that it was affected by aspects of the twin situation especially when twins committed crimes together.

This interesting idea could be applied to other areas of twin research. Use of this technique could possibly provide explanations for differences in frequency rates for behavioral disorders among twin samples.

ADOPTION STUDIES

Additional support for a genetic component to criminality comes from several adoption studies. Crowe (1975) found that when 37 persons born to female offenders and later adopted were compared to 37 controls also adopted but born to noncriminal mothers, there were 7 versus 1 with adult convictions (see Table 48). A later study by Cadoret (1978) provided similar results. In his study of adopted-away offspring of biological parents with antisocial personality, Cadoret utilized data from 246 adoptees ranging in age from 10 to 37 years. Diagnosis of antisocial personality disorder was made on the basis of psychiatric records and/or personal interview. Eighteen adopted children were

Table 48. Arrest Records of 37 Adult Probands Born to Female Criminal Offenders Compared to Age-Matched Controls

	Probands	Controls
Subjects with adult arrest	7	2
Adult conviction	7	1
Multiple arrests	4	0
Multiple convictions	2	0
Felons	3	0
Incarcerations		
Juvenile	3	0
Adult	4	0
Total subjects incarcerated	6	0[a]
N	37	37

Note. Adapted from "An Adoptive Study of Psychopathy: Preliminary Results from Arrest Records and Psychiatric Hospital Records" by R. R. Crowe, 1975, in R. R. Fieve, D. Rosenthal, & H. Brill (Ed.), *Genetic Research in Psychiatry.* Baltimore: The Johns Hopkins University Press.
[a]$p < .05$.

found who had been separated at birth from an antisocial biological parent, placed in a permanent adoptive home, and who had no contact with either biological parent or other members of the biological parents' families. These 18 experimental adoptees were matched by age, sex, age of biological mother at birth of the child, and time spent in a foster home prior to permanent adoption, to control adoptees who had biological parents with no records of behavioral disorders. Cadoret reports that 4 of the 18 experimental adoptees were diagnosed as having antisocial personality disorder. None of the control group was given that diagnosis. This difference was significant $(p < .05)$.

Schulsinger (1972), using the Danish Adoption Registry, found a relationship between biological relatives with symptoms of psychopathy (antisocial behavior) and similar behavior patterns in their adopted-away offspring. Schulsinger's study design was as follows: Fifty-seven index cases of psychopathic adoptees formed the experimental group (40 males, 17 females; average age = 36). These were matched by sex, age of first placement into adoptive home, and social class of adopting family to nonpsychopathic-adoptee controls. The incidence of mental disorders was then established in the adoptive and biological first-degree relatives of the experimental and control groups.

The results of these comparisons revealed no difference in the amount of any form of mental illness (including psychopathy) among adoptive relatives of the experimental $(N = 131)$ and control groups $(N = 133)$.

However, comparisons between the two groups with regard to affected biological relatives resulted in several differences. Overall rates of mental illness were higher among biological relatives of psychopaths (19%, $N = 305$) than among relatives of controls (13%, $N = 285$). Among family members, evidence of psychopathy was noted in 3.9% of the experimental group and in 1.4% of the controls. When the comparisons were restricted to biological fathers of both groups, the results were that 9.3% of fathers of affected adoptees (5/54) and only 1.8% of fathers of control adoptees (1/56) proved to have had symptoms of psychopathy.

Thus, there does seem to be a stronger predisposition for psychopathic traits in biological relatives of psychopathic adoptees. In contrast, there is no evidence that the adoptive families of psychopaths differ in amount of psychopathology in any comparison among family members when compared to the adoptive families of nonpsychopathic, normal adoptees.

Hutchings and Mednick (1977) also used the Danish adoption registry and checked the criminal convictions of 1,145 males adopted in Copenhagen between 1927 and 1941. They were also able to check the

Table 49. *Percentage of Adoptive Sons Convicted of Criminal Offenses Broken Down by Parent Type*

	Noncriminal biological parent	Criminal biological parent
Noncriminal adoptive parent	13.5%	20.0%
	(N = 2492)	(N = 1226)
Criminal adoptive parent	14.7%	24.5%
	(N = 204)	(N = 143)

Note. Adapted from "Genetic Influences in Criminal Behavior" by S. A. Mednick, W. F. Gabrielli, & B. Hutchings, 1983, in K. T. VanDusen & S. A. Mednick (Eds.), *Prospective Studies of Crime and Delinquency*, Hingham, MA: Martinus Nyhoff.

criminal-record status of many of the biological fathers of these adoptees. However, for some of these adoptees, the mother had not named the putative father, or had named several possibilities. In still other cases, no record was available for the father; thus a full accounting was not possible. The noncriminal adoptees were matched to the criminal ones by age and social status of adoptive father. Omitting minor offenses for either father or son, Mednick, Gabrielli, and Hutchings (1983) reported the results shown in Table 49. When neither the biological nor the adoptive father had a criminal record, 13.5% of the sons became criminals. This base rate was only raised to 14.7% when the adoptive father had a criminal record. (Such records were based either on the result of crime committed after the adoption had taken place, or, in some cases, when the adoptive father had not had a criminal conviction for 5 years prior to the adoption). In contrast, when the biological father had a criminal record but the adoptive father did not, 20% of the adopted sons had a criminal record. The parent/offspring similarity was increased further to 24.5% when the adoptive father and biological father both had criminal records, suggesting the strong possibility of an interaction between genetic and environmental influences.

One of the more interesting findings is illustrated in Figure 16, in which the percentage of adopted-away sons who committed either property offenses or violent crimes is plotted as a function of the amount of recidivism in their respective biological fathers. Among the biological fathers having several convictions, the probability that their adopted-away sons would have a history of property offenses increased noticeably. No such trend was noted for sons' history of violent crimes. This finding seems to run counter to some popular notions that, if criminality is influenced by genetic factors, it is probably through the inheritance of an unstable, excitable temperament that would put one

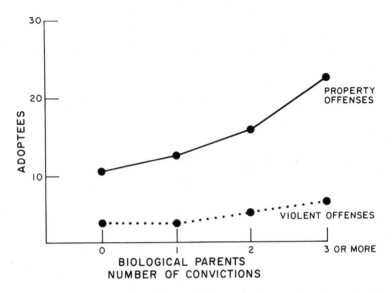

Figure 16. Percentage of male adoptee property offenders and violent offenders by number of convictions in biological father. *Note.* From "Genetic Influences in Criminal Behavior" by S. A. Mednick, W. F. Gabrielli, & B. Hutchings, 1983, in K. T. VanDusen & S. A. Mednick (Eds.), *Prospective Studies of Crime and Delinquency*, Hingham, MA: Martinus Nyhoff. Copyright 1983 by Martinus Nyhoff. Reprinted by permission.

at higher risk for committing violent acts. However, these data are more in keeping with the speculations by Mednick and Eysenck that what may be inherited is simply faulty impulse control, rather than violent tendencies.

Bohman (1978), in direct contrast to the preceding investigation, found little evidence for a predisposition toward criminality when he compared police records of Swedish adoptees born to biological parents with long-standing histories of criminality, and adopted controls whose birthparents had no criminal record. However, in a reanalysis of these data, he and his co-investigators (Bohman, Cloninger, Sigvardsson & von Knorring, 1982; Cloninger, Sigvardsson, Bohman, & von Knorring, 1982) report certain findings that do support a genetic hypothesis. For example, these investigators found that alcoholic and nonalcoholic criminals differed: the alcoholic ones often had committed violent offenses, whereas the nonalcoholic criminals had more frequent records of petty property offenses. This latter group were more likely to have biological parents with histories of petty crimes but no alcoholism. In alcoholics, the risk of crime increased with the severity of alcohol abuse but was not correlated with criminality in their biological parents. Unstable preadoptive placement increased the

Table 50. *Criminality in Male Adoptees by Status of Adoptive and Biological Parents' Predisposition to Crime*

	Low-risk biological status	High-risk biological status
Low-risk adoptive status	2.9% ($N = 666$)	12.1% ($N = 66$)
High-risk adoptive status	6.7% ($N = 120$)	40% ($N = 10$)

Note. Adapted from "Predisposition to Petty Criminality in Swedish Adoptees. II. Cross-Fostering Analysis of Gene–Environment Interaction" by C. R. Cloninger, S. Sigvardsson, M. Bohman, & A. L. von Knorring, 1982, *Archives of General Psychiatry, 39.*

risk for petty crimes, whereas low social status increased the risk for alcohol-related crimes (Bohman *et al.*, 1982). These data permitted an analysis of "cross-fostering" (i.e., adoptive parents and biological parents could each be classified as high and low in criminality, and the incidence of petty criminality in male adoptees in the four cells could be compared). The results are shown in Table 50. It can be seen that not only did a genetic predisposition raise the risk, but the environmental one did also (though only about half as much). Most interesting was the very large increase in risk when both biological and adoptive parents had criminal records. The adoptees were between 23 and 43 years of age when this information was collected. The minimum offense was one that had a jail sentence or fine equivalent to 60-days' income.

This analysis was also performed in the 913 adopted women in the sample (Sigvardsson, Cloninger, Bohman, & von Knorring 1982). In women, but not in men, prolonged institutional care and urban living increased the risk of criminality. However, multiple temporary placements and low social status did not increase the risk for women, as it did for men. Petty crime and alcohol abuse again had different predictors and there was, as in the males, a much higher risk for adoptees when both biological and adoptive parents had criminal records (11.1%—both versus 0.5—neither; 2.9%—criminal biological parents and 2.2%—criminal adoptive parents).

PREDISPOSING INFLUENCES

As a result of his analyses, Mednick has further addressed the question of what constitutes a predisposition toward crime and has gone somewhat beyond the ideas of Eysenck. In addition to impaired social learning, he proposes a theory that implicates abnormal function of the autonomic nervous system as witnessed by a slower recovery after stress. Mednick believes that this causes psychopaths to be deficient in emotional responsiveness and, hence, callous. Further, he feels that, because of autonomic system abnormalities, these individuals are unable to anticipate negative consequences of their behavior and, therefore, more easily succumb to temptation. Finally, he postulates that they fail to learn from punishment. He provides evidence that these attributes do not apply to all criminals but more often to the so-called habitual criminal whose rate of recidivism is higher than average (Mednick & Volavka 1980; Mednick et al., 1982).

On the basis of the available evidence, it does seem that conclusive and precise statements about the heritable nature of criminal tendencies are premature. Nor can we say very much yet about the suspected interplay between such tendencies if they exist and the environmental circumstances that may encourage or suppress them. However, the studies reviewed here suggest that both a genetic component and environmental factors are quite likely important.

It is probably the case that any inconsistency in the evidence for the heritability of criminal behaviors may be in part explained by the fact that quite a bit of difference exists among studies in the way the phenotypes are defined. If this continues, little progress can be expected in research into the heritable aspects of these behaviors. In the future, care should be taken to define even more clearly what constitutes criminal, psychopathic, or antisocial behavior and to diagnose relatives as affected only when the criterion used is in strict accordance with that of the proband.

We have one more reservation about the evidence collected to date. In most adoption studies, the authors report that the adoptive parents were not informed about the status of the biological parents. However, one wonders whether they or others who come in contact with the adopted child might not in some instances have heard rumors about the identity of the child's biological parents or noted a physical similarity between the child and someone known to them. This could easily occur in smaller communities and could bias the treatment of an adopted child. Of course, this criticism would apply to the adoption study technique in general, regardless of which behavioral phenotype was under study.

CHAPTER 11

Huntington's Chorea, Alzheimer's Disease

HUNTINGTON'S CHOREA

Huntington's chorea has long been recognized as a specific, highly heritable disorder and is often used as a textbook example of a disease that is inherited as an autosomal dominant single-gene abnormality. It has been estimated to occur in 54.3 persons per million in the U.S. It is more tragic than senility or other degenerative conditions because of the early onset of symptoms (frequently in the fourth decade of life) and because it often destroys the personality completely. Although symptoms most often begin between 30 and 40 years of age, it has been known to start in adolescence or the early 20s. Initial signs include muscle discoordination that is expressed by choreic movements, facial ticks and, later, personality changes that may lead to temporary misdiagnosis. As the disease progresses, both the mental and motor deterioration become progressively worse. The mental deterioration assumes the form of dementia. Thus, memory is impaired as is the ability to think and reason clearly. These changes are frequently accompanied by symptoms of depression. In the final stage, the patient is in constant, jerky movement, totally unable to take care of bodily functions and may need to be nursed professionally.

   Some authors distinguish a juvenile type, based on very early age of onset of symptoms, but individuals with this type seem to occur in families affected with the adult type of disease, so that they are probably not suffering from a different genetic entity. However, it has been suggested that there may well be an additional sex-linked factor operating in these younger affected cases, because Bird, Caro, and Pilling (1974) found that affected sons of affected fathers died significantly younger. Every child of an affected parent has a 50-50 chance of being affected and, because the symptoms do not begin until middle age, the eventual victim will not know if he or she is affected until the age of establishing a family is usually past, by which time most have had children. The uncertainty of whether the disease has been passed on to the offspring adds to the psychological burden. To facilitate an early decision not to have children, research was directed toward early diagnosis by electromyographic studies. It was hoped that some abnormality of muscle function could be detected before it became apparent in behavior. To date, however, this research has not yielded any reliable method for early detection. Myrianthopoulos (1966) has reviewed many of the earlier studies. Recently, there has been much research activity devoted to the identification of a genetic marker for Huntington's disease. In fact, Gusella et al. (1983) reported that the gene for Huntington's disease is located on the short arm of chromosome 4.

They report the results of a study done in a large Huntington's disease family living along the shores of Lake Maracaibo, Venezuela. This pedigree contained information on more than 3,000 individuals dating back to the early 1800s. It was ascertained that all Huntington's disease patients in this family have inherited the defective gene from a common ancestor, and therefore it was possible to identify the lineage relationship with a high degree of certainty.

Much work, however, remains to be done. The authors indicate that the chromosomal localization of the Huntington's disease gene is only the first step in using recombinant DNA technology to identify the primary genetic defect in this disorder.

However, the linkage information does permit the identification of individuals carrying the gene before they show any symptoms. It requires having enough information about an individual's family to establish the linkage phase, but once that is done, much more accurate estimates of the probability of being a carrier of the gene can be calculated.

This finding for Huntington's disease represents one of the first successful applications of gene mapping techniques to the study of abnormal behavior. Much work is currently underway using this technique to help clarify the genetics of many different behavioral disorders. The next decade should, therefore, be a particularly exciting one for research using these methods.

Alzheimer's Disease (Presenile Dementia)

In 1906, Alois Alzheimer reported the first case of the disease that has since been named after him (McMenemey 1970). In its early phase, it resembles the disorder of old age, senile dementia, except that onset of symptoms occurs at a much earlier age, sometimes as early as age 40. The first sign of the disorder is impairment of memory for recent events. Gradually awareness of time and place become faulty, the patient's thought processes become impaired, while the quality of speech and motor skills also slowly worsen. Finally the patient can no longer care for his or her needs and ultimately will be bedridden, often without any recognition of family or friends or awareness of surroundings. Some patients may develop seizures or spasticity. Because Alzheimer's patients may continue to live for several years, they can become a terrible burden on the family.

Clinically, Alzheimer's disease cannot be distinguished from Pick's disease, which seems to be inherited as an autosomal dominant and which is reportedly much more rare. The differential diagnosis is based on pathological and histological findings: there is more brain atrophy in Pick's disease, whereas in Alzheimer's, there are silver-staining aggregates of abnormal cells called "plaques" throughout the cortex as well as a specific type of degeneration of nerve cells with enlarged neurofibrillary tangles. No sharp distinction can be drawn between Alzheimer's disease and senile dementia, other than the age of onset because the latter type of disorder shows similar signs of brain

Table 51. Alzheimer's and Senile Dementia in Relatives of 326 Hospitalized Patients with Alzheimer's and Senile Dementia

	Incidence (%)	
	Alzheimer's dementia	Senile dementia
Alzheimer's dementia (97 probands)		
Sibs	3.33%	.5%
Offspring	1.6%	.8%
Parents	1.4%	2.8%
Senile dementia (229 probands)		
Sibs	.4%	3.4%
Offspring	2.2%	3.2%
Parents	—	2.2%

Note. Adapted from "The Inheritance of Senile Psychoses" by J. Constantinides, G. Garrone, & J. de Ajuriaguerra, *Encephale, 51.*

Table 52. Common Causes of Symptoms of Dementia

Toxic Substances
  Barbiturate intoxication
  Alcoholism
  Multiple drug administration
  Metabolic disorders
  Potassium loss from self-purgation
  Other electrolyte disturbance
  Hepatic disease
  Porphyria
Nutritional Factors
  Undernutrition (compounded by prolonged neglect and self-isolation)
  Chronic malabsorption syndrome
  Vitamin B_{12} deficiency
  Nicotinic acid encephalopathy
Infectious Agents
  Chronic respiratory infection with cardiac decompensation
  Pulmonary tuberculosis
  Bacterial endocarditis
Endocrine Diseases
  Myxedema
  Pituitary insufficiency
  Addison's disease
Brain Diseases
  Slowly growing cerebral tumor (e.g., frontal meningioma)
  Multiple cerebral emboli
  Normal pressure hydrocephalus

---

degeneration at autopsy. In fact, these two conditions may be genetically related as the results shown in Table 51 suggest.

Although Alzheimer's disease was thought for many years to be an autosomal dominant disorder, it is now more frequently classified as a multifactorial disorder in which the effects of modifying genes and perhaps environmental variables are critical factors in the expression of the symptoms. Family studies are complicated by the variable age of onset and the probability that family members may have died before their symptoms were properly recognized. No estimate of the incidence of Alzheimer's or Pick's disease has been reported.

To further complicate the matter of diagnosing Alzheimer's disease, symptoms similar to those found in Alzheimer's patients might easily be caused by a host of other dementing conditions, some of which are listed in Table 52.

CHAPTER 12

Psychiatric Problems of Childhood

THE DIAGNOSIS AND INVESTIGATION OF PSYCHIATRIC PROBLEMS OF CHILDHOOD

Many physical illnesses are the same in children and adults, whereas other illnesses are limited to one age period, that is, they occur mainly or exclusively in childhood or almost exclusively at a later age. Finally, there are diseases such as diabetes that have both a juvenile and an adult form that differ in certain respects. What is the situation regarding psychiatric problems in childhood?

Over the years, it has become increasingly clear that many behavior or psychiatric disorders of children are not simply juvenile versions of adult psychiatric syndromes but rather are quite distinct entities that can be easily differentiated with regard to symptomatology, treatment, and prognosis. We have already suggested in earlier chapters that childhood problems are often not prognostic of adult disorders. In other words, not all problem children become problem adults, and this provides yet another type of evidence for the unique nature of children's problems.

Examples of some unique categories of childhood syndromes that have been the subject of genetic analyses include stuttering, the hyperactive child syndrome, autism, often referred to as childhood schizophrenia, Tourette's syndrome, and specific learning disabilities. There are, however, other disorders of childhood that seem similar in nature to adult syndromes. For example, nightmares and night terrors, although seen more frequently in children, appear to be quite similar to the corresponding clinical entities that manifest in adults. The symptoms of mild (or neurotic) depression, anorexia nervosa, phobic reactions, and anxiety also seem to be common to both age groups. Finally, there is mounting evidence that the syndromes of conduct disorder in childhood and adult antisocial personality disorder are often age-specific manifestations of the same underlying disorder.

Spitz (1946) and Bowlby (1960) made famous the idea that separation from the mother could produce a depression even in infants and very young children. Lefkowitz and Burton (1978) discussed whether or not a specific disorder exists that can be called childhood depression and conclude that there is no agreement in the literature on this question. On the other hand, the DSM-III has recognized the growing consensus that children can suffer from major depression and suggest using the same criteria for all ages. In the past, because of the difficulty of diagnosing the condition in children, this diagnosis was rarely made. Recently, however, effective semistructured interviews and rating forms have been developed (for example, the K-SADS-P: Schedule for Affective Disorders and Schizophrenia for School Age Children by Puig-Antich & Chambers). These new diagnostics are more precise. They provide clear criteria that have been developed to apply to children.

At an intuitive level, it seems reasonable to link hyperactivity in children with manic behavior in adults; however, as Stewart and Morrison (1973), have reported, there is no evidence that hyperactive children are at higher risk for this form of adult affective disorder. Further, when those researchers studied families of hyperactive children, they found no increased propensity for affective disorder in relatives of the affected children.

One way to establish whether childhood abnormalities are similar in kind to adult abnormalities is, in fact, to see whether they are precursors of the adult disorder. How much continuity is there? There have been a number of studies that have asked this question, usually by looking back toward the childhood of adult patients. These will only be reviewed briefly because we have already touched on this topic in some of the previous chapters.

Mellsop (1972) compared 284 adult psychiatric patients and 332 controls, all of whom had been referred as children to a psychiatric service in Melbourne and found no variables in the records of children that predicted adult status. Waldron (1976) found some continuity of maladjustment in a small study of persons seen as children for school phobia and other neurotic symptoms.

Morris, Escoll, and Wexler (1956) reported that of 66 children who had been inpatients before the age of 15 at the Pennsylvania State Hospital because of aggressive behavior, 12 were diagnosed psychotic as adults, whereas another 12 had criminal records. Eleven others had spent time in mental hospitals, and only 15 were considered well adjusted. Watt, Stolorow, Lubensky, and McClelland (1970) concluded from a study of school records that preschizophrenic boys differed from controls by being disagreeable and unstable, whereas such girls were more likely to be shy and overinhibited. Cass and Thomas (1979), however, found only small correlations between childhood variables and ratings of adult adjustment when following up 200 cases from a university child guidance clinic.

INCIDENCE OF CHILDHOOD DISORDERS

It is difficult to form an opinion on the incidence of childhood abnormalities. Achenbach and Edelbrock (1981) reported on the incidence of various problem behaviors in normal and disturbed children, as reported by their parents. These authors noted that a number of behaviors that were mildly troublesome to parents were reported equally often for children not referred to mental health services as for those who were. However, other behaviors such as severe depression and obvious signs of psychosis did delineate the two groups. We can get an idea of the frequency of serious abnormality from a study by Baldwin, Robertson, and Satin (1971) who reported that in Northeast Scotland, the area around Aberdeen, the incidence of "reported deviant behaviour" in children aged 2 to 16 years was 1.8% for boys and 0.6% for girls. These figures included court cases.

In the following chapters, possible heritable influences on each of the preceding childhood behavioral problems will be discussed. Before doing so, it is necessary to review the DSM-III classification scheme for childhood problem behaviors. The DSM-I devoted very little attention to them. The DSM-II devoted somewhat more, and in the DSM-III a considerably expanded treatment was included. These categories are listed in Table 53. The same five multiaxial approach used in the adult classification system is employed in the children's section of the DSM-III. Axis I is for specifying the major categories of children's psychiatric problems, Axis 2 is for specific developmental problems, and Axis 3 is

Table 53. Major Child and Adolescent Diagnostic Categories of the DSM-III

Axis 1

Mental Retardation
  Mild mental retardation
  Moderate mental retardation
  Severe mental retardation
  Profound mental retardation
Attention Deficit Disorder
  With hyperactivity
  Without hyperactivity
  Residual type
Conduct Disorder
  Undersocialized, aggressive
  Undersocialized, nonaggressive
  Socialized, aggressive
  Socialized, nonaggressive
Anxiety Disorders
  Separation anxiety disorder
  Avoidant disorder
  Overanxious disorder
Other Disorders
  Reactive attachment disorder of infancy
  Schizoid disorder
  Elective mutism
  Oppositional disorder
  Identity disorder

Eating Disorders
  Anorexia nervosa
  Bulimia
  Pica
  Rumination disorder of infancy
  Atypical eating disorder
Stereotyped Movement Disorders
  Transient tic disorder
  Chronic motor tic disorder
  Tourette's disorder
Other Disorders with Physical Manifestations
  Stuttering
  Functional enuresis
  Functional encopresis
  Sleepwalking disorder
  Sleep terror disorder
Pervasive Developmental Disorders
  Infantile autism
  Childhood onset pervasive developmental disorder
  Atypical

Axis II

Developmental reading disorder
Developmental arithmetic disorder
Developmental language disorder
Developmental articulation disorder
Mixed specific developmental disorder
Atypical specific developmental disorder

Axis III

Physical disorders and conditions, whether or not
these have immediate psychiatric implications. It is
obvious, for instance, that diabetes or blindness
would complicate the treatment of most childhood
problems.

(continued)

Table 53. (Cont.)

Axis IV. Severity of Psychosocial Stressors

Code	Term	
1	None	(e.g., no apparent psychosocial stressor)
2	Minimal	(e.g., Vacation)
3	Mild	(e.g., New School Term)
4	Moderate	(e.g., Birth of sibling)
5	Severe	(e.g., Parents divorcing, serious illness)
6	Extreme	(e.g., Death of parent)
7	Catastrophic	(e.g., Serious accident resulting in multiple family deaths)

Axis V. Highest Level of Adaptive Functioning in Past Year

Levels

1 Superior—Very effective in social relations, use of leisure time, and school activities
2 Very Good—Better than average functioning in the above endeavors
3 Good—No more than mild impairment in one of the above
4 Fair—Moderate impairment in one category or some impairment in more than one
5 Poor—Marked impairment in one category or moderate impairment in more than one

Note. Adapted from *Diagnostic and Statistical Manual of Mental Disorders* (3rd ed.) by the American Psychiatric Association, 1980.

for physical illnesses, whether or not these have specific psychiatric implications. (It is, for instance, obvious that diabetes would complicate the treatment of any childhood problem.) Finally, Axis 4 is for noting the severity of psychological stressors, whereas on Axis 5 one rates the highest level of adaptive functioning during the past year.

CHECKLISTS AND PERSONALITY TESTS FOR USE WITH CHILDREN

Just as for adults, there have been several past attempts to develop classification schemes of the various forms of childhood psychopathology by using multivariate analysis. The data used are most frequently behaviors noted in problem children seen in child guidance clinics or from similar data bases gathered from other sources (Collins, Maxwell, & Cameron, 1962; Dreger, 1964; Jenkins, 1966; Kolvin *et al.*, 1975; Peterson, 1961; Quay 1972; Stott, 1974; Rodin, Lucas, & Simson

1963). From this information, a number of checklists and rating scales have recently been derived (see Achenbach & Edelbrock, 1979, and Dreger, 1981, for reviews of this research area). In addition, a general discussion of such methods as well as individual chapters devoted to measures assessing for specific disorders can be found in Mash and Terdal (1981).

To some extent, multivariate analyses of behaviors has led to rather broad diagnostic groupings, which are not likely to be useful for genetic analysis. In fact, most genetic studies of childhood disorders have focused on very narrow entities, such as enuresis or Tourette's syndrome. Regardless of whether they were derived by multivariate techniques or other means, most checklists or scales for use with children are to be filled in by adults. Aside from the fact that some children might be too young to read fairly difficult text, children are often not able to answer many questions about their own behavior. All the problems encountered with adults, such as "faking good" or bad, plus lack of insight or having no basis for comparison are magnified when dealing with children, and in general, the younger the child, the more serious the problem. For this reason, very few personality questionnaires given directly to children are generally accepted. Instead, there are a number of devices for use by parents, guardians, teachers, or mental health professionals. One teacher's checklist, for example, called the Bristol Social Adjustment Guides, was developed by Stott (1974) to assess motivational and other problems associated with learning problems in school.

Hodges, Kline, Stern, Cytryn, and McKnew (1981) and Hodges, McKnew, Cytryn, Stern, and Kline (1982) have published a structured interview guide for use with children, the Child Assessment Schedule (CAS) Diagnostic Interview. They report the interscorer agreements shown in Table 54 based on a sample of 87 children with a mean age of 10 years. The interview is reported to take about one hour.

Another rating form to be used by teachers is the Conners Teacher Rating Scale (1969). It was constructed specifically to evaluate hyperactivity and aggression in schoolchildren. A short form of it is the Iowa Conners Teacher's Rating Scale (Loney & Milich, 1981).

Kovacs and Beck (1977) provide a Child Depression Inventory with 27 items that children between ages 8 and 13 answer while the items are read to them and interpreted to some extent when necessary. This method of administration has not been used very often and should be explored more.

Rimland developed a checklist for autism in 1971 and expanded it

Table 54. Percentage Scoring Agreement between Raters for CAS Variables

Variable	Scoring agreement
All CAS response items	0.91
Content areas	
School	0.94
Friends	0.97
Activities	0.96
Family	0.97
Fears	0.98
Worries	0.93
Self-Image	0.92
Mood	0.90
Somatic concerns	0.94
Expression of anger	0.86
Observational judgments by interviewer	0.90
Symptom complexes	
Attention deficit with hyperactivity	0.89
Attention deficit without hyperactivity	0.89
Undersocialized conduct disorder—aggressive	0.94
Undersocialized conduct disorder—nonaggressive	0.96
Socialized conduct disorder—aggressive	0.97
Socialized conduct disorder—nonaggressive	0.96
Separation anxiety	0.94
Overanxious	0.91
Oppositional	0.94
Depression	0.92

Note. From "The Development of a Child Assessment Interview for Research and Clinical Use" by K. Hodges, J. Kline, L. Stern, L. Cytryn, and D. McKnew, 1981, *Journal of Abnormal Child Psychology, 10.* Copyright 1981 by Plenum Press. Reprinted by permission.

into a chapter for a book edited by Davids (1974). Another questionnaire focusing especially on autistic children is the Children's Handicaps, Behaviours and Skills (HBS) Schedule constructed by Wing and Gould (1978). A third diagnostic system for autism is the Childhood Autism Rating Scale (CARS), developed by Shopler, Reichler, and DeVillis and Daley (1980).

In childhood disorders, one must grapple with the problem that we have very few clear standards for what is normal and what is abnormal in children. Often, children display behaviors some parents find undesirable, even abnormal, that most children engage in at one time or another. Therefore, data from control children are absolutely necessary in the development of any valid assessment of children's psychiatric problems.

Achenbach (1978) published a Child Behavior Profile based on a checklist of behaviors that was in turn used by a group at the University of Minnesota as a basis for the construction of a psychiatric classification system (Solis, Neuchterlein, Garmezy, Devine, & Schaefer, 1981). Achenbach's scheme was designed primarily to diagnose problems seen in children referred to child guidance clinics; therefore, it is less useful for more extreme problems such as autism, which are usually referred to facilities other than guidance clinics.

Achenbach's checklist was used to obtain a data base from a study in which parents of 1,300 children, referred to 1 of 28 mental health facilities, and parents of another 1,300 control children reported on the degree to which their child showed 118 behavior problems and 20 social competence behaviors. The data were analyzed not just for the difference between the two groups but also for socioeconomic status, sex, race, and age. The incidence at each age is reported for four groups: the "clinical" boys and girls and the control boys and girls. We will occasionally refer to these figures in the pages that immediately follow.

Wirt, Seat, and Broen (1977) published the Personality Inventory for Children, and Wirt, Lachar, Klinedinst, and Seat (1977) provided the manual for it. This inventory was designed in a manner analogous to the MMPI: it has scales constructed by using criterion groups as well as "rational" scales based on theoretical ideas. There are 600 items to be answered by an adult informant, usually a parent. The scales are listed in Table 55. Additional information about reliability and validity is provided in Wirt and Lachar (1981). A profile sheet with normed scores is provided which helps in evaluating responses. A sample of "normal" children of about 100 boys and 100 girls at each age level from 5 1/2 to 16 1/2 was obtained from the Minneapolis public schools for a total of 2,390 children. This was supplemented with responses from mothers of children being seen for nonpsychological reasons at the Hennepin County Medical Center in Minneapolis. Automated computer interpretation is also available.

Lachar, Gdowski, and Snyder (1982) have recently factor analyzed the 313 inventory items of the clinical profile scales. A number of solutions were considered. A six factor solution led to four dimensions that were named: Undisciplined/Poor Self-Control, Social Incompetence, Internalization/Somatic Symptoms, and Cognitive Development. These broad categories are somewhat like the ones obtained by Dreger, which we will discuss next. Use of these four dimensions

Table 55. *The Profile Scales of the Personality Inventory*
for Children

Validity and Screening scales	Supplemental scales
Lie	Adolescent maladjustment
F	Aggression
Defensiveness	Asocial behavior
Adjustment	Cerebral dysfunction
Clinical scales	Delinquency prediction
Achievement	Ego strength
Intellectual screening	Excitement
Development	Externalization
Somatic concern	Infrequency
Depression	Introversion-extraversion
Family relations	K
Delinquency	Learning disability prediction
Withdrawal	Reality distortion
Anxiety	Sex role
Psychosis	Social desirability
Hyperactivity	Somatization
Social skills	

Note. From *The Personality Inventory for Children* by R. D. Wirt, P. D. Seat, &
W. E. Broen, Jr., 1977. Copyright 1977 by the Western Psychological Services.
Reprinted by permission.

permitted remarkably accurate separation of six groups of individuals:
(1) delinquent; (2) hyperactive; (3) cerebral dysfunction; (4) somatizing;
(5) retarded; and (6) psychotic. The scales developed to assess these four
dimensions have high reliabilities.

In developing the Children's Behavioral Classification Project
(CBCP), Dreger has been engaged in an ambitious effort to develop a
rational basis for classifying children. Parents of 1,278 children re-
sponded to a list of 274 statements that were descriptive of behaviors
in terms as concrete as possible, limiting the need for inferences. Of
the children, 455 were from child guidance clinics or private mental
health practitioners. In 1981, Dreger reported on factor analyses of the
CBCP inventory at three levels of specificity. The first-order analysis
resulted in 30 factors that were rather narrow, such as disturbed sleep
and dreams, clumsiness, displayed anxiety, and the like. The second-
order analysis reduced these 30 narrow groupings to 9 broader factors,
whereas the third-order analysis led to 4 factors in which the 9 factors
of the previous analysis appeared in various combinations. These 4
factors are compared to three other classifications in Table 56. Some of
the second-order factors that define the four CBCP categories do not
seem to fit in too well however.

Table 56. *Third-Order Factors Derived from the CBCP Compared with Other Classification Systems*

Factor	Achenbach's Child Behavior Profile	DSM-III
I. Acting-out aggressiveness with retardation	Learning problems Conduct disorder	Mental retardation Specific developmental disorders
II. Psychosis versus with-drawing confusion	—	Conduct disorder Pervasive developmental disorders
III. Explosive aggressiveness with muscle problems	Socialized aggressive Immaturity	Socialized aggressive
IV. Anxiety turned inward	Anxiety-withdrawal	Anxiety disorder

Note. Adapted from "First, Second and Third-order Factors from the Children's Behavioral Classification Project Instrument and an Attempt at Rapprochement" by R. M. Dreger, 1981, *Journal of Abnormal Psychology, 49.*

Of course, all of the problems encountered when one attempts to diagnose children are further aggravated when dealing with infants and toddlers. For a longitudinal study at New York University, Thomas, Chess, Birch, Hertzig, and Konn (1963) and Thomas, Chess, and Birch (1968) constructed questionnaires for measuring temperament in babies. They focus on the following nine characteristics: (1) activity; (2) rhythmicity; (3) approach/withdrawal; (4) adaptability; (5) intensity; (6) mood; (7) persistence; (8) distractability; and (9) threshold of excitation. In a past symposium (Rutter, 1982c), various participants discussed the extent to which these childhood characteristics are enduring and predictive of later adjustment as well as the amount of overlap between the terms *temperament* and *personality* and whether temperament is more genetically determined than personality.

Carey has developed questionnaires for use with parents to assess temperament at four age levels: infants, toddlers, 3–7-year-olds, and middle childhood (8–12). These are based on the ideas of the New York longitudinal study of Thomas *et al.* (1963, 1968) and Thomas and Chess (1977).

Hubert, Wacha, Peters-Martin, and Gandour (1982) have reviewed the instruments available for the study of early childhood temperament traits and find none of them psychometrically adequate. They also discuss the conceptual issues, some of which contribute to the deficiencies of the instruments. However, Thomas and Chess (1968) do report some predictability between temperament measures taken in the first two years of life and later problem behavior in school-aged children. Because these temperament traits appear so early in life, it would be interesting to make family comparisons in twin pairs, among siblings, and possibly between parental personality traits and temperament measures in children. However, at the present time, very little research of this sort has been done.

CHAPTER 13

Infantile Autism

One of the most puzzling types of abnormal development, which manifests itself soon after birth, is infantile autism. This condition, first described by Kanner (1943) and to which Rimland (1964), Wing (1966), and Coleman (1976), among others, have devoted entire books, is characterized by the following symptoms: lack of eye contact with other persons, absence of social development, and a noticeable "noncuddling," rigid body position when being held. In addition, there is an obvious failure to develop appropriate language (with deficiencies of communicative speech being the most striking example of this language deficiency) and an insistence on sameness in the environment that is most often exhibited by ritualistic, repetitive, and compulsive behaviors. Age of onset is usually before 30 months of age, and very probably the condition is present at birth (Ornitz & Ritvo, 1976).

Although autistic children are frequently also mentally retarded, this characteristic should not be regarded as essential in making the diagnosis or in describing the syndrome. In some cases, the peculiar behavior of an autistic child, especially the delayed language development, may lead to a low score on an intelligence test. However, retesting—often with a different test—sometimes leads to a higher estimate of intelligence.

Even though mental retardation is not a diagnostic feature of autism, it may be difficult at times to draw a sharp distinction between autism and mental retardation. This makes a precise determination of the incidence of autism a matter of judgment. Rutter and Hersov (1976) estimated the incidence to be very low: around 2 in every 10,000 children. In calculating this figure, they used a restrictive definition of autism similar to the initial view of infantile autism that differentiated it rather sharply from mental retardation. In recent years, the requirement of average intelligence has most often been dropped. In fact, the DSM-III states that about 40% of children with the disorder have an IQ below 50 (see Table 57 for DSM-III criteria).

It is also stated in certain sources that infantile autism is more common in the upper socioeconomic classes. This impression could be due to the fact that children from such families are more likely to be studied extensively, whereas children from lower class families are more likely to be simply seen as mentally retarded and are perhaps sooner sent off to institutions for the retarded. Contrary to this social class hypothesis, in Sweden, the class distribution of 20 autistic children from Goteburg was similar to that of a control sample (Gillberg & Schaumann, 1982). Other data collected recently also fail to uphold the positive correlation between autism and social class. Therefore, the earlier data were probably reflective of a bias toward diagnosing autism less frequently in lower class children.

Material included in DSM-III states that infantile autism "may be associated with known organic conditions, such as maternal rubella or phenylketonuria" (p. 87). This suggests that it is a condition that can have multiple origins, in which case it is unlikely that it forms a single genetic entity.

Several times during the last 20 years, researchers have posed the following question: "Is autism different from dysphasia, or as it is sometimes called, delayed language development?" Bartak, Rutter, and

Table 57. DSM-III Criteria for Autism and Childhood-Onset Pervasive Developmental Disorder

Infantile Autism

A. Onset before 30 months of age
B. Pervasive lack of responsiveness to other people (autism)
C. Gross deficits in language development
D. If speech is present, peculiar speech patterns such as immediate and delayed echolalia, metaphorical language, pronominal reversal
E. Bizarre responses to various aspects of the environment, e.g., resistance to change, peculiar interest in or attachments to animate or inanimate objects
F. Absence of delusions, hallucinations, loosening of assocations, and incoherence as in schizophrenia

Note. From *Diagnostic and Statistical Manual of Mental Disorders* (3rd ed.), pp. 89–90, by the American Psychiatric Association, 1980. Copyright 1980 by the American Psychiatric Association. Reprinted by permission.

Table 58. Presence of Symptoms in Autistic and Dysphasic Boys

	Percentage with symptom		Differences rank-ordered (1 = largest difference)
	Autistic	"Dysphasic"	
Defects of articulation	53	91	7
Pronoun reversal (you-I)	58	17	6
Echolalia	100	26	1
Stereotyped utterances	63	9	2
Inappropriate remarks	32	0	8
Spontaneous regular speech	26	74	4
Regularly gives account of activities in answer to questions	37	78	6
Imaginative play	21	74	3
Use of gesture, other than pointing	11	57	5
N	19	23	

Note. Adapted from "A Comparative Study of Infantile Autism and Specific Developmental Receptive Language Disorder: I. The children" by L. Bartak, M. Rutter, & A. Cox, 1975, British Journal of Psychiatry, 126.

Cox (1975) compared 19 autistic boys with 23 boys with developmental receptive dysphasia, all with an IQ of at least 70. Some of the results are shown in Table 58.

It appears that in contrast to the dysphasics, the autistic children much less frequently used language for communication and much more frequently utilized echolalic, sterotyped, or inappropriate speech high in obsessional or ritualistic behaviors. They also scored lower on three Wechsler subtests: comprehension, similarities, and vocabulary. The authors conclude that a language disability probably is necessary but not sufficient for the development of autism. In a companion paper (Cox, Rutter, Newman, & Bartak, 1975), the authors examined personality characteristics of the parents for the two groups. They found no differences and expressed their belief that it seems unlikely that autism develops as a consequence of the parents' personality. Earlier research, especially by Kanner, often cited parents as being cold and unresponsive and seen as contributing to the child's lack of contact.

Rutter (1967) mentions that even though autism is very rare, 2% of the siblings of autistic children are also affected and emphasizes that this is 50 times the rate in the general population. The low frequency of the disorder suggests the occurrence of the condition in relatives of the proband would be extremely rare, even if it were entirely hereditary in origin. This makes the usual comparison of incidence rates in various relatives of a proband virtually useless as a genetic tool. There is yet another experimental impediment to the study of infantile autism. To wit: the behavior of an autistic individual is such that reproduction is highly unlikely. Follow-up studies of autistic individuals suggest that about 60 to 80% remain institutionalized for life. The remainder, although less affected as adults, still have problems in making social adjustments and holding jobs. On the whole, these individuals rarely marry. Thus, the most feasible genetic study is the classical comparison of MZ and DZ twins. Folstein and Rutter (1977b), using a variety of British sources, found 21 same-sex twin pairs with at least one proband diagnosed as autistic. Among these individuals there were 10 DZ twin pairs, none of which was concordant. This lack of concordance seems to rule out the possibility of an infectious or intrauterine condition as the critical factor in the expression of the disease. Of the 11 MZ pairs studied, 4 were concordant (see Table 59). This suggests a fairly high heritability (using Falconer's formula, $h^2 = .72$).

In four of the seven cases of discordant MZ twins, the authors found five features known to be associated with brain injury: multiple congenital anomalies, neonatal convulsions, perinatal apnea, severe febrile illness, and pathologically narrow umbilical cord. In each of these MZ pairs, the autistic child, but not the co-twin, had experienced one or more of the previously mentioned traumas. However, physiological trauma does not adequately explain the etiology of this disorder. Among the MZ twins concordant for autism, a history of biological insult could usually only be ascertained for one member of each twin pair. Thus, the evidence seems to point to a syndrome that is under strong biological influence, some of which is likely to be of a heritable nature.

Other evidence for a familial influence on the expression of autism has been reported from several sources. Smaller scale twin studies, usually consisting of reports of concordancy in one MZ twin pair or discordancy in a DZ pair, support a familial hypothesis (earlier reports are reviewed in Rimland, 1964; later reports include Eshkevari, 1977; McQuaid, 1975; Stabenau, 1977). Actual family studies have been attempted only infrequently. This small body of literature has been reviewed by Coleman and Rimland (1976). They conclude that there is most likely a small familial/genetic subtype of autism, distinct from the more general type of autism associated with several different kinds of physiological trauma. The authors suggest that the genetic pattern of the heritable subtype is probably autosomal recessive in nature.

That there is heterogeneity within the general syndrome that we

Table 59. A Twin Study of Infantile Autism

	Concordance rate		Significance level of MZ − DZ
	MZ pairs	DZ pairs	Difference[a]
Concordance for autism	36% (4/11)	0% (0/10)	$p = .055$

Note. Adapted from "Infantile Autism: A Genetic Study of 21 Twin Pairs" by S. Folstein & M. Rutter, 1977, Journal of Child Psychology and Psychiatry, 18.
[a]Using Fischers Exact Test.

call infantile autism has become quite well documented in recent years. Within the last 5 years, positive evidence for association between autism and the following conditions has been reported: herpes simplex virus (Peterson & Torrey, 1976); minor physical anomalies (Waldrop & Halverson, 1971; Walker, 1977); perinatal complications (Peterson & Torrey, 1976); parental preconception exposure to chemicals (Walker, 1976); abnormal dermatoglyphic patterns (Walker, 1976); subtle neurological abnormalities as indicated by aberrant EEG patterns and pneumonencephalographic data (Stewart & Gath, 1978) and the Fragile X syndrome (Brown et al., 1982; Meryash, Szymanski, & Gerald, 1982).

A different sort of evidence for the familial nature of a certain proportion of infantile autism comes from research carried out at the Indiana University Medical School. When DeMyer (1979) compared learning, speech, and physical defects among siblings of autistic children and siblings of a control group, it was found that siblings of autistic children tended to have a great incidence of such defects (36% among siblings of autistic children and 21% among siblings of controls). About 69% of the extended families of the autistic probands were reported to have a member with one of the previously mentioned defects, compared to about 30% in the control families. This led to the conclusion that infantile autism is somehow associated with the larger class of neurological handicaps that results in severe learning disorders, and that the learning problems are the causal nexus of all the other symptoms. Their point of view comes directly from 15 years of work studying autistic children and following their development. However, many other researchers in the field do not agree with this cognitive-disability definition of the syndrome. Lowe, Tanaka, Seashore, Young, and Cohen (1980) screened 65 children with autism or atypical childhood psychosis for phenylketonuria and discovered three affected children. Two of these had autistic-like symptoms. One wonders how many other children may have been misdiagnosed as autistic, or to put it another way: how many children have, by virtue of autistic-like symptoms, been diagnosed autistic before other syndromes had been ruled out?

Because of its rare nature, infantile autism will probably remain an etiological puzzle longer than some of the other more frequently observed behavioral disorders. It will remain a focus of interest for many researchers, however, because of its extremely early onset, its notably bizarre symptomatology, and, of course, for its terribly pernicious effects on patient and family. Similarities in behavior has led to speculation that infantile autism may be due to a temporal lobe abnormality similar to the Kluver-Bucy syndrome, or a hippocampal abnormality similar to that noted in cases of Korsakoff's psychosis. Future studies using dynamic computer-generated displays of brain function may permit testing such ideas.

OTHER FORMS OF CHILDHOOD PSYCHOSES?

A number of other types of psychotic disorders have been proposed to occur in children. Many of these were probably just based on erroneous diagnosis or seriously retarded and/or brain-damaged children. Rutter (1968) endorsed a classification proposed by Eisenberg (1972). Eisenberg proposed that psychotic symptoms with an age of onset in early adolescence or just before puberty should probably be classified as schizophrenia. This type of early-onset adult schizophrenia generally continues on into adult life. Many psychotic conditions occurring at earlier ages are often associated with progressive brain disease, as shown by neurological tests. Often, such a child may resemble an autistic one, so that frequently no definitive diagnosis can be made. Eisenberg concludes by stating that classical autism, as described by Kanner, has symptoms that appear shortly after birth and are not associated with brain disease.

Other researchers are more inclined to combine autism and general childhood psychoses into one diagnostic class. This complex category is then sometimes characterized as being the childhood variant of adult schizophrenia. Fish, for example, (1977) described childhood symptoms of persons who later were diagnosed schizophrenic. Bender (1947) also espoused the concept of "childhood" schizophrenia, where childhood refers to elementary-school age or even earlier. She describes these children as ranging from moderately retarded to low normal, with an average IQ around 70, and physically clumsy. The particular symptoms are not especially characteristic of autism,however. Also, no mention is made of the lack of communicative language or of the fear of change to the environment. Finally, Bender notes that a substantial number of these childhood schizophrenics became socially independent as adults. To date, there is much diversity of opinion about whether a childhood version of schizophrenia exists, and if it does, just how much overlap exists between that condition and autism. In the face of this confusing state of affairs, it is probably wise to treat autism as an entity separate from that of any form of schizophrenia.

CHAPTER 14

Specific Reading Disability

A child usually begins formal lessons in reading between the ages of 5 and 7 years. Initially, it is difficult to learn the arbitrary associations of symbol and sound and even more difficult to remember that combinations of alphabetic characters are capable of representing an unlimited number of words. Although most children have mastered the complex mechanics of reading after 2 or 3 years of schooling, and some even earlier, as many as 25% have not (Bryant & McLoughlin, 1972). For some of this population, deficits in the acquisition of reading skills can be attributed to mental retardation, to congenital or traumatic brain damage, to emotional disturbance, to peripheral sensory dysfunction, or to cultural or educational deprivation.

There remains, however, a group of children whose reading problems cannot be associated with specific etiological antecedents. Poor reading is a pervasive handicap that interferes with all other aspects of their education. The disability of these children has been described by several terms including *developmental dyslexia, congenital word blindness,* and *strephosymbolia. Specific reading disability* (SRD) and more simply, *reading disability,* are currently popular terms.

Even though a full understanding is lacking, U.S. Public Law 94-142 gave the following definition of learning disabilities:

> Those who have a disorder in one or more of the basic psychological processes involved in understanding or in using language, spoken or written, which disorder may manifest itself in imperfect ability to listen, think, speak, read, write, spell, or do mathematical calculations. (*Federal Register,* 1977, Section 121a. vol. 5, p. 9)

In spite of the well-known nature of the problem, the diagnosis of true dyslexia is difficult. In common with other disorders thought to be (in part) genetic in origin, dyslexia is frequently diagnosed on the basis of the occurrence of similar problems in relatives. Attempts to develop specific psychological tests for dyslexia have not yet been successful. It is clear that a single test will not do. Recent efforts to develop better diagnostic methods have used batteries including a wide variety of tests. One example is a study by Naidoo (1972) in which the use of a battery of 34 indicators resulted in division of the children into a number of groups. Several of the groups showed evidence of brain damage; one group might have been formed by hereditary cases because dyslexic problems were found in many of the children's relatives; in another group, at least one relative was left-handed, and the children exhibited crossed laterality. Another example is a study by Mattis, French, and Rapin (1975) who described three groups: dyslexics with a family history of dyslexia, brain-damaged dyslexics, and normal readers with brain damage. The search for an adequate genetic model and the refinement of diagnostic criteria continue as new ideas from cognitive psychology are introduced into test batteries.

INCIDENCE

Estimates from several countries of the incidence of reading disability have varied from less than 1% to more than 20% of school-aged children (Critchley, 1970; Goldberg & Schiffman, 1972). In English-speaking countries, estimates typically range between 5 and 10% of children in school (Benton & Pearl, 1978).

In a study by Berger, Yule, and Rutter (1975), the incidence of reading disability was compared in two areas: the Isle of Wight and an inner district ("borough") in London.

Using a normal sample, the regression of reading level on IQ was calculated, and using this regression, an overall incidence of 14.4% was found for the London boys and 5.1% for the London girls. For the Isle of Wight sample, these figures were 5.6 and 2.1%. If poor readers with lower intelligence are included, the figures are substantially higher: 22.2% for boys and 15.6% for girls in London and 10.5 and 6.1% in the Isle of Wight.

The majority of reading-disabled children are male; ratios of 3 or 4 males for each affected female are often reported. The frequency of reading disability and the pervasive effects that a handicap of this sort implies for individuals living in highly literate societies renders this disorder a matter of considerable concern.

Fundamental to all definitions of reading disability is the presence of a pronounced deficit in reading and written language skills in children of normal intelligence. That is, the acquisition of these skills is inconsistent with the child's age, educational exposure, and apparent intellectual potential. However, both the severity of the reading disorder and the constellation of traits associated with it may vary from one individual to another. Visual-spatial disorientation, impaired capacity for intersensory integration, poor motor coordination, verbal processing deficits, impaired temporal sequencing ability, and attentional deficits are often considered to be causally related to the disorder (see Critchley, 1970; Vellutino, 1980). Other investigators have proposed "constitutional" explanations, including delayed or atypical cerebral dominance (Corballis & Beal, 1976; Orton, 1937; Sladen, 1972; Zurif & Carson, 1970); localized dysfunction associated with specific neurological lesions (Drew, 1956); or theories invoking maturational lags in neurological development (Satz, Rardin, & Ross, 1971). Often implicit in the "constitutional" theories is a proposed organic and probable genetic origin for specific reading disability.

Specific reading disability is a particularly suitable phenotype for behavioral genetic analysis for three reasons. First, there is general agreement that the primary symptom of reading disability is reading failure that cannot be explained by an obvious environmental influence. Second, the incidence of the disorder is quite high. Finally, familial incidence of reading disability has been consistently reported over many years and from studies done in several countries.

As early as 1905, it had been reported in the scientific literature that congenital word blindness was often a familial trait. Stephenson (1907) postulated the first specific genetic theory of dyslexia. Based on a three-generation pedigree of a single family in which six cases appeared, he suggested a recessive mode of inheritance. According to Critchley (1970), between 1905 and 1910 several reports of multiple occurrence of dyslexia within a single family group were cited in the scientific literature. Marshall and Ferguson (1939) reported similar findings in a family over three generations.

Numerous reports of reading disability aggregating in family groups have followed the first flurry of observations noted earlier in the century. In the more recent literature, Finucci (1978), Michael-Smith, Morgenstern, and Karp (1969) Drew (1956), and Lenneberg (1967) have illustrated the familial nature of reading disability with pedigrees showing affected relatives in one or more generations. Wolf (1967) described deficiencies in the fathers and brothers of 32 learning-disabled boys, but found the mothers and sisters to be relatively unaffected. In a sample of 65 reading-disabled children at a counseling

clinic, Záhálkóva, Vrzal, and Kloboukova (1972) reported familial incidence in 29 cases and evidence of familial incidence complicated by
encephalopathology in an additional 27 cases.

There have been relatively few twin studies, but observations of
twins strongly support the hypothesis of genetic factors in reading
disability (see Table 60). Hermann and colleagues (Hermann, 1959;
Hermann & Norrie, 1958) reported 100% concordance in 9 identical
twin pairs, 21% concordance in 19 pairs of same-sex fraternal twins,
and 54.5% concordance in 11 pairs of different-sex fraternal twins.
Bakwin (1973b) found a history of reading disability in 14.5% of the
school records of 328 twin pairs. The incidences among the identical
and fraternal twins were equivalent. Identical twin pairs were concordant for the disability (i.e., both individuals affected) in 84% of the
pairs, but only 29% of the same-sex fraternal pairs were concordant for
reading deficiencies. Bakwin's report was the first twin study that did
not yield 100% concordance in identical twins. The finding that 16%
of the identical twin pairs were discordant is not a serious refutation of
possible genetic involvement, however, because Bakwin's diagnoses
were made on the basis of a survey of school records and milder disabilities may not always have been recorded. Also, the lack of complete concordance among some of the identical twin pairs could indicate that environmental factors, as well as heredity, influence the
expression of the disability. Whatever the cause of discordance among
MZ twin pairs, no purely environmental theory can easily account for
the difference noted in rates of concordance between identical and
fraternal twin pairs. It is this consistently higher concordance of identical twin pairs compared to that of fraternal pairs that constitutes for
most researchers in this area the most compelling evidence that there

Table 60. Reading Disability Twin Studies

	Total number of twin pairs	MZ		DZ	
		Concordant	Discordant	Concordant	Discordant
Hermann & Norrie (1958) and Zerbin-Rudin (1967)	51	17	0	12	22
Bakwin (1973)	62	26	5	9	22
Total	113	43	5	21	44

is an important heritable component in the etiology of reading disability.

One of the earliest large-scale family studies of specific reading disability was reported from Scandinavia (Hallgren, 1950). Between 1947 and 1950, Hallgren systematically studied 116 reading-disabled children from Stockholm schools and also collected data on the relatives of these children. His monograph was the first major work to present a statistical approach to the genetics of reading disability.

Among the families of the reading-disabled children, Hallgren found an additional 160 reading-disabled individuals that were first-degree relatives of a proband, and these cases were labeled "secondary cases."

From observations of his primary and secondary cases of reading disability, he concluded that reading disability was not transmitted as either a sex-linked dominant or a sex-linked recessive trait.

Hallgren argued that the absence of consanguinity, the presence of a probable direct line of descent through three generations in 29 families (probable, because reading disability could not be absolutely confirmed in grandparents of probands), and the presence of at least one affected parent in 83% of the cases supported a monogenic autosomal dominant mode of inheritance.

In proposing this mode of transmission, however, Hallgren disregarded the fact that 10% of his family histories contained no secondary cases. He explained that the 7% of families in which neither parent was affected simply indicated "incomplete manifestation of the dominant gene owing to modifying genes or to environmental factors" (Hallgren, p. 197). He then applied a genetic analysis to the families in which only one parent was affected. The Mendelian ratios obtained for males did not differ significantly from expected values for single-gene inheritance. However, the ratios obtained for females did not fit a monogenic hypothesis. Hallgren argued that the poor fit in the case of females might signify *sex-limited* inheritance with the disorder appearing in males far more frequently.

Several criticisms of Hallgren's work have been made (see Foch, DeFries, McClearn, & Singer, 1977, for a discussion). In summary, there are two major flaws in this study. First, Hallgren's description of diagnostic classification and of the families creates the impression that he was reluctant to diagnose reading disability, unless there was evidence of the disorder in at least one other member of the family. This must be considered as a possible source of bias toward a genetic hypothesis. Second, because ascertainment was not done blindly, the detection of reading disability in one family member could have easily biased one toward positive diagnosis of the disorder in other family members. For example, no strict protocol was followed during the interviews of parents, and Hallgren admitted that his questions were sometimes suggestive.

In a later study, Symmes and Rapaport (1972) propose a theory concerning the inheritance of reading disability based on a study of 108 reading-disabled children. Fifty-four of these children were eliminated from analysis because they were considered to be at a high risk for brain damage. They report that of the 54 remaining subjects (1 female, 53 males), all were superior in visuospatial skills, when compared to the performance of normal children. Past studies suggest that spatial ability may be inherited through a sex-linked recessive mechanism (see Stafford, 1961). Symmes and Rapaport postulate that the same gene is responsible for reading disability. Females would need two doses of the recessive allele (one on each X chromosome) to manifest the trait, whereas males—having only one X chromosome—would need only one. They believe this would account for the low frequency of girls in their sample. However, other studies of reading-disabled children have not noted any tendency for affected individuals to possess superior spatial ability.

Sex-influenced models of inheritance have been proposed by several researchers (e.g., Sladen, 1970, 1972; Záhálkóva et al., 1972). Sladen (1970) applied an unusual model to Hallgren's data. Her analysis presumed that the trait is not sex-linked but autosomal and that it shows reduced penetrance in males (e.g. is not always expressed when a single allele for the disorder is present) but is essentially recessive in females; therefore, most female probands would be homozygous for reading disability. If only homozygous females and a large proportion of homozygous males were selected as probands in Hallgren's sample, the gene would have been carried by both parents. Sladen proposed that this would account for the relatively smaller sex ratio in the secondary cases, which Hallgren found. Assuming the incidence of female reading disability to be 2% in the total population (i.e., 4% in females) and assuming a sex ratio of four affected males for each affected female, Sladen estimated that the frequency of the allele was 20%. For an autosomal single-gene model under conditions of random mating and neutral selection, the population proportions for females would be as follows: 64% homozygous, normal phenotype; 32% heterozygous, apparently normal phenotype; and 4% homozygous, reading-disabled phenotype. Males would also be 64% homozygous normal and 4% homozygous reading disabled. Of the 32% of males who are heterozygous, 20% would be normal and 12% would be reading disabled.

Thus, the total number of reading-disabled males would be four times the number of females. The proposed reduced penetrance is purely hypothetical. However, Sladen's model accounts for Hallgren's secondary cases fairly well, and it can explain the presence of a genetically influenced form of reading disability among the offspring of unaffected parents. Lewitter, DeFries, and Elston (1980) have published data suggesting that, in females, reading disability may often take the form of a recessive-gene disorder. But even if this proves to be correct, females make up such a small proportion of all reading-disabled individuals that a continued search for the causes of reading disability in general is necessary.

Several researchers, noting the unequal distribution of reading disability between the sexes and the different degrees of severity manifested within the syndrome, have contended that a single-gene model of inheritance is much too simplistic. These investigators (including Vogel & Kruger, 1967; Bannatyne, 1971; and Finucci, 1978) propose that reading disability is a polygenic trait. Sladen (1970), on the other hand, has criticized the polygenic models by arguing that the "integrity" of the trait within families indicates that transmission follows a single-gene mode.

An alternative to polygenic theories that has the added advantage of also explaining the large variation found in the severity of symptomatology from one reading-disabled individual to another must also be considered.

There is a strong possibility that reading disability may not be a unitary disorder at all.In a similar manner to the various etiologically distinct disorders subsumed under the category of mental retardation, there may well be several distinct types of reading disabilities. It is generally reported that all children diagnosed as reading disabled do not present identical symptoms. Ingram (1970) postulated three subcategories: (1) children with visuospatial difficulties; (2) children with speech-sound difficulties; and (3) children with both types of deficiencies.

Johnson and Myklebust (1967) suggested that there are two distinct types of SRD, namely visual and auditory. Boder (1971) has described what she believes to be three distinct subcategories of reading disability. These subtypes are identified by various types of characteristic spelling errors.

The most recent evidence that reading disability may not be a unitary disorder comes from research done at the Institute for Behavioral Genetics at the University of Colorado. This confirmation was based on evidence from the largest family study of reading disability to date. In this project, 125 reading-disabled children, their parents, and siblings were tested on a battery of reading-related measures. In addition, 125 matched control families were also tested (a total of 1,044 individuals participated in this study). Reading deficits were found in the probands, their siblings, and parents. These deficits were of sufficient magnitude to conclusively demonstrate the familial nature of the disorder (DeFries, Singer, Foch, & Lewitter, 1978). When the Colorado Family Reading Study data were subjected to several types of genetic analyses, the authors found very little evidence for sex linkage or for any type of single-gene mode of inheritance of reading disability in general. By utilizing techniques that permit the investigation of patterns of gene segregation in two-generation families (Elston & Yelverton, 1975), these researchers concluded that their data best support the hypothesis that reading disability is a genetically heterogeneous disorder (Lewitter et al., 1980). Thus, future etiological research should include differential diagnoses that define subtypes of the disorder. These subtypes could then be analyzed separately with regard to mode of transmission in families.

This hypothesis of heterogeneity has recently been reinforced by the result of a study that links a genetic marker on chromosome 15 to a specific manifestation of reading disability. Smith, Kimberling, Pennington and Lubs (1983) reported that among a small group of families in which reading disability is transmitted in a pattern consistent with an autosomal dominant mode of transmission, there is evidence of an association between the marker and the disorder, often over several generations.

CHAPTER 15

Hyperactivity, Conduct Disorder, Attention Deficits, and the Concept of Minimal Brain Dysfunction

Minimal brain dysfunction (MBD) has been described as a syndrome that includes a very broad spectrum of deviant behaviors. It is almost without exception a childhood diagnosis. The typical MBD child is thought to display symptoms of overactivity, impulsivity, clumsiness, and school-learning problems. In addition, aggressiveness, disobedience, and delinquent behavior are often cited as being associated with the syndrome. However, the MBD child is usually defined within the normal range of intelligence, thus eliminating the mentally retarded from this diagnostic category. The concept is losing its popularity because in most cases there is no evidence of any brain damage, which is seemingly invoked because of similarity in behavior of these children to patients with known brain damage.

Although elements from the complex of behaviors just described are frequently noted in many children, most do not display all the symptoms. Therefore, in recent years, many professionals have concluded that MBD is an overly broad category and that classifications using more narrowly defined syndromes can and should be made.

Rutter (1982a) discusses the syndrome of MBD and concludes that this concept has been used in two ways. First, it has been proposed that

MBD lies on a continuum with actual (more severe) brain damage in children, but in some of these children there are no lasting psychological effects unless the physical trauma is quite severe (Rutter, 1981). Because even gross damage does not produce a homogeneous symptom cluster, Rutter suggests that one should not expect the presumed minimal dysfunction to have uniform consequences. The second way in which MBD has been conceptualized is as a much rarer type of dysfunction suggestive of a genetic disorder. Rutter concludes that this possibility exists but that it is supported only by very sparse evidence. He cautions that it may be better not to use the term *minimal brain dysfunction* because it suggests a cause that may not exist. Rather one should use more discretely defined categories such as *hyperactivity, conduct disorder,* or *learning disability.* In the following discussion, we will utilize these more specific terms.

HYPERACTIVE CHILD SYNDROME

The classical hyperactive child syndrome (also referred to as hyperkinesis, impulse disorder, attentional deficit disorder with hyperactivity, or, simply, hyperactivity) is characterized by deviance from the norm in attention span, activity level, and, often in degree of social compliance. This syndrome is one of the most common behavioral disorders diagnosed in children. In the United States, most prevalence estimates range between 4 and 10% of the school-age population. However, there are individual reports as low as 1.4% and as high as 15%. A range of 5 to 20% has been noted in the Netherlands (Prechtl & Stemmer, 1962), and an extremely low rate of 0.1% was reported from a cross-sectional study of the total population of children aged 10 to 11 living on the Isle of Wight (Rutter, Graham, & Yule, 1970). The male-to-female ratios noted in these reports most frequently range from 4:1 to 9:1.

Achenback and Edelbrock (1981) found rather high percentages of children who have engaged in behaviors that are considered indicative of hyperactivity. This was true both for the children referred to mental health centers and for the "normal" children. The figures were high at all ages and substantially higher for boys than for girls. Figure 17 displays some of these results.

There is much diversity in the way individual symptoms are expressed among affected children. This variation has led some researchers to question whether the hyperactive child syndrome is unitary or a collection of diverse disorders. This interindividual variability in symptoms often causes diagnostic confusion. Routh (1980) notes

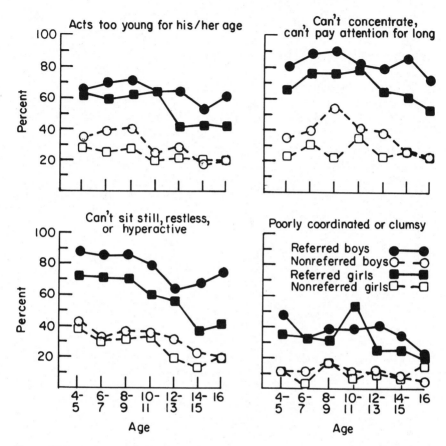

Figure 17. Percentage of children referred for psychological help and control children for whom items of a hyperactivity scale were reported. *Note.* From "Behavioral Problems and Competencies Reported by Parents of Normal and Disturbed Children Aged Four through Sixteen" by T. M. Achenbach & C. S. Edelbrock, 1981, *Monographs of the Society for Research in Child Development, 46.* Copyright 1981 by the Society for Research in Child Development. Reprinted by permission.

that based on a review of the literature, 10 of the most frequently cited symptoms, besides the increased activity level, are perceptual-motor impairments, emotional lability, general coordination deficits, disorders of attention, impulsivity, disorders of memory and thinking, specific learning disabilities, disorders of speech and hearing, and soft neurologic signs that include electroencephalographic irregularities. There are very few hyperactive children who display *all* of these symptoms, however.

In the same report, Routh also mentions that hyperactivity was once defined, in a lighthearted manner as "those aspects of a person's behavior which annoy the observer." Some hyperactive children may be more aggressive than comparison control children, but recent research suggests that many hyperactive children are not hyperaggressive. The prevailing opinion among researchers in the field, reflected in the nomenclature of the latest edition of the DSM-III, is that hyperactivity (or, "attention deficit disorder with hyperactivity" as it is referred to in DSM-III) is distinctly different from the disorder in which cardinal symptoms involve aggressive or destructive acts and that is labeled "conduct disorder" in DSM-III. Many of the symptoms of hyperactivity are, of course, related to the age of the affected individual. Certain symptoms often appear with the first 2 to 3 years of life, and negative sequelae have been noted even into adolescence and adulthood (Ackerman, Dykman, & Petero, 1977; Borland & Hechtman, 1976; Hoy, Weiss, Minde, & Cohen, 1978; Huessy, Cohen, Blair, & Rood, 1978; Stewart & Gath, 1978; Weiss, Hechtman, & Perlman, 1978). Table 61 enumerates the DSM-III criteria for this disorder.

The early symptoms are most likely to include overactivity, reduced need for sleep, and hyperexcitability. It has been suggested that to a certain extent hyperactivity may be nothing more than the mismatch of parental expectations of how a child should behave and how the actual behavior is expressed. Parents who expect their child to play quietly and take 3-hour naps twice a day may perceive an active child who takes one short nap as "hyperactive." This same child might not be considered remarkable at all by parents whose expectations are in keeping with the child's particular habits. This conflict between parental expectations and a child's actual behavior probably results in a certain amount of overdiagnosis of this disorder. However, there is a core group of children whose activity level is so deviant from the norm that there would be little disagreement among parents or professionals in classifying them as abnormal with regard to level and quality of activity. As these children mature over the first 9 years of life, the discrepancy between their behavior and that of normal age-mates usually becomes more marked. Stewart and Gath (1978) noted that the age at which diagnoses are most easily made is around the time a child is in the second to fourth grades in school. Along with the core symptom of overactivity, the school-aged hyperactive child is likely to exhibit several of the following secondary symptoms as well: attention deficits, impulsivity, specific learning disabilities, memory deficits, and perceptual-motor problems, including general clumsiness. The residual symptoms noted most frequently in late adolescence and adulthood include restlessness, frequent treatment for "nervousness," and impulsive behavior. These habits seemingly lead to the increased

Table 61. Diagnostic Criteria For Attention Deficit Disorder with Hyperactivity (DSM-III)

The child displays, for his or her mental and chronological age, signs of developmentally inappropriate inattention, impulsivity, and hyperactivity. The signs must be reported by adults in the child's environment, such as parents and teachers. Because the symptoms are typically variable, they may not be observed directly by the clinician. When the reports of teachers and parents conflict, primary consideration should be given to the teacher reports because of greater familiarity with age-appropriate norms. Symptoms typically worsen in situations that require self-application, as in the classroom. Signs of the disorder may be absent when the child is in a new or a one-to-one situation.

The number of symptoms specified is for children between the ages of 8 and 10, the peak age range for referral. In younger children, more severe forms of the symptoms and a greater number of symptoms are usually present. The opposite is true of older children.

A. *Inattention.* At least three of the following:
   1. Often fails to finish things he or she starts
   2. Often doesn't seem to listen
   3. Easily distracted
   4. Has difficulty concentrating on schoolwork or other tasks requiring sustained attention
   5. Has difficulty sticking to play activity
B. *Impulsivity.* At least three of the following:
   1. Often acts before thinking
   2. Shifts excessively from one activity to another
   3. Has difficultly organizing work (not due to cognitive impairment)
   4. Needs a lot of supervision
   5. Frequently calls out in class
   6. Has difficulty awaiting turn in games or group situations
C. *Hyperactivity.* At least two of the following:
   1. Runs about or climbs on things excessively
   2. Has difficulty sitting still or fidgets excessively
   3. Has difficulty staying seated
   4. Moves about excessively during sleep
   5. Is always "on the go" or acts as if "driven by a motor"
D. Onset before the age of seven
E. Duration of at least six months
F. Not due to schizophrenia, affective disorder, or severe or profound mental retardation

Note. From *Diagnostic and Statistical Manual of Mental Disorders* (3rd ed.), pp. 43–44, by the American Psychiatric Association, 1980. Copyright 1980 by the American Psychiatric Association. Reprinted by permission.

academic, professional, emotional, and social problems that are frequently reported by individuals who were hyperactive as children. (In recent years, several studies of hyperactives as adults have been published. A short review of this work can be found in Weiss *et al.*, 1978.)

Because mothers of hyperactive children often report in retrospect that their children were very difficult even as babies, it has been suggested that this syndrome is constitutional in nature and that early signs are present soon after birth. Ross and Ross (1976) characterize these precursory signs as relating to irregularity in physiological and psychological functioning and to a general activity level much higher than that of normal age-mates. A longitudinal study of the so-called "difficult" infant and later incidence of hyperactive behavior has been reported by Thomas, Chess, and Birch (1968). The authors provide evidence that infants of the temperament type just described are, indeed, at a much higher risk for behavioral and learning problems than are infants of other temperament types. Most researchers in the field explain this phenomenon as a result of interaction of constitutional variables and the strained parent–child relationship that develops as parents attempt to deal with a child having that particular temperament type (Ross & Ross, 1976).

Several investigations have suggested an association between hyperactive behavior and the presence of mild congenital physical abnormalities (minor physical anomalies). These anomalies include high arched palate, epicanthal folds, abnormal positioning or configuration of the ears, wide spacing of the eyes, abnormalities of fingers or toes, and a single palmar crease in each hand. Evidence that signs of this sort are linked to heightened risk for hyperactivity comes from studies by Waldrop, Pedersen, and Bell (1968) and Steg and Rapoport (1975).

Evidence associating the hyperactive child syndrome to some form of brain dysfunction is present in the work of Lucas, Rodin, & Simson (1965), Werry (1972), and Stevens, Sachdev, and Milstein (1968). These studies implicate such factors as abnormal EEG readings, poor general coordination, and mild choreoathetoid movements of the arms.

Although the existence of overt symptoms of brain damage in some hyperactive children has been reported, most cases of hyperactivity exhibit no evidence of this sort. Yet, many professionals in the fields of child psychiatry and psychology continue to classify the hyperactive child syndrome as a form of "minimal brain damage." This convention can most likely be traced to the infamous encephalitis epidemic of 1918 in the United States. A frequent residual effect of encephalitis contracted at this time was a behavior pattern similar to that noted in hyperactive children. After convalescence, many stricken individuals underwent extreme behavioral changes, including heightened irritability, impulsivity, overactivity, and deficits in attention (Ebaugh, 1923). Children thus affected were especially difficult to manage in a schoolroom environment. Soon after these reports on encephalitis-related behavior changes were published, other researchers noted that the same group of behavioral problems occurred quite often in children who had experienced anoxia at birth, as well as in children and adults who had suffered certain types of head injuries. Thus, this group of symptoms became associated with several types of brain damage. This notion was extended by Strauss and Lehtinen (1947) by using the following logic: on occasion, mild injury to the brain could occur and not have been detected. This trauma might still result in the symptoms of impulsivity, overactivity, and deficits in attention noted so frequently as sequels to encephalitis, anoxia, and other identifiable injury to the brain. Thus, Strauss and Lehtinen hypothesized that given this particular set of behavioral signs, brain damage could be inferred. In this way, the syndrome of minimal brain damage (or dysfunction) was introduced. The hyperactive child syndrome was used as a prime example of the new concept of inferred brain damage. Minimal brain damage was, from its inception, a broadly inclusive diagnostic class. Clements (1966), in a review of the literature on the topic, listed 99 characteristic symptoms. By the 1970s, it became apparent that the syndrome was too diffuse and ill-defined to be helpful in either diagnosis or treatment. As noted earlier, this classification, minimal brain dysfunction, is falling out of favor among contemporary clinicians and researchers.

Inheritance of Hyperactivity

Investigations of possible heritable components of the syndrome of hyperactivity had begun in earnest by about 1970. A logical basis for these studies had been established by earlier studies indicating that laboratory mice could be selectively bred for both high and low activity levels (McClearn, 1973) and that there was evidence for a genetic component to normal activity level in humans as established by twin studies (Vandenberg, 1969; Willerman, 1973). Further, when parents of hyperactive children were asked to think in retrospect about their childhood, many recalled that they were considered overly active as children.

Among those studies made of hyperactive children and their relatives, one of the first was a twin study by Lopez (1965). Although evidence was presented suggesting a heritable influence (100% concordance in four pairs of monozygotic twins and 17% in six pairs of dizygotic twins), the study was flawed by several weaknesses in methodology, rendering any conclusion questionable. This, unfortunately, is the only attempt that has been made to study clinically defined hyperactivity among twins.

Several family studies have been reported in the last 15 years, however. Morrison and Stewart (1971) found a trend toward hyperactivity occurring in two generations of family members. In comparing families of hyperactive children and matched control children, they noted that 20% of the hyperactive children had a parent who had been hyperactive as a child, whereas only 5% of the control children had parents reporting childhood hyperactivity. Further, combining first- and second-degree relatives who were hyperactive and making a comparison between affected and control families yielded a significant difference in incidence of hyperactivity ($p < .001$). The authors note that, in addition to a heightened incidence of hyperactivity, family members of hyperactive children had a higher rate of psychiatric disorder in general. Especially notable was the incidence of alcoholism, sociopathy, and hysteria among family members of hyperactive children. A study by Cantwell (1972) corroborated most of the major findings of the Morrison and Stewart study. When comparing families of hyperactive and control children, Cantwell found that among the parents of the hyperactive children 10% had been diagnosed as hyperactive in childhood. In contrast, only 2% of the parents of control children had been similarly diagnosed. A second comparison revealed that 45% of the parents of hyperactive children had been formally diagnosed as having a psychiatric disorder (most frequently alcoholism or sociopathy in fathers and hysteria in the mothers), whereas only 18% of parents of controls had any established histories of psychiatric disorders. A third study by Singer, Stewart, and Pulaski (1981) revealed further evidence that when the families of hyperactive children are compared to families of control children (in this case children referred for reading problems), there is a significantly greater amount of hyperactivity seen among family members of hyperactive children. This latter study once again notes that a significant difference in rates of alcoholism and sociopathy was found between adult family members of hyperactive children and family members of the reading-disabled control children. All of the family studies just reviewed were based on information obtained from intact families. None, therefore, provide data by which to separate overall familial influence into components of heritable and environmental variance. Nor do they permit one to draw inferences about the exact relationship between hyperactivity in childhood and other adult-onset psychiatric disorders.

A method that does yield information about the amount of heritable variance associated with the syndrome of hyperactivity is the adoption method. Only a very few studies of this general type have been made. Morrison and Stewart (1973), using a so-called partial-adoption design, collected data on 35 hyperactive children who had been permanently placed by the age of 2.5 years into adoptive homes. These children had had no contact with their biological parents since birth. Data collected were in the form of interviews with the adoptive parents of these children. A control group was devised of hyperactive children being reared by their own biological parents. Results suggest that the biological parents of hyperactive children reported a significantly higher rate of childhood hyperactivity among first- and second-degree relatives in their families than did the adoptive parents of hyperactive children. Again, the adult behavior disorders of sociopathy, alcoholism, and hysteria were far more prevalent among the biological relatives of hyperactive children studied than among the relatives of the adoptive parents participating in the study. Cantwell (1972), in an almost identically designed study, corroborated these results. Both of these studies emphasize the importance of familial influence. However, in both studies, the fact that the comparison of biological and adoptive similarities were made on two different sets of hyperactive children prevents drawing strong conclusions about the relative importance of shared heredity and shared familial environment in the expression of hyperactivity.

A study comparing the number of times that full-sibling pairs and half-sibling pairs were concordant for the diagnosis of minimal brain dysfunction was reported by Safer (1973). The half-siblings in the study, in each case, had the maternal parent in common and were reared together. Safer noted that there was a significantly higher concordance rate among the full-sibling pairs than among the half-siblings. His data reveal that 10 of 19 full-sibling pairs were diagnosed as having minimal brain dysfunction. This phenomenon occurred in only 2 of the 22 pairs of half-siblings. Although these data again suggest a heritable component to the hyperactive syndrome, a direct estimate of the importance of heritable factors must await further studies of hyperactive twins or studies utilizing a full adoption design.

Another line of research related to inherited factors of hyperactivity has been employed several times. Studies of this type have attempted to describe the specific genetic mechanism associated with the syndrome, given that it has a heritable component. For example, Morrison and Stewart (1974) suggest that the preponderance of males among hyperactive children precludes a simple pattern of autosomal genetic transmission. Simple recessive inheritance seems unlikely in view of all the evidence for frequent occurrence of the disorder from parent to child. Cantwell (1972) and Omenn (1973) make an argument against sex-linked inheritance on the basis of the large number of fathers and sons who seem affected.

One study of chromosomal structure in hyperactive children has been reported to date (Warren, Karduck, Bussaratid, Stewart, & Sly 1971). No evidence for anomalous chromosomal characteristics was noted.

In an ingenious application of Slater's (1966) method of distinguishing between polygenic inheritance and a mode of inheritance involving a major dominant gene with decreased penetrance, Morrison and Stewart (1974) made the following comparison. Secondary cases of hyperactivity were noted among family members of 12 hyperactive children. These cases were then examined to see if, in any given family, most of the cases had occurred in the maternal or paternal relatives. If a unidirectional pattern of transmission (e.g., most cases in either paternal or maternal relatives) was most frequent, this would be evidence for a major gene influence rather than a polygenic influence. If, on the other hand, secondary cases were found in each family with similar frequencies among maternal and paternal relatives, polygenic inheritance seems more likely. Morrison and Stewart reported that, among the 12 families, relatives affected with hyperactivity and other types of adult psychiatric disorders as well were found on both sides of the families. Those results, of course, must be interpreted carefully as this research method does not permit speculation about the strength or even the presence of any inherited factor. On the basis of this study, one can only say that *if* there is a heritable component to hyperactivity, it would be most likely polygenic in nature.

Cunningham, Cadoret, Loftus, and Edwards (1975) reported the results of studies in which 59 adoptees with mentally ill biological parents were compared to 54 adoptees with normal biological parents. The ages of the adoptees ranged from 12 to 24 years. Even though most of them were too young to express adult psychiatric illness, 22 of the group with the mentally ill parents had received psychiatric treatment. Hyperactivity was the diagnosis in 8 of these cases. In at least 5 cases, the nature of the disorder in the adoptee was similar to that in the ill parent. On the other hand, only 8 of the adoptees with normal biological parents had received psychiatric treatment. Of these, one was diagnosed as possibly hyperactive, and the others exhibited a variety of undiagnosed behavioral problems.

Borland and Hechtman (1976) compared children of 20 men who, themselves, had been treated for hyperactivity with the children of their nonhyperactive brothers. Only two of the children of the first group were considered hyperactive, a rather low figure, whereas none of the children in the second group were hyperactive. Invoking an environmental hypothesis, one might speculate that the treatment of the hyperactivity had been rather successful in preventing cultural transmission to the children. However, the sample size in this study was too small to allow any generalization to be drawn from the results. In another similar study, Welner, Welner, Stewart, Palkes, and Wish (1977) found 11 out of 42 brothers of hyperactive boys but only 5 out of 54 brothers of controls diagnosed hyperactive.

Laboratory Tests for Hyperactivity?

At present there is no laboratory test for hyperactivity. However, some children with such a diagnosis have abnormal EEGs. The abnormalities include either epileptiform or slow wave patterns; some also have lower resting levels of autonomic nervous system indexes such as the galvanic skin resistance, heart, and breathing rate. Finally, there is a tendency for children with abnormalities such as these to be more responsive to stimulant drug therapy (Cantwell, 1982). This may mean that there are several types of hyperactive children and that they may eventually be distinguished by laboratory techniques.

CONDUCT DISORDER

A complicating factor in any research on the heritable nature of hyperactivity is its similarity to another childhood disorder—conduct disorder. Conduct disorder is characterized, not so much by overactivity or attention deficit, as by overly aggressive behavior. Some children seem to display traits of both disorders, whereas others display more purely hyperactive behavior or mostly symptoms of conduct disorder.

It was noted earlier, in the chapter on criminality, that there is evidence suggestive of a hereditary factor. Is there similar evidence regarding juvenile delinquency?

Nearly two-thirds of all persons arrested in the United States are between 13 and 30 years of age (Cline 1980). The fact that the incidence of arrests decreases after age 16 guarantees by itself that many juvenile delinquents do no go on to a life of crime. This results in the somewhat paradoxical fact that although most delinquents do not become criminals, many adult offenders were juvenile delinquents (Robins, 1978; West & Farrington, 1977). Glueck and Glueck (1940) followed up 1,000 delinquent boys and found a decrease in arrests as the boys grew up, but for those who had committed more serious crimes, such as theft or violence, the decrease was less marked. These authors ascribed these facts mainly to unfavorable social and home conditions. This is the predominant view of criminologists, and it seems certain that such factors play a major role. However, because very many children grow up under such bad conditions, one can still question why only some of these children become delinquent. The diagnostic term favored today to describe the behavior of difficult children is *conduct disorder*. It occurs more often in males than in females.

Very little research has been done that relates to the differential diagnostic problem that sometimes occurs in children who are both aggressive and highly active. However, Stewart, DeBlois, and Cummins (1980) suggest that, if families of purely hyperactive children are compared to families of a group of children with mixed symptoms (i.e., hyperactivity *and* aggressive behavior), the families of the mixed group have a significantly higher incidence of psychopathology. This finding has been confirmed by other studies (Sandberg, Rutter, & Taylor, 1978; Singer *et al.*, 1981). Of course, all of these studies were conducted using intact families, so the familial resemblance could as easily result from shared environmental factors as from genetic influence. However, they do suggest that hyperactivity should probably be considered as a separate syndrome from conduct disorder.

Another diagnostic problem, although somewhat more semantic than substantive, is related to differentiating between conduct disorder and juvenile delinquency. Most habitual juvenile offenders fit into the category of conduct disorder. DSM-III defines conduct disorder as behavior marked by acts against others, and/or their possessions, and/or society in general. Often these acts are aggressive (inflicting physical harm, stealing, arson) but not always. In some children, conduct disorder is displayed in a nonaggressive manner. Behaviors associated with this form include cheating, lying, sexual misconduct (excluding forcible rape), truancy, curfew violations, and running away. Symptoms should have their onset by age 15 and often appear much earlier.

Perhaps the best study of conduct disorder is a retrospective one published in book form in 1966, by Lee Robins, entitled *Deviant Children Grow Up* (Robins, 1966). Robins details the clinical history and adult life-styles of over 500 children seen at a child guidance clinic in St. Louis. Although this was not a study of heritable influences, Robins notes that the families of children who were diagnosed at the clinic as having what would presently be called a conduct disorder frequently contained parents and siblings who were antisocial, who engaged in criminal activities, who drank excessively, and who had a very high incidence of diagnosed psychiatric problems. Each of these characteristics was found at a significantly higher rate in the families of children with conduct disorders than in a control group reared in the same neighborhood.

In addition, Robins found that among male children with conduct disorders, more than half were later diagnosed as sociopathic (antisocial) adults. This trend is so often noted in longitudinal studies of antisocial personality and conduct disorder that many researchers believe that conduct disorder could be considered the juvenile counterpart of a lifelong personality disorder that in the adult is now referred to as "antisocial personality disorder."

Whether this seemingly early-onset personality disorder is under a genetic influence has yet to be established. However, when viewed from this perspective, the genetic studies of adult criminality and antisocial personality discussed earlier in this book may be relevant to a study of the heredity of conduct disorder as well. One adoption study, in particular, was designed in such a way as to be quite germane to investigations of the heredity of conduct disorder. This longitudinal study is being conducted in Sweden by Bohman and Sigvardsson (1980). They are studying a cohort of 624 children, a portion of which had biological parents with criminal records. The children were either adopted at an early age, placed in foster homes, or ultimately kept by their biological mothers. The children were 15 years of age the last time data were collected. In general, at this age, the adopted children were very unremarkable with regard to developmental problems, although there had been evidence of maladjustment and nervous problems in this group at age 11. At that time, there were several significant differences noted when this group was compared to classmates living with their biological parents. At age 15, however, most dimensions of maladjustment noted were found only in the foster children and in children kept by their biological mothers, whereas the adoptees were, by and large, well adjusted.

There was only one exception to the very normal picture portrayed by the 15-year-old adoptees. That is the fact that an association seems to emerge at age 15 between biological mothers who had criminal records or a history of alcohol abuse, and socialization problems in their adopted-away or fostered children. This association is intriguing for two reasons. The first is that no parent/child association of this type was found at age 11. The second is that the association at age 15 is specifically between children and their biological *mothers*. (As with the age-11 data, no association was found at age 15 between criminality or alcoholism in fathers and any abnormal behavior in their biological offspring.) In these mothers who had records of having engaged in criminal behavior or who had a history of alcohol abuse, there was a trend for their biological adopted-away children to score significantly *lower* than other adoptees in measures of psychomotor activity and contact with peers ($p < .05$). In addition, children of such mothers who were placed in foster homes were significantly more withdrawn, less motivated in school, and had a reduced ability to concentrate than were other foster children. As Bohman and Sigvardsson suggest, these results could indicate a genetic association between mothers and their offspring. Perhaps mothers with antisocial tendencies transmit biological factors to their children that predispose them to behavior that seems poorly socialized. This finding might also reflect the fact that, in general, females who express criminal and alcoholic tendencies are suffering from a much more severe form of pathology than are males who display the same symptoms. Of course, the children were not displaying any obvious signs of serious conduct disorder, and had they done so, one would expect symptoms to be fairly obvious by age 15. Therefore, whatever this relationship might prove to be between biological mothers with criminal tendencies and their offspring, we can conclude that the results of this study do not point to any strongly inherited association between psychopathic or criminal tendencies in parents and conduct disorder in their offspring. The topic of early childhood predictors of delinquency and criminal behaviors is a very interesting one, indeed, and although it does not in any direct way relate to possible genetic factors, it is currently an active area of research (For discussion of such early predictors, see Loeber & Dishion, 1983).

In summary, conduct disorder is a form of behavioral abnormality that clusters with antisocial personality. These two disorders often occur in several members of the same family group. Whether they do so because of direct genetic factors has not yet been established.

CHAPTER 16

Stuttering

Stuttering consists of the interruption in the flow of speech and blocking of the pronunciation of certain sounds, which is frequent enough to cause problems for the speaker. The diagnostic criteria noted in DSM-III (1980) are as follows:

> Frequent repetitions or prolongations of sounds, syllables, or words or frequent, unusual hesitations and pauses that disrupt the rhythmic flow of speech.

Stuttering has an incidence in the general population of well over 1%, with an appreciably higher frequency in males than in females. Although probably aggravated by environmental factors, as will be noted, there are strong indications that there is a genetic component. Johnson (1959) found no relationship between stuttering and any obvious form of birth injury. Nor does it seem to occur more frequently in twins than in the general population (Beach & Fransalla, 1968). Kay (1964) found stuttering in 6.3% of female relatives of 175 male probands and in 18.2% of male relatives of those male probands. The same study revealed that stuttering occurred in 12.9% of female relatives of 38 female probands and in 27.5% of male relatives of those female probands. Among only first-degree relatives of the entire proband set, 20% of the parents and sibs reportedly had problems with stuttering.

Bloodstein (1969) summarized nine studies comparing the frequency of stuttering in the families of diagnosed stutterers and nonstutterer controls. In all studies, there were many fewer stutterers in the families of the nonstutterers. Adding the results from all 2,010 families in these studies, there were other stutterers in 55.6% of the families of stutterers and only 14.3% of the families of the nonstutterers. Bloodstein reports that in this study, the incidence of stuttering seemed somewhat increased in twins as compared to singletons.

Andrews, Harris, Garside, and Kay (1964) reported the following percentages for incidence of stuttering among relatives of male stutterers: mothers 6.3, fathers 17.6, sisters 6.4, and brothers 18.7. And for female stutterers: mothers 8.3, fathers 25.7, sisters 19.4, and brothers 29.9. For all stutterers, the incidence for uncles and aunts was 4.7. These data are from two large British surveys. It is clear that the incidence of stutterers is higher among relatives of female stutterers. Such a pattern is frequently found for traits that are less common in females than males. As noted in Chapter 4, it is usually thought that this particular pattern is due to a sex-influenced differential threshold for expression of the disorder in which the female has to have a stronger genetic predisposition to phenotypically display the trait than does the male. Stuttering is not sex-linked, however, because there are many cases of father–son transmission. The trait has often been said to be "sex-limited." The term *sex-limited* is frequently used in an imprecise manner. It was introduced to distinguish a type of sex-influenced inheritance from sex-linked inheritance. In sex linkage, the trait in question is influenced by a gene on the X chromosome so that sons, who always receive their one X chromosome from the mother, never from the father, could not inherit a sex-linked trait from the father. Sex-limited inheritance, on the other hand, occurs when a trait is not expressed in one sex because other factors related to being male or female prevent its being incorporated into the phenotype. Thus, the type of baldness common in men is rare in women, who are protected by female sex hormones. By the same token, should cancer of the uterus prove to have a hereditary factor, then men could inherit this predisposition (and pass it on to offspring), but they would not express it. When the term *sex-limited* is used more loosely, it often refers to a trait with significantly higher frequency in one sex than in the other. Specifically, it is often used for traits such as reading problems, antisocial behavior, hysteria, stuttering, and the like that are more prevalent in one sex than in the other.

Stuttering, in all probability, cannot be due to a fully penetrant major gene, whether dominant or recessive, because the incidence figures in relatives are too low. If it were due to a single dominant gene, we would usually expect that if one parent were affected, then 50% of the children would also be affected. If the condition is due to a simple recessive gene, we would expect both parents of an affected individual to be carriers or one to be a carrier and one affected. Using an incidence in the population of 4% stutterers, we would then expect 32% to be carriers. Phenotypically, therefore, about 21.3% of the parents of stutterers should be affected.

We obtain this estimate using the Hardy-Weinberg rule that AA + 2Aa + aa are the frequencies of the three genotypes (Falconer, 1965). Using only parents capable of having affected offspring, one can generate the following table, where (AA) denotes an individual who is a stutterer and (Aa) denotes a phenotypically normal individual who carries a single allele for the trait of stuttering.

		Mother's genotype	
		AA (4)	Aa (32)
Father's genotype	AA (4)	16	128
	Aa (32)	128	1024

From this diagram, we can see that out of the total 1,296 (the sum of all four cells) matings, there would be 256 in which an affected parent married a carrier (128 + 128) and 16 in which both parents are affected. Therefore, the total number of affected parents would be 272 out of 1296, which is 21% or roughly one-fifth. By similar reasoning, we would expect that of the siblings of a stutterer, one-third should be affected. Both of these expected figures are considerably higher than the incidences observed in survey studies.

Although simple single-gene hypotheses have been effectively ruled out, data from twin studies suggest a substantial genetic contribution to stuttering (for a survey, see Luchsinger & Arnold, 1965). Many of the studies to date have been done in German-speaking countries. In an American study by Nelson, Hunter, and Walter (1945), of 131 fraternal twin pairs studied only 2 were concordant, whereas of the 69 identical pairs in their sample, 68 were concordant. These figures are almost too good to be true. The near perfect concordance for the identical twins would suggest that environmental influences are virtually nil. This seems implausible, especially in view of the fact that other twin studies do not report such high levels of MZ concordance. In addition, the fraternal concordance is so low that it would be difficult to hypothesize a genetic theory that would fit this observation.

In a past study, Howie (1981) examined 17 pairs of MZ twins (12 male and 5 female) and 13 pairs of DZ twins (9 male and 4 female). In this research, conducted in Australia, she found concordances of .77 and .32 for the MZ and DZ pairs, respectively. Speech samples were analyzed for the presence of six types of symptoms. MZ and DZ intra-

Table 62. Intraclass Correlations for Various
Types of Speech Disruption in MZ and
Same-Sexed DZ Twins

	Intraclass correlation	
Symptom	MZ twins	DZ twins
Blocks	.55	−.02
Prolongations	.25	.02
Syllable repetitions	.38	.09
Word repetitions	.41	.01
Phrase repetitions	.27	−.15
Interjections	.83	.52
All symptoms	.67	−.09

Note. From "Interpair Similarity in Frequency of Disfluen-
cy in Monozygotic and Dizygotic Twin Pairs Containing
Stutterers" by P. M. Howie, 1981, Behavior Genetics, 11.
Copyright 1981 by Plenum Press. Reprinted by permission.

class correlations for each of the six types of speech disruption are
shown in Table 62.

In other reports, Kidd (1977, 1980) has published the results of a
series of genetic studies of stuttering. His data on frequency of stuttering in relatives of probands are in rather good agreement with those
mentioned earlier in the Andrews et al. (1964) study. Kidd's data are
noted in Table 63. Upon reviewing these data, it is obvious that in both
studies, the incidence of stuttering is higher in relatives of female than
male stutterers but lower in general in females than in males.

Kidd also found that no simple Mendelian model fit the data, but a

Table 63. Stuttering among First-Degree
Relatives of Adult Stutterers (Frequency Rates)

	Male probands	Female probands
Fathers	18%	20%
Mothers	5%	12%
Brothers	20%	23%
Sisters	4%	12%
Sons	22%	36%
Daughters	9%	17%

Note. From "Genetic Models of Stuttering" by K. K. Kidd, 1980,
Journal of Fluency Disorders, 5. Copyright 1980 by Elsevier
Scientific Publishers. Reprinted by Permission.

multifactorial or polygenic model with different thresholds for the two sexes gave a good fit to the data. In it, the male lifetime prevalence rate was 4%, and for females it was 2%. When fit to a multifactorial model, 86% of the variance in the data set would seem to be genetic. A model with a single major locus was also tried and gave a good fit as well. In a subsequent analysis of these data, Cox, Kramer, and Kidd (1984) found that the pattern of transmission could not be adequately explained by a major locus hypothesis. They could not, however, reject the polygenic hypothesis.

In summary, data from most research suggests that stuttering may well have a genetic component, although the phenotypic frequencies of the disorder in relatives are not compatible with a single-gene mode of transmission. Probably more likely is a multifactorial-polygenic explanation, especially one that invokes a sex-influenced threshold for expression of the disorder. As with many disorders, it is possible that stuttering is etiologically heterogeneous. Cox, et al. (1984) state that although the most parsimonious explanation for the transmission of stuttering is a multifactorial-polygenic pattern, a proportion of cases could be due to simple genetic mechanisms or environmental factors.

CHAPTER 17

Other Disorders of Childhood

DISORDERS OF EATING

Although described more than a century ago (Gull, 1874), it is only in recent years that the attention of the mental health professions and the general public has become focused on two abnormal eating patterns: anorexia nervosa and bulimia. These disorders are frequently included in literature devoted to childhood problems because both most often originate early in adolescence, although they may persist into adult life. Anorexia nervosa is described in the DSM-III (1980, pp. 67–68) as follows:

> The essential features are intense fear of becoming obese, disturbance of body image, significant weight loss, refusal to maintain normal body weight, and amenorrhea (in females). The disturbance cannot be accounted for by a known physical disorder. (The term "anorexia" is a misnomer, because loss of appetite is usually rare until late in the illness).
>
> Individuals with this disorder say they "feel fat" when they are of normal weight or even emaciated. They are preoccupied with their body size and often gaze at themselves in a mirror. At least 25% of their original body weight is lost, and a minimal normal weight for age and height is not maintained. The weight loss is usually accomplished by a reduction in total food intake, with a disproportionate decrease in high carbohydrate and fat-containing foods, self-induced vomiting, use of laxatives or diuretics, and extensive exercising. The individual usually comes to medical attention when weight loss becomes significant. When it becomes profound, physical signs such as hypothermia, dependent edema, bradycardia, hypotension, lanugo (neonatallike hair), and a variety of metabolic changes occur. Amenorrhea often appears before noticeable weight loss has occurred.

Anorexia nervosa occurs mainly in females between the ages of 12 and 18, with an incidence of perhaps 4 per 1,000. To forestall death by starvation, hospitalization is sometimes required. The disorder is probably more common in Western countries with their concern for fashionable looks and relatively abundant food, although little is known about the incidence in various non-Western countries. Socioeconomic factors have not often been studied, although Crisp believes the disorder to be more common in upper social class families (Crisp, 1970; Crisp, Palmer, & Kalvey, 1976). The absence of reports from Eastern European countries may reflect different conceptions of psychiatry as much as differences in occurrence of the disorder. Table 64 summarizes the DSM-III diagnostic criteria for anorexia nervosa.

An interesting idea was proposed by Young (1975) that related both anorexia nervosa and the Klein-Levin syndrome to a basic endocrine imbalance. The Kleine-Levin syndrome is mainly found in adolescent boys and consists in attacks of sleep or drowsiness that last several days at a time, in which the individual sleeps up to 20 hours a day, often only rising to go to the bathroom or to eat. It is frequently accompanied by eating large amounts of particularly sweet foods. Young suggests that anorexia nervosa and the Kleine-Levin syndrome may be opposite poles of a disturbance of sex hormones due to immaturity of hypothalamic regulation. He supports this hypothesis by experimental work with rats. Although it is an intriguing idea, much more evidence, especially in humans, is required before the theory can be seriously considered.

Bulimia is defined in the DSM-III (1980, pp. 69–70) as follows:

> The essential features are episodic binge eating accompanied by an awareness that the eating pattern is abnormal, fear of not being able to stop

Table 64. DSM-III Diagnostic criteria for Anorexia Nervosa

A. Intense fear of becoming obese, which does not diminish as weight loss progresses
B. Disturbance of body image, e.g., claiming to "feel fat" even when emaciated
C. Weight loss of at least 25% of original body weight or, if under 18 years of age, weight loss from original body weight plus projected weight gain expected from growth charts may be combined to make the 25%
D. Refusal to maintain body weight over a minimal normal weight for age and height
E. No known physical illness that would account for the weight loss

eating voluntarily, and depressed mood and self-deprecating thoughts following the eating binges. The bulimic episodes are not due to Anorexia Nervosa or any known physical disorder. Eating binges may be planned. The food consumed during a binge often has a high caloric content, a sweet taste, and a texture that facilitates rapid eating. The food is usually eaten as inconspicuously as possible, or secretly. The food is usually gobbled down quite rapidly, with little chewing. Once eating has begun, additional food may be sought to continue the binge, and often there is a feeling of loss of control or inability to stop eating. A binge is usually terminated by abdominal pain, sleep, social interruption, or induced vomiting. Vomiting decreases the physical pain of abdominal distention, allowing either continued eating or termination of the binge, and often reduces post-binge anguish. Although eating binges may be pleasurable, disparaging self-criticism and a depressed mood follow. Individuals with bulimia usually exhibit great concern about their weight and make repeated attempts to control it by dieting, vomiting, or the use of cathartics or diuretics. Frequent weight fluctuations due to alternating binges and fasts are common. Often these individuals feel that their life is dominated by conflicts about eating.

Table 65 summarizes the DSM-III diagnostic criteria for bulimia. Just as with anorexia nervosa, bulimia is predominantly seen in females and most often in young women. There does not seem to be the same degree of disturbed body image as in anorexia; thus patients maintain more normal body weight. If it becomes chronic, bulimia can have very serious negative effects on the gastrointestinal system.

Anorexia and bulimia, although distinct, can occur together. Some clinicians believe that it is particularly frequent among ambitious young teenage girls who are high achievers, at least by the standards of their peers. In fact, both disorders may be the exaggerated reaction of vulnerable young females to much more general concerns about control of weight through dieting.

There is evidence from several studies that patients with anorexia nervosa often have depressive symptoms (Cantwell, Sturzenberger, Burroughs, Salkin, & Green, 1977; Crisp, Hsu, Harding, & Hartshorn, 1980; Eckert, Goldberg, Halmi, Casper, & Davis, 1982; Gershon et al., 1982b). Similarly, depression is frequently noted in bulimia (Hudson, Laffer, & Pope, 1982; Pyle, Mitchell, & Eckert, 1981; Nogami & Yabana, 1977; Russell, 1979).

Hudson et al. (1982) studied the first-degree relatives of 14 patients with anorexia nervosa, 55 patients with bulimia, and 20 patients with both disorders and found an incidence of affective disorders similar to that for relatives of patients with bipolar disorder. This suggests that anorexia nervosa and bulimia may be genetically related to affective disorder. The authors also report dexamethasone suppression results in

Table 65. DSM-III Diagnostic Criteria for Bulimia

A.   Recurrent episodes of binge eating (rapid consumption of a large amount of food in a discrete period of time, usually less than 2 hours).
B.   At least three of the following:
   1.   Consumption of high-caloric, easily ingested food during a binge
   2.   Inconspicuous eating during a binge
   3.   Termination of such eating episodes by abdominal pain, sleep, social interruption, or self-induced vomiting
   4.   Repeated attempts to lose weight by severely restrictive diets, self-induced vomiting, or use of cathartics or diuretics
   5.   Frequent weight fluctuations greater than 10 pounds due to alternating binges and fasts
C.   Awareness that the eating pattern is abnormal and fear of not being able to stop eating voluntarily.
D.   Depressed mood and self-deprecating thoughts following eating binges.
E.   The bulimic episodes are not due to anorexia nervosa or any known physical disorder.

Note. From *Diagnostic and Statistical Manual of Mental Disorders* (3rd ed.), p. 71, by the American Psychiatric Association, 1980. Copyright 1980 by the American Psychiatric Association. Reprinted by permission.

anorexics and bulimics similar to those in patients with primary depression. They also report some success in treatment of eating disorders with antidepressants. These findings are very intriguing and strongly suggest the need for further research regarding the possible connection between affective disorders and the eating disorders.

SLEEP-RELATED DISORDERS

Several types of sleep disturbance or sleep-related behaviors have been traditionally included in many psychiatric classification systems. Of those that the DSM-III recognizes, at least two seem to have familial, perhaps, hereditary, factors.

The study of sleep disturbances such as sleepwalking (somnambulism) and night terrors was begun very early in this century. However, with the advent of devices such as the electroencephalograph (EEG) to monitor brain activity, the recent research in this area is quite different in nature from the older studies. One fact that has been established by this modern research is that unlike most dream-related activity, sleepwalking and night terrors occur in nonrapid-eye-movement (NREM) sleep. Further, both of these disturbances are most likely to occur when an individual is producing electroencephalographic activity in which slow, high-amplitude delta waves predominate. This feature is also uncharacteristic of normal dream states.

As most sleepwalking and night terrors begin in childhood, they will be discussed as childhood disorders. It should be noted, however, that they often persist into adulthood. Further, on occasion, these behavioral disorders are expressed for the first time in adults. However, this circumstance is quite rare.

The essential features of sleepwalking include repeated attempts to get out of bed during sleep and walk around (often in the process, the sleepwalker will engage in other activities such as talking, dressing, eating, and urinating). The sleepwalker presents a blank, staring face. The eyes, however, are usually open. There is an obvious unresponsiveness to others and a lack of normal coordination. It is very difficult to waken a sleepwalker during one of these episodes. Also, upon awakening, it is most usual for the affected individual to have amnesia for events that occurred during the episode. Table 66 summarizes the DSM-III criteria for diagnosing the disorder of sleepwalking.

Sleepwalkers usually exhibit symptoms for the first time between the ages of 6 and 12. Sleepwalking most often remits during midadolescence (around age 15) but may be reexpressed in adulthood, especially during times of psychological stress. It is estimated that as many as 15% of all children will have isolated episodes of this nature, and

Table 66. DSM-III Diagnostic Criteria for Sleepwalking Disorder

A.	There are repeated episodes of arising from bed during sleep and walking about for several minutes to a half hour, usually occurring between 30 and 200 minutes after onset of sleep (the interval of sleep that typically contains EEG delta activity, Sleep Stages 3 and 4).
B.	While sleepwalking, the individual has a blank, staring face; is relatively unresponsive to the efforts of others to influence the sleepwalking or to communicate with him or her; and can be wakened only with great difficulty.
C.	Upon awakening (either from the sleeping episode or the next morning), the individual has amnesia for the route traversed and for what happened during the episode.
D.	Within several minutes of awakening from the sleepwalking episode, there is no impairment of mental activity or behavior (although there may initially be a short period of confusion or disorientation).
E.	There is no evidence that the episode occurred during REM sleep or that there is abnormal electrical brain activity during sleep.

Note. From *Diagnostic and Statistical Manual of Mental Disorders* (3rd ed.), p. 84, by the American Psychiatric Association, 1980. Copyright 1980 by the American Psychiatric Association. Reprinted by permission.

sleepwalking is often associated with symptoms of enuresis. The disorder seems equally prevalent in females and males. Among affected children, there seem to be few complications associated with sleepwalking. The exception to this rule, of course, is the obvious physical peril of accidents while sleepwalking. Many children will exhibit a number of episodes of sleepwalking over a period of several years and yet display no other signs of psychological disturbance. However, sleepwalking behavior in adults is more frequently associated with life stress and maladaptive behavior patterns (Kales, et al., 1980a). This is especially true of subjects in whom sleepwalking began after the age of 10 years and for whom there was no family history of sleepwalking. This finding suggests the possibility of there being two variants of the disorder: an early-onset familial type and a later-onset type that occurs sporadically and principally in response to stress.

It has recently been suggested that the early-onset familial type of sleepwalking might be one manifestation of a more complex disorder, sharing the same hereditary predisposition. The second manner in which this proposed complex disorder manifests is in symptoms of severe nightmarelike dreams referred to as "night terrors" (Kales *et al.*, 1980b). Night terrors are episodic, sleep-related experiences that share with sleepwalking the fact that they occur in deep, NREM sleep in which delta wave EEG activity predominates. The sufferers seem to be abruptly awakened from this deep sleep for a period of usually 1 to 10 minutes. This awakening, which is not related to any disturbance in the sleeper's environment, is frequently accompanied by panicky screams, disorientation, confusion, and obvious anxiety. In addition, sympathetic nervous system arousal is usually denoted by such signs as tachycardia, rapid breathing, sweating, piloerection, and dilated pupils. The episodes most frequently terminate within 10 minutes, although until termination, efforts to arouse and comfort the affected individual meet with little success. After awakening, the individual may recount fragmentary dream images of a frightening nature, often involving a creature who by some action interferes with the breathing process of the sufferer. (Thus, the older name for this disorder was "incubus dreams," as an incubus is a legendary creature who kills by sucking the breath out of its victims.) As a rule, by morning, there is total amnesia for an episode that occurred in sleep during the night. Studies in which the vital signs were monitored prior to the onset of a night terror episode reveal that heart rate and breathing rate, by dropping below the normal rate for deep stages of sleep, will often herald the onset of a night terror episode. The DSM-III criteria for night terrors are summarized in Table 67.

Table 67. DSM-III Diagnostic Criteria for Sleep Terror Disorder

---

A. Repeated episodes of abrupt awakening (lasting 1 to 10 minutes) from sleep, usually occurring between 30 and 200 minutes after onset of sleep (the interval of sleep that typically contains EEG delta activity, Sleep Stages 3 and 4) and usually beginning with a panicky scream.
B. Intense anxiety during the episode and at least three of the following signs of autonomic arousal:
    1. Tachycardia
    2. Rapid breathing
    3. Dilated pupils
    4. Sweating
    5. Piloerection
C. Relative unresponsiveness to efforts of others to comfort the individual during the episode and, almost invariably, confusion, disorientation, and perseverative motor movements (e.g., picking at pillow).
D. No evidence that the episode occurred during REM sleep or of abnormal electrical brain activity during sleep.

Note. From *Diagnostic and Statistical Manual of Mental Disorders* (3rd ed.), p. 86, by the American Psychiatric Association, 1980. Copyright 1980 by the American Psychiatric Association. Reprinted by permission.

There is no associated psychopathology with the expression of this disorder when it occurs in childhood. However, in adults who continue to manifest signs of night terrors or who begin to exhibit signs of night terrors for the first time in adulthood, the disorder is often associated with anxiety disorder.

Prevalence rates among children for the disorder are usually reported as being between 1 and 4%. The disorder can be distinguished from the far more prevalent form of simple nightmares that occur in rapid eye movement sleep by the fact that, in common nightmares, the anxiety is usually far milder, and there are fewer signs of sympathetic nervous system arousal. Finally, a simple nightmare usually can be recounted vividly and in great detail. In contrast, the recall of a night terror episode is disjointed, fragmentary, and lacking in any detail.

The familial aspects of both childhood-onset sleepwalking and childhood-onset night terrors have been established by several researchers. Kales *et al.* (1980c) found that 80% of 25 sleepwalking probands and 96% of 27 probands with night terrors had one or more relatives with histories of sleepwalking, night terrors or both, suggesting a genetic predisposition. Possible genetic factors have been reported by Bakwin (1970) who found 9 out of 19 MZ twin pairs but only 1 out of 14 DZ twin pairs concordant for sleepwalking. Abe and Shimakawa (1966b) also report family data consistent with a genetic influence. Hallstrom (1972) reported the occurrence of night terrors among

three individuals in three consecutive generations of a particular family pedigree, and on that basis, posited a possible dominant mode of
inheritance.

A paper by Kales *et al.* (1980b), in which 25 sleepwalking probands
and 25 night terror sufferers and their respective families were studied,
reiterates the familial nature of these disorders. The probands had all
been referred for treatment of their disorders to a specific clinic. Kales
and co-workers found one or both disorders clustering in many of the
families investigated. In all, 80% of the pedigrees of sleepwalking probands revealed at least one affected relative. Ninety-six percent of the
night terror pedigrees were similarly loaded. In many families, both
disorders were noted. The authors report that the overlap within families for these two disorders was calculated by cross-correlational analysis and yielded a value of $r = .89$.

This same data set was subjected to segregation analysis, the results of which provided little evidence for any major gene effect. However, the pedigree findings are in accord with a two-threshold multifactorial model of inheritance. Specifically, the investigators suggest that
sleepwalking is the milder variant of a composite disorder, whereas
night terrors are expressed only in those individuals who are more
seriously affected. Of course, as discussed earlier in Chapter 4, the fit of
a data set to this particular model does not provide sufficient evidence
of a heritable component to a disorder. It does imply that there is a
strong familial factor that, if of genetic origin, will likely be non-
Mendelian in nature. The high frequency of occurrence of both disorders in single pedigrees further suggests that there are etiological similarities between these two sleep disturbances.

Not all sleep disorders have a typical age of onset in childhood. For
example, a fairly common affliction in adults is excessive sleeping (as
defined by the number of hours out of each 24-hour period one spends
sleeping). This characteristic is often referred to as hypersomnia and is
frequently noted among individuals suffering from clinical depression.
Somewhat paradoxically, an inability to sleep (insomnia) is also a frequently reported symptom of depression. Another rare sleep disorder
with age of onset usually in adulthood is narcolepsy. This disorder is
characterized by brief, uncontrollable episodes of sleep in the midst of
daily activity. Many victims of narcolepsy have suffered repeated accidents related to episodes of the disorder that have taken place while
operating machinery or driving. The incidence of narcolepsy is quoted
as 3 per 10,000. It has been established that narcolepsy is unrelated to
epilepsy and is, in fact, most successfully treated with central nervous
system stimulants, whicn, in general, tend to exacerbate seizure ac-

tivity. Both hypersomnia and narcolepsy have been reported to be familial (Kessler, Guilleminault, & Dement, 1974) and have been studied frequently in recent years (Roth, 1978a). Leckman and Gershon (1976) suggests that these two conditions are manifestations of a single, multiple-threshold disorder with a sizable genetic component. Sours (1963) suggested that sleepwalking and nightmares were also more common in individuals who suffer from narcolepsy. A particularly striking symptom in some narcoleptic individuals is called "catalepsy," which consists of a sudden loss of muscle tone leading to an inability to move. It seems to be brought on by laughter, joy, surprise, or amusement. It usually leads to a fall and sometimes resulting physical injury. There is no loss of consciousness, however, and it should not be confused with an epileptic attack.

Functional Enuresis and Functional Encopresis

Another sleep-related problem is bedwetting, or functional enuresis. Actually, this is so common in young children up to about age 6 that it should not be considered abnormal. Most data reveal that the occurrence is markedly lower in children older than age 7, however, and continues to decrease until by 12 years of age it is very uncommon.

A 1971 report (Series 11, Number 108) from the National Center for Health Statistics for the U.S. Department of Health, Education and Welfare reported the following population incidence figures for enuresis: 21% for 6-year-olds and 10.4% for 11-year-old children. The DSM-III criteria for this disorder are noted in Table 68. There may be a period of reoccurrence during the first year of school or as the result of other disturbing factors, such as prolonged absence of a parent, a move to another city, and the like. Rutter, Yule, and Graham (1973) reported very similar percentages from England: 9% in boys and 5 to 7% in girls, aged 9 to 10. These figures in 14-year-olds were 3% and 1.7%, respectively. Peckham (1973) reported that of 12,232 children in an 1958 English birth cohort seen at age 11, 4% were enuretic at ages 7 and 11, 7% at age 7 but not at age 11, and 75% of those enuretic at age 11 had also been enuretic at age 7, whereas one-third of those wetting at age 7 were still doing so at age 11. This suggests that enuresis frequently may be a persistent problem, at least for a substantial number of those affected at age 7.

No single theory about the causes of enuresis is generally accepted; physical as well as emotional ones are being advanced. Similarly, many different methods of treatment are being used.

Table 68. DSM-III Diagnostic Criteria for Functional Enuresis

A. Repeated involuntary voiding of urine by day or at night
B. At least two such events per month for children between the ages of 5 and 6 and at least one event per month for older children
C. Not due to a physical disorder, such as diabetes or a seizure disorder

Note. From *Diagnostic and Statistical Manual of Mental Disorders* (3rd ed.), p. 80, by the American Psychiatric Association, 1980. Copyright 1980 by the American Psychiatric Association. Reprinted by permission.

Table 69. DSM-III Diagnostic Criteria for Functional Encopresis

A. Repeated voluntary or involuntary passage of feces of normal or near-normal consistency into places not appropriate for that purpose in the individual's own sociocultural setting
B. At least one such event a month after the age of 4
C. Not due to a physical disorder, such as aganglionic megacolon

Note. From *Diagnostic and Statistical Manual of Mental Disorders* (3rd ed.), p. 82, by the American Psychiatric Association, 1980. Copyright 1980 by the American Psychiatric Association. Reprinted by permission.

A number of investigations agree on the fact that enuresis runs in families. Shields (1954) found 4/6 MZ but 0/10 DZ twins concordant. Bakwin (1961) found that about 70% of all cases had a similarly affected first-degree relative. Hallgren (1960) and Bakwin (1973) reported significantly higher concordance rates for MZ than for DZ twins. Finally, Kaffman (1962) found that among Kibbutz children who are reared to a considerable extent apart from their parents, the relatives of enuretic children still showed a higher incidence of bedwetting than relatives of dry children, in spite of the lack of common sleeping quarters. In contrast to enuresis, there is no evidence of familial occurrence for the much rarer abnormality of encopresis (repeated voluntary or involuntary passage of feces into inappropriate places). Table 69 contains the DSM-III criteria for diagnosing encopresis.

OTHER DISORDERS OF CHILDHOOD

Multiple Tics and Gilles de la Tourette Syndrome

Multiple tics is a disorder of childhood in which the cardinal symptoms are abnormal and inappropriate muscle movements. The word *tique* comes from the French and was used originally in veterinary medicine to describe stereotypic movements made by horses when physically restrained (Corbett, 1971). Tics have been described as quick, frequently repeated movements of circumscribed groups of muscles, serving no apparent purpose. However, tics are different in several ways from the stereotypic movements associated with other neurological and psychiatric disorders, including autism. These latter movements include such behaviors as hair pulling, twirling, grimacing, finger flicking or repetition of a specific sound and are all more complex (often involving the coordination of two or more muscle systems) and lack the convulsive quality that is characteristic of tic behaviors.

The age of onset of multiple tics is most often during the childhood years, with symptoms almost always being expressed for the first time between 2 and 16 years of age. Far more males than females are affected. The DSM-III criteria for the syndrome of multiple tics are noted in Table 70.

In general, it is thought that there are a number of different etiological factors associated with the expression of multiple tics. A proportion can be explained on the basis of association with overt signs of brain damage. In some children, the symptoms seem to be an expression of an underlying neurotic condition, as they are associated with high levels of anxiety. One theory explains multiple tics as being a conditioned behavior that originally was a direct reaction to stress.

Until very recently, little or no research had been done on the genetic aspects of multiple tics, with the exception of studies by Zausmer (1954) and Torup (1962). Both of these authors reported a high incidence of brain damage in relatives of ticquers and thus a possible familial relationship between the two disorders.

In a more recent study, Abe and Oda (1980) found an incidence rate for tic behavior of 20% in children of parents who had themselves had tics, whereas the incidence was 10% in a control group of children.

Table 70. DSM-III Diagnostic Criteria for Chronic Motor Tic Disorder

A. Presence of recurrent, involuntary, repetitive, rapid, purposeless movements (tics) involving no more than three muscle groups at any one time
B. Unvarying intensity of the tics over weeks or months
C. Ability to suppress the movements voluntarily for minutes to hours
D. Duration of at least 1 year

Note. From *Diagnostic and Statistical Manual of Mental Disorders* (3rd ed.), p. 75, by the American Psychiatric Association, 1980. Copyright 1980 by the American Psyciatric Association. Reprinted by permission.

Gilles de la Tourette syndrome is a rare chronic tic-related syndrome with onset in childhood. The age range for expression of first symptoms is the same as that for multiple tics (i.e., 2–16 years of age). The cardinal symptoms of Tourette syndrome are multiple motor tics of the kind described previously, plus so-called "vocal" tics. Especially notable in this disorder are facial-motor tics that frequently include tongue thrusting, jaw snapping, and blinking. Vocal tics are defined as including stuttering and nonverbal utterances such as clicks, yelps, barks, sniffs, coughs, groans, and grunts. In addition, the associated symptom of coprolalia (the inappropriate utterance of obscenities) is often reported. DSM-III criteria for Gilles de la Tourette syndrome are listed in Table 71.

The first description of this disorder was made by Gilles de la Tourette in 1885 in a French journal. From that time to the present, the disorder has always seemed to affect more males than females. (The sex ratio has been reported as being about four affected males to every affected female). The disorder has been considered to be exceptionally rare. Prevalence information drawn from a 1976 edition of an international registry devoted to Tourette syndrome (Abuzzhab & Anderson, 1974), suggested that only 485 cases existed, worldwide, at that time. More recent studies have estimated higher prevalence rates, approaching 1/2,000 in males and 1/5,000 in females.

Several studies have also been published suggesting that Tourette syndrome, although quite rare in the general population, does cluster in families. A review of this literature, based mostly on collections of case histories of individual probands or on samples drawn from clinic populations, can be found in Wilson, Garron, and Klawans (1978). Increasingly, investigators of Tourette syndrome are suggesting that this disorder is likely to be a more serious manifestation of the disorder of

Table 71. DSM-III Diagnostic Criteria for Tourette's Disorder

A.   Age at onset between 2 and 15 years
B.   Presence of recurrent, involuntary, repetitive, rapid, purposeless motor movements affecting multiple muscle groups
C.   Multiple vocal tics
D.   Ability to suppress movements voluntarily for minutes to hours
E.   Variations in the intensity of the symptoms over weeks or months
F.   Duration of more than 1 year

Note. From *Diagnostic and Statistical Manual of Mental Disorders* (3rd ed.), p. 77, by the American Psychiatric Association, 1980. Copyright 1980 by the American Psychiatric Association. Reprinted by permission.

multiple tics. For example, Wilson *et al.* (1978) note that in their re-view of studies, 30% of individuals affected with Tourette syndrome had a positive extended family history of either multiple tics or Tour-ette syndrome, whereas the frequency of tics in the general population is approximately 10%. However, as the authors point out, the studies of the family history consider extended families and several relatives si-multaneously, so that it would not be unreasonable to find that 30% of family aggregates in the general population might by chance have a positive family history for a disorder with a prevalence rate of 10%.

Kidd, Prusoff, and Cohen (1980) collected data by questionnaire on the incidence of Tourette syndrome and multiple tics in 231 relatives of 66 Tourette syndrome probands. For male probands, they found the following percentages: fathers 23%, mothers 13%, brothers 16%, sis-ters 9%, and for female probands: fathers 33%, mothers 11%, brothers 46%, sisters 19%. Although these researchers noted the same lower overall incidence in females found by others, the condition is clearly not X-linked because of the high proportion of cases involving father-to-son transmission. The strikingly higher incidence of affected male relatives of female probands argues for a differential threshold for females, so that those affected have more genes, or a greater "genetic loading," for the disease. By implication, therefore, their relatives have a greater probability of also being affected.

In a later study, Pauls, Cohen, Heimbuch, Detlor, and Kidd (1981) examined the hypothesis that multiple tics represent a milder form of Tourette syndrome in the families of Tourette cases. They found that the patterns in these families were consistent with that hypothesis but pointed out that their results did not suggest that all tics were etiologi-cally related to Tourette syndrome.

All of these studies were done using a family history method in which not all relatives were interviewed. Thus, the risk rates noted among the relatives would be expected to be underestimates of the true rates. Recently, Pauls, Kruger, Leckman, Cohen, & Kidd (1984) re-ported preliminary results from a study where almost all relatives of the probands had been directly interviewed. They found that 10.7% of first-degree relatives had Tourette syndrome and an additional 18.5% of first-degree relatives had chronic multiple tics. In addition, in the majority of families, at least one of the parents was affected with either tics or Tourette syndrome. This pattern is consistent with an auto-somal dominant mode of transmission.

The fact that symptoms of Tourette syndrome are frequently al-leviated by anticonvulsants or antipsychotic medication (specifically the drug Haloperidol) provides additional clues for an underlying bio-chemical/genetic abnormality. Much research is currently underway in an attempt to understand this disorder.

In addition to multiple tics, there may be other associated behaviors. Shapiro and Shapiro (1982) have written an historical account of the condition as well as a summary of research in the field. Although the patients show the normal range of intelligence, they often do more poorly on the performance subtests of the Wechsler tests of intelligence than on the verbal tests. These authors report that perhaps as many as half of all Tourette patients may show "soft" signs of organicity. They also note that abnormal EEGs are often associated with the disorder. Shapiro, Shapiro, Brunn, and Sweet (1978) noted that Tourettelike symptoms are occasionally associated with overt neurological disorders.

The rare nature of Tourette syndrome makes it difficult to establish good cross-cultural incidence figures. However, it has been reported in Japan (Nomura & Segawa, 1979) and among the Hong Kong Chinese. In general, for these populations, fewer females are affected, but those tend to show a stronger family history. Thus, these sex difference trends seem to be constant across ethnic groups.

Shapiro et al. (1978) describe the complex interaction of genetic and environmental factors in Tourette children, and from that perspective, the condition can be viewed as a prototype of many childhood disorders. For example, the constant psychological tension the patients live under and the relief medication gives are only two concrete examples of how one's environment can and does influence a disorder that is probably determined principally by biogenic factors.

Tourette syndrome is a good example of what is commonly referred to as an "orphan" disorder. This term is used these days to describe a disease entity that is so rare that very few resources are allocated for research into its cause and treatment. Like Tourette syndrome, however, many "orphan" disorders are very debilitating and result in untold hours of human suffering. Because it is so rare, it is probable that research progress in understanding Tourette syndrome will be made rather slowly.

CEREBRAL PALSY

This congenital motor defect can be distinguished from progressive neuromuscular dystrophies and lesions of the spinal cord. Reported incidences vary from 1 to 5 per 1000.

Although cerebral palsy is generally thought to be a result of ante- or perinatal problems, especially anoxia, there frequently is no indication of a difficult birth, and Sarason (1949) as well as Cruickshank and Raus (1955) have suggested that a genetic component often plays a role. They generated this hypothesis from the findings that often when there is more than one affected child in a family the children tend to have the same subtype: athetosis, spasticity, ataxia: diplegia, hemiplegia, and the like. Although it is often assumed, there is no necessity to view birth trauma and genetic factors as mutually exclusive. It is possible that the mother is genetically predisposed to have difficult deliveries. The problem of cerebral palsy is complicated by the fact that perhaps as many as 50% of those affected are seriously retarded with IQs below 70. However, many cerebral-palsied individuals suffer no mental impairment whatsoever. In these individuals, the attendant psychological ramifications of having to cope with physical handicaps are the only behavioral sequelae associated with the disorder.

References

Abe, K., & Oda, N. (1980). Incidence of tics in the offspring of childhood tiquers: A controlled follow-up study. *Developmental Medicine and Child Neurology, 22,* 649–653.

Abe, K., & Shimikawa, M. (1966). Genetic and developmental aspects of sleeptalking and teeth-grinding. *Acta Paedopsychiatrica* (Basel), *33.* (a)

Abe, K., & Shimakawa, M. (1966). Predisposition to sleepwalking. *Psychiatrie, Neurologie und Medizinische Psychologie* (Basel), *152,* 306–312. (b)

Abuzzhad, F., & Anderson, F. (1974). Gilles de la Tourette's syndrome. *Clinical Neurology and Neurosurgery, 1,* 66–74.

Achenbach, T. M. (1966). The classification of children's psychiatric symptoms: A factor-analytic study. *Psychological Monographs, 80* (7, Whole No. 615).

Achenbach, T. M. (1978). The Child Behavior Profile: An empirically based system for assessing children's behavioral problems and competencies. *International Journal of Mental Health, 7,* 24–42. (a)

Achenbach, T. M. (1978). The Child Behavior Profile: 1. Boys aged 6 through 11. *Journal of Consulting and Clinical Psychology, 46,* 759–776. (b)

Achenbach, T. M., & Edelbrock, C. S. (1978). The classification of child psychopathology: A review and analysis of empirical efforts. *Psychological Bulletin, 85,* 1275–1301.

Achenbach, T. M., & Edelbrock, C. S. (1979). The Child Behavior Profile: II. Boys aged 12–16 and girls aged 6–11 and 12–16. *Journal of Consulting and Clinical Psychology, 47,* 223–233.

Achenbach, T. M., & Edelbrock, C. S. (1981). Behavioral problems and competencies reported by parents of normal and disturbed children aged four through sixteen. *Monographs of the Society for Research in Child Development, 46* (Serial number 188).

Ackerman, P., Dykman, T., & Petero, J. (1977). Teenage status of hyperactive and nonhyperactive learning disabled boys. *American Journal of Orthopsychiatry, 47,* 577–96.

Agras, W. S., Sylvester, D. & Oliveau, D. (1969). The epidemiology of common fears and phobias. *Comprehensive Psychiatry, 10,* 151–56.

Ahern, F. M., & Johnson, R. C. (1973). Inherited uterine inadequacy: An alternate explanation for a portion of cases of defect. *Behavior Genetics, 3,* 1–12.

Akiskal, H. S. (1983). Dysthymic disorder: Psychopathology of proposed chronic depressive subtypes. *American Journal of Psychiatry, 140,* 11–20.

Akiskal, H. S., Hirschfeld, R. M. A., & Yerevanian, B. I. (1983). The relationship of personality to affective disorders. *Archives of General Psychiatry, 40,* 801–810.

Alexander, F. G., & Selesnick, S. T. (1966). *The history of psychiatry.* New York: Harper & Row.

Allan, W., Herndon, C. N., & Dudley, F. C. (1944). Some examples of the inheritance of mental deficiency: Apparently sex-linked idiocy and microcephaly. *American Journal of Mental Deficiency, 48,* 325–334.

Allen, G. (1976). Scope and methodology of twin studies. *Acta Genetic Medicae et Gemellologiae* (Rome), *25,* 79.

Allen, G., Harvald, B., & Shields, J. (1967). Measures of twin concordance. *Acta Genetica, 17,* 475–481.

Allport, G. W., & Odbert, H. S. (1936). Trait names, a psychological study. *Psychological Monographs, 47* (1, Whole No. 211).

American Psychiatric Association. (1980). *Diagnostic and statistical manual of mental disorders* (3rd ed.). Washington, DC: American Psychiatric Association.

Anderson, V. E. (1982). Family studies of epilepsy. In V. E. Anderson, W. A. Hauser, J. K. Penry, & C. F. Sing (Eds.), *Genetic basis of the epilepsies* (pp. 103–112). New York: Raven Press.

Andreasen, N. C. (1982). Negative v. positive schizophrenia. Definitions and validation. *Archives of General Psychiatry, 39,* 789–794.

Andrews, G., Harris, M., Garside, R., & Kay, D. (1964). *The syndrome of stuttering* (Clinics in Developmental Medicine, No. 17). London: Heinemann.

Angst, J. (1966). *Zur Aetiologie und Nosologie endogener depressiver Psychosen.* Berlin: Springer.

Angst, J., Frey, R., Lohmeyer, B., & Zerbin-Rudin, E. (1980). Bipolar manic-depressive psychoses: Results of a genetic investigation. *Human Genetics, 55,* 237–254.

Armstrong, M. D., & Tyler, F. H. (1955). Studies on phenylketonuria: Restricted phenylalanine intake. *Journal of Clinical Investigations, 34,* 565–580.

Asano, N. (1967). Study of manic-depressive psychosis. In H. Mitsuda (Ed.), *Clinical genetics in psychiatry.* Tokyo: Igaku Shoin.

Avery, D. & Lubrano, A. (1979). Depression treated with imipramine and ECT: The Carolina study reconsidered. *American Journal of Psychiatry, 136,* 559–562.

Bailey, N. T. J. (1961). *Introduction to the mathematical theory of genetic linkage.* Oxford: Clarendon Press.

Bakwin, H. (1961). Enuresis in children. *Journal of Pediatrics, 58,* 806–819.

Bakwin, H. (1970). Sleepwalking in twins. *The Lancet, 2,* 446–447.

Bakwin, H. (1973). The genetics of bedwetting. In I. Kolvin, R. MacKeith, & S. R. Meadow (Eds.), *Bladder control and enuresis* (Clinics in Developmental Medicine, Nos. 48/49). London: Heinemann. (a)

Bakwin, H. (1973). Reading disability in twins. *Developmental Medicine and Child Neurology, 15,* 184–187. (b)

Baldwin, J. A. (Ed.). (1971). *Aspects of the epidemiology of mental illness: Studies in record linkage.* Boston: Little, Brown.

Baldwin, J. A., Robertson, N. C., & Satin, D. G. (1971). The incidence of reported deviant behaviour in children. In J. A. Baldwin (Ed.), *Aspects of the epidemiology of mental illness: Studies in record linkage.* Boston: Little, Brown.

Bannatyne, A. (1971). *Language, reading and learning disabilities.* Springfield, IL: C. C Thomas.

Barnard, J. S. (1972). *The future of marriage.* New York: World.

Baron, M. (1980). Genetic models of affective disorder: Application to twin data. *Acta Geneticae Medicae et Gemellologiae* (Rome), *29*, 289–294.

Barslund, I., & Danielsen, J. (1963). Temporal epilepsy in monozygotic twins. *Epilepsia, 4*, 138–150.

Bartak, L., Rutter, M., & Cox, A. (1975). A comparative study of infantile autism and specific developmental receptive language disorder: I. The children. *British Journal of Psychiatry, 126*, 127–145.

Barth, D. S., Sutherling, W., Engel, J., & Beatty, J. (1982). Neuromagnetic localization of epileptiform spike activity in the human brain. *Science, 218*, 891–894.

Beach, H. R., & Fransalla, F. (1968). *Research and experiment in stuttering.* London: Pergamon Press.

Beauchamp, D. E. (1980). *Beyond alcoholism. Alcohol and public health policy.* Philadelphia: Temple University Press.

Bech, P. (1981). Rating scales for affective disorders: Their validity and consistency. *Acta Psychiatrica Scandinavica*, Suppl. 295.

Beck-Mannagetta, G., & Janz, D. (1982). Febrile convulsions in offspring of epileptic probands. *In* V. E. Anderson, W. A. Hauser, J. K. Penry, & E. F. Sing (eds.), *Genetic basis of the epilepsies* (pp. 145–150). New York: Raven Press.

Becker, W. C. (1959). *Journal of Nervous and Mental Disorder, 219,* 442.

Beers, C. W. (1920). *A mind that found itself.* New York: Longmans, Green. (originally published 1905)

Bender, L. (1947). Childhood schizophrenia: Clinical study of one hundred schizophrenic children. *American Journal of Orthopsychiatry, 17*, 40–56.

Benton, A. L., & Pearl, D. (Eds.). (1978). *Dyslexia: An appraisal of current knowledge.* New York: Oxford University Press.

Berger, H. (1929). Über das Elektrenkephalogramm des Menschen. *Archive der Psychiatrie, 87*, 527–570.

Berger, M., Yule, W., & Rutter, M. (1975). Attainment and adjustment in two geographical areas. I: The prevalence of specific reading retardation. *British Journal of Psychiatry, 126*, 510–19.

Bert, J., Kripke, D. F., & Rhodes, J. (1970). Electroencephalogram of the mature chimpanzee: Twenty-four recordings. *Electroencephalography and Clinical Neurophysiology, 28*, 368–373.

Bertelsen, A., Harvald, B., & Hauge, M. (1977). A Danish twin study of manic-depressive disorder. *British Journal of Psychiatry, 130*, 330–351.

Bickel, H. (1954). The effects of a phenylalanine—free and phenylalanine—poor diet in phenylpyruvic oligophrenia. *Experiments in Medicine and Surgery, 12*, 112–118.

Bielski, R. J., & Friedel, R. O. (1976). Prediction of tricyclic antidepressant response. *Archives of General Psychiatry, 33*, 1479–1489.

Bird, E. D., Caro., & Pilling, J. B. (1974). A sex related factor in the inheritance of Huntington's chorea. *Annals of Human Genetics, 37*, 255–260.

Black, A. (1974). The natural history of obsessional neuroses. In H. R. Beech (Ed.), *Obsessional states.* London: Methuen.

Bleuler, E. (1950). *Dementia praecox or the group of schizophrenias.* New York: International Universities Press. (originally published in 1911)

Bloodstein, O. (1969). *A handbook of stuttering.* Chicago: National Easter Seal Society for Crippled Children and Adults.

Bock, R. D., & Kolakowski, D. (1973). Further evidence of sex-linked major gene influence in twins' spatial visualizing ability. *American Journal of Human Genetics, 25,* 1–14.

Boder, E. (1971). Developmental dyslexia: Prevailing diagnostic concepts and a new diagnostic approach through patterns of reading and spelling. In H. R. Myklebust (Ed.), *Progress in learning disabilities* (Vol. 2). New York: Grune & Stratton.

Bohman, M. (1978). Some genetic aspects of alcoholism and criminality: A population of adoptees. *Archives of General Psychiatry, 35,* 269–76.

Bohman, M., & Sigvardsson, S. (1980). A prospective, longitudinal study of children registered for adoption. *Acta Psychiatrica Scandinavica, 61,* 339–355.

Bohman, M., Sigvardsson, S., & Cloninger, R. (1981). Maternal inheritance of alcohol abuse. *Archives of General Psychiatry, 38,* 965–969.

Bohman, M., Cloninger, C. R., Sigvardsson, S., & von Knorring, A. L. (1982). Predisposition to petty criminality in Swedish adoptees. I. Genetic and environmental heterogeneity. *Archives of General Psychiatry, 39,* 1233–1241.

Böök, J. A. (1953). A genetic and neuropsychiatric investigation of a north-Swedish population, with special regard to schizophrenia and mental deficiency. *Human Heredity, 4,* 1–100.

Böök, J. A. (1957). Genetical investigation in a north Swedish population: The offspring of first-cousin marriages. *Annals of Human Genetics, 21,* 191–221.

Borland, B. L., & Hechtman, H. K. (1976). Hyperactive boys and their brothers: A 25 year follow up study. *Archives of General Psychiatry, 33,* 669–675.

Botstein, D., White, R. L., Skolnick, M., & Davis, R. W. (1980). Construction of a genetic linkage map in man using restriction fragment length polymorphisms. *American Journal of Human Genetics, 32,* 314.

Bower, E. M., Shellhammer, T. A., & Daily, J. M. (1960). School characteristics of male adolescents who later became schizophrenic. *American Journal of Orthopsychiatry, 30,* 712–729.

Bowlby, J. (1942). *Personality and mental illness, an essay in psychiatric diagnosis.* New York: Emerson House.

Bowlby, J. (1960). Grief and mourning in infancy and early childhood. *Psychoanalytic Study of the Child, 15,* 9–52.

Bowman, K. M. (1934). A study of the prepsychotic personality in certain psychoses. *American Journal of Orthopsychiatry, 4,* 473–498.

Braconi, Z. (1961). Le psiconeurosi e le psicosi nei gemelli. *Acta Geneticae Medicae et Gemellologia* (Rome), *10.*

Bray, P. F., Wiser, W. C., Wood, M. C., & Pusey, S. B. (1965). Hereditary characteristics of familial temporal-central focal epilepsy. *Pediatrics, 36,* 207–211.

Broadbent, D. E., Cooper, P. F., Fitzgerald, P., & Parkes, K. R. (1982). The Cognitive Failures Questionnaire (CFQ) and its correlates. *British Journal of Clinical Psychology, 21,* 1–16.

Brockington, I. F., Kendell, R. E., & Wainwright, S. (1980). Depressed patients with schizophrenic or paranoid symptoms. *Psychological Medicine, 10,* 665–675.

Broen, W. E. (1969). *Schizophrenia: research and theory.* New York: Academic Press.

Brown, F. N. (1942). Heredity in the psychoneuroses. *Proceedings of the Royal Society of Medicine, 35,* 785–790.

Brown, G. W., & Harris, T. (1978). *Social origins of depression: A study of psychiatric disorders in women.* New York: The Free Press.

Brown, W. T., Jenkins, E. C., Friedman, E., Brooks, J., Wisniewski, K., Raguthu, S., & French, J. (1982). Autism is associated with the Fragile X syndrome. *Journal of autism and developmental disorders, 12,* 303–308.

Bruell, J. H. (1967). Evolution and heterosis. In J. Hirsch (Ed.), *Behavior genetic analysis.* New York: McGraw-Hill, 1967.

Bruhova, S., & Roth, B. (1972). Heredofamilial aspects of narcolepsy and hypersomnia. *Archives Suisses de Neurologie, Neurochirurgie et de Psychiatrie, 110,* 45–54.

Bryant, N. D., & McLoughlin, J. A. (1972). Subject variables: Definition, incidence, characteristics, and correlates (Leadership Training Institute in Learning Disabilities, Proj. No. 127145). Washington, DC: U.S. Office of Education.

Buchsbaum, M. S., & Haier, R. J. (1983). Psychopathology: Biological approaches. In M. R. Rosenzweig & L. W. Porter (Eds.), *Annual Review of Psychology,* Volume 34.

Buchsbaum, M. S., & Rieder, R. O. (1979). Biologic heterogeneity and psychiatric research: Platelet MAO activity as a case study. *Archives of General Psychiatry, 36,* 1163–1169.

Buglas, D., Clarke, J., Henderson, A. S., Kreitman, N., & Presley, A. S. (1977). A study of agoraphobic housewives. *Psychological Medicine, 7,* 73–86.

Burns, L. E., & Thorpe, G. L. (1977). Fears and clinical phobias: Epidemiological aspects and the national survey of agoraphobics. *Journal of International Medical Research, 5,* Supplement 1, 132–139.

Buros, O. K. (Ed.) (1965). *The sixth mental measurements yearbook.* Highland Park, NJ: Gryphon Press.

Burton, R. (1924). *The anatomy of melancholy.* New York: Empire State Book Company. (Facsimile reprint of Oxford edition, 1621)

Cadoret, R. J. (1978). Psychopathology in adopted-away offspring of biologic mothers with antisocial behavior. *Archives of General Psychiatry, 35,* 176–189.

Cadoret, R. J. (1976). Evidence for genetic inheritance of primary affective disorder in adoptees. Unpublished manuscript. Cited in L. Willerman, 1979, *The psychology of group and individual differences.* San Francisco: W. H. Freeman.

Cadoret, R. J., & Gath, A. (1976, October). Biologic correlates of hyperactivity: Evidence for a genetic factor. Paper presented at the meeting of the Society for Life History Research in Psychopathology, Fort Worth, Texas.

Cadoret, R. J., & Tanna, V. L. 1977. Genetics of affective disorders. In G. Usdin (Ed.), *Depression: Clinical, biological and psychological perspectives* (pp. 104–121). New York: Brunner/Mazel.

Cannings, C., & Thompson, E. A. (1977). Ascertainment in the sequential sampling of pedigrees. *Clinical Genetics, 12,* 208.

Cantú, J. M., Saglia, H. E., Medina, M., Gonzalez-Diddi, M., Morato, T., Moreno, M. E., & Perez-Palacios, G. (1976). Inherited congenital normofunctional testicular hyperplasia and mental deficiency. *Human Genetics, 33,* 23–33.

Cantwell, D. P. (1972). Psychiatric illness in the families of hyperactive children. *Archives of General Psychiatry, 27,* 414–417.

Cantwell, D. P. (1975). Familial-genetic research with hyperactive children. In D. P. Cantwell (Ed.), *The hyperactive child.* Holliswood, NY: Spectrum.

Cantwell, D. F. (1982). A model for the investigation of psychiatric disorders of childhood: Its application in genetic studies of the hyperkinetic syndrome. In S. I. Harrison & J. F. McDermott (Eds.), *New directions in childhood psychopathology* (Vol. 2). New York: International Universities Press.

Cantwell, D. P., Sturzenberger, S., Burroughs, J., Salkin, B., & Green, J. D. (1977). Anorexia nervosa: An affective disorder? *Archives of General Psychiatry, 34,* 1087–1093.

Carey, G. (1978). A clinical–genetic study of obsessional and phobic states. Doctoral dissertation, University of Minnesota.

Carey, W. B., & McDevitt, S. C. (1978). Revision of the Infant Temperament Questionnaire. *Pediatrics, 61,* 735–739.

Carpenter, W. T., Strauss, J. S., & Bartko, J. J. (1973). Flexible system for the diagnosis of schizophrenia: Report from the WHO Pilot Study of Schizophrenia. *Science, 182,* 1275–1278.

Carroll, B. J., Feinberg, M., Creden, J. F., Tarika, J., Abala, A. A., Haskett, R. F., James, N. M., Kronfol, Z., Lohr, N., Steiner, M., deVigne, J. P., & Young, E. (1981). A specific laboratory test for the diagnosis of melancholia. *Archives of General Psychiatry, 38,* 15–22.

Carter, C. H. (1970). *Handbook of mental retardation syndromes* (2nd ed.). Springfield, IL: Charles C Thomas.

Carter, M., & Watts, C. A. H. (1971). Possible biological advantages among schizophrenics' relatives. *British Journal of Psychiatry, 118,* 453–460.

Cass, L. K., & Thomas, C. B. (1979). *Childhood pathology and later adjustment. The question of prediction.* New York: Wiley.

Cattell, R. B., Eber, H. W., & Taksuoka, M. M. *Handbook for Sixteen Personality Factor Questionnaire.* Champaign, IL: Institute for Personality and Ability Testing, 1970.

Cavalli-Sforza, L. L., & Feldman, M. W. (1973). Cultural versus biological inheritance: Phenotypic transmission from parent to children (A theory of the effect of parental phenotypes on children's phenotype). *American Journal of Human Genetics, 25,* 618.

Cavalli-Sforza, L. L., & Kidd, K. K. (1971). Genetic models for schizophrenia. *Neurological Research Program Bulletin, 10,* 406.

Chess, S., Korn, S. J., & Fernandez, P. G. (1971). *Psychiatric disorders of children with congenital rubella.* New York: Brunner/Mazel.

Chodoff, P., & Lyons, H. (1958). Hysteria, the hysterical personality and "hysterical" conversion. *American Journal of Psychiatry, 114,* 734–740.

Christensen, A. L. (1974). *Luria's neuropsychological investigation.* Copenhagen: Munksgaard.

Christiansen, K. O. (1977). A review of studies of criminality among twins. In S. A. Mednick & K. O. Christiansen (Eds.), *Biosocial bases of criminal behavior.* New York: Gardner Press.

Christiansen, K. O. (1968). Threshold of tolerance in various population groups illustrated by results from a Danish criminological twin study. In A. V. S. Reuck & R. Porter (Eds.), *The mentally abnormal offender.* Boston: Little, Brown.

Chu, F. D., & Trotter, S. (1974). *The madness establishment* (Ralph Nader's Study Group Report on the National Institute of Mental Health). New York: Grossman Publishers.

Clements, S. D. (1966). *Minimal Brain Dysfunction in Children—Terminology and identification.* (U.S.P.H.S. Pub. No. 1415). Washington, DC: U.S. Government Printing Office.

Clifford, C. A., Fulker, D. W., & Murray, R. M. (1981). A genetic and environmental analysis of obsessionality in normal twins. In L. Gedda, P. Parisi, & W. E. Nance (Eds.), *Twin Research 3, Part B. Intelligence, personality, and development.* New York: Alan R. Liss.

Cline, H. F. (1980). Criminal behavior over the life span. In O. G. Brim & J. Kagan (Eds.), *Constancy and change in human development.* pp. 641–674. Cambridge, MA: Harvard University Press.

Cloninger, C. R., Reich, T., & Guze, S. B. (1975). The multifactorial model of disease transmission: II. Sex differences in the familial transmission of sociopathy (antisocial personality). *British Journal of Psychiatry, 127,* 11–22. (a)

Cloninger, C. R., Reich, T., &Guze, S. B. (1975). The multifactorial model of disease transmission: III. Familial relationships between sociopathy and hysteria (Briquet's syndrome). *British Journal of Psychiatry, 127,* 23–32. (b)

Cloninger, C. R., Rice, J., Reich, T. (1979). Multifactorial inheritance with cultural transmission and assortative mating. II. A general model of combined polygenic and cultural inheritance. *American Journal of Human Genetics, 31,* 176. (a)

Cloninger, C. R., Rice, J., & Reich, T. (1979). Multifactorial inheritance with cultural transmission and assortative mating. III. Family structure and the analysis of separation experiments. *American Journal of Human Genetics, 31,* 366. (b)

Cloninger, C. R., Sigvardsson, S., Bohman, M., & von Knorring, A. L. (1982). Predisposition to petty criminality in Swedish adoptees. II. Cross-fostering analysis of gene–environment interaction. *Archives of General Psychiatry, 39,* 1242–1247.

Cohen, M. E., Badal, D. W., Kilpatrick, A., Reed, A., & White, P. (1951). The high familial prevalence of neurocirculatory asthenia (anxiety neurosis, effort syndrome). *American Journal of Human Genetics, 3,* 126–158.

Cohen, T., Block, N., Flum, Y., Kadar, M., & Goldschmidt, E. (1963). School attainments in an immigrant village. In E. Goldschmidt (Ed.), *The genetics of migrant and isolate populations.* Baltimore: Williams & Wilkins.

Coleman, M. (Ed.). (1976). *The autistic syndromes.* Amsterdam: North-Holland.

Coleman, M., & Rimland, B. (1976). Familial autism. In M. Coleman (Ed.), *The autistic syndromes.* Amsterdam: North-Holland.

Collier, J. (1928). Lumleian lectures on epilepsy. *Lancet, 1,* 587, 642–687.

Colligan, R. C., Osborne, D., Swenson. W. M., & Offord, K. P. (1983). *The MMPI: A contemporary normative study.* New York: Praeger.

Collins, I. F., Maxwell, A. E., & Cameron, K. (1962). A factor analysis of some childhood psychiatric clinic data. *Journal of Mental Science, 108,* 274–285.

Committee on Interstate and Foreign Commerce. (1953). *Health inquiry.* Department of Commerce, Washington, DC: Government Printing Office.

Comrey, A. L. (1970). *Comrey Personality Scales.* San Diego, CA: Educational and Industrial Testing Service.

Conneally, M. P., & Rivas, M. L. (1980). Linkage analysis in man. In H. Harris & K. Hirschborn (Eds.), *Advances in human genetics* (Vol. 10) (pp. 209–266). New York: Plenum Press.

Conners, C. K. (1969). A teacher rating scale for use in drug studies with children. *American Journal of Psychiatry, 126,* 885–888.

Conners, C. K. (1973). Rating scales for use in drug studies with children. *Psychopharmacology Bulletin, Special issue, Pharmacotherapy of children,* 28–84.

Constantinides, J., Garrone, G., & Ajuriaguerra, J. de. (1962). The inheritance of senile psychoses. *Encephale, 51,* 301–344.

Cooper, J. E. (1970). The Leyton Obsessional Inventory. *Psychological Medicine, 1,* 48–64. (a)

Cooper, J. E. (1970). Use of a procedure for standarding psychiatric diagnosis. In Hare, E. H., & Wing, J. K. (Eds.), *Psychiatric epidemiology.* London: Oxford University Press. (b)

Cooper, J. E., Kendell, R. E., Gurland, B. J., Sharpe, L., Copeland, J. R. M., & Simon, R. (1972). *Psychiatric Diagnosis in New York and London* (Maudsley Monograph No. 20). London: Oxford University Press.

Corballis, M. C., & Beal, I. L. (1976). *The psychology of left and right.* Hillsdale, NJ: Lawrence Erlbaum.

Corbett, J. A. (1971). The nature of tics and Gilles de la Tourette's syndrome. *Journal of Psychosomatic Research, 15,* 403–407.

Cowdry, R. W., & Goodwin, F. K. (1978). Amine neurotransmitter studies and psychiatric illness: Toward more meaningful diagnostic concepts. In R. L. Spitzer & D. F. Klein (Eds.), *Critical issues in psychiatric diagnosis*. New York: Raven Press.

Cox, A., Rutter, M., Newman, S., & Bartak, L. (1975). A comparative study of infantile autism and specific developmental receptive language disorder: II. Parental characteristics. *British Journal of Psychiatry, 126*, 146–159.

Cox, N. J., Kramer, P. L., & Kidd, K. K. (1984). Segregation analysis of stuttering. *Journal of Genetic Epidemiology, 1*, 245–253.

Crago, M. A. (1972). Psychopathology in married couples. *Psychological Bulletin, 77*, 114–128.

Craik, W. H., & Slater, E. (1945). Folie à deux in uniovular twins reared apart. *Brain, 68*, 213–221.

Crifo, S. (1973). Shiver-audiometry in the conditioned guinea pig (simplified Anderson-Wedenberg test). *Acta Oto-Laryngologica, 75*, 38–44.

Crisp, A. H. (1970). Anorexia nervosa: "Feeding disorder," "nervous malnutrition," or "weight phobia"? *World Review of Nutrition and Diet, 12*, 452–504.

Crisp, A. H., Palmer, R. L., & Kalvey, T. S. (1976). How common is anorexia nervosa? A prevalence study. *British Journal of Psychiatry, 128*, 549–554.

Crisp, A. H., Jones, M. G., & Slater, P. (1978). The Middlesex Hospital Questionnaire: A validity study. *British Journal of Medical Psychology, 51*, 269–280.

Crisp, A. H., Hsu, L. K. G., Harding, B., & Hartshorn, J. (1980). Clinical features of anorexia nervosa. *Journal of Psychosomatic Research, 24*, 179–91.

Critchley, M. (1970). *Developmental dyslexia*. London: Heinemann, 1970.

Crittenden, L. B. (1961). An interpretation of familial aggregation based on multiple genetic and environmental factors. *Annals of the New York Academy of Sciences, 91*, 769.

Crome, L., Tymms, V., & Woolf, L. I. (1962). A chemical investigation of the defects of myelination in phenylketonuria. *Journal of Neurology, Neurosurgery and Psychiatry, 25*.

Crook, M. N. (1937). Intra-family relationships in personality test performance. *Psychological Record, 1*, 479–502.

Crowe, R. R. (1975). An adoptive study of psychopathy: Preliminary results from arrest records and psychiatric hospital records. In R. R. Fieve, D. Rosenthal, & H. Brill (Eds.), *Genetic research in psychiatry*. Baltimore: The Johns Hopkins University Press.

Crowe, R. R., Noyes, R., Pauls, D. L., & Slymen, D. (1983). A family study of anxiety disorder. *Archives of General Psychiatry, 40*, 1065–1069.

Crowe, R., Pauls, D., Slymen, D., & Noyes, R. (1980). A family study of anxiety neurosis. *Archives of General Psychiatry, 37*, 77–79.

Crown, S., & Crisp, A. H. (1966). A short clinical diagnostic self-rating score for psychoneurotic patients: The Middlesex Hospital Questionnaire (MHQ). *British Journal of Psychiatry, 112*, 917–923.

Crown, S., & Crisp, A. H. (1970). *Manual of the Middlesex Hospital Questionnaire*. Barnstaple, England: Psychological Test Publications.

Cruickshank, W. M., & Raus, S. (Eds). (1955). *Cerebral palsy, its individual and community problems*. Syracuse, NY: Syracuse University Press.

Crumpacker, D. W., Cederlof, F., Friberg, L., Kimberling, W. J., Sorensen, S., Vandenberg, S. G., Williams, J. S., McClearn, G. E., Grever, B., Iyer, H., Krier, M. J., Pedersen, N. L., Price, R. A., & Roulette, I. (1979). A twin methodology for the study of genetic and environmental control of variation in human smoking behavior. *Acta Geneticae Medicae et Gemellologiae, 28*, 173–195.

Cunningham, L., Cadoret, R. J., Loftus, R., & Edwards, J. E. (1975). Studies of adoptees from psychiatrically disturbed biological parents. *British Journal of Psychiatry, 126*, 534–549.

DaFonseca, A. F. (1959). *Analise heredo-clinica des perturbacoes affectivas*, Ph.d. dissertation, Universidade do Porto, Portugal.

Dahlstrom, W. G., Welsh, G. S., & Dahlstrom, L. E. (1975). *An MMPI handbook: Vol. II. Research applications* (Rev. ed.). Minneapolis: University of Minnesota Press.

Dalgaard, O. S. and Kringlen, E. A. (1976). A Norwegian twin study of criminality *British Journal of Criminology, 16*, 213–232.

Daly, D. D., & Yoss, R. E. (1959). A family with narcolepsy. *Proceedings of the Staff Meetings of the Mayo Clinic, 34*, 313–320.

Dasberg, H., & Shalif, I. (1978). On the validity of the Middlesex Hospital Questionnaire: A comparison of diagnostic self-ratings in psychiatric out-patients, general practice patients, and "normals" based on the Hebrew version. *British Journal of Medical Psychology, 51*, 281–289.

Davids, A. (Eds.) (1974). Child personality and psychopathology (Vol. I). New York: Wiley.

Davis, H., & Davis, P. A. (1936). Action potentials of the brain. *Archives of Neurology and Psychiatry, 36*, 1214–12224.

Davis, J. G., Silverberg, G., Williams, M. K., Spiro, A., & Shapiro, L. R. (1982). A new X-linked recessive mental retardation syndrome with progressive spastic quadriplegia. *American Journal of Human Genetics, 34*, 75A.

Davison, B. C. C. (1969). *Severe mental defect: The contribution by X-linked or sex-limited gene mutation.* M.D. thesis, The Queen's University of Belfast.

DeFries, J., Singer, S., Foch, T., & Lewitter, F. (1978). Familial nature of reading disability. *British Journal of Psychiatry, 132*, 361–367.

DeFries, J. C., Johnson, R. C., Kuse, A. R., McClearn, G. E., Polovina, J., Vandenberg, S. G., & Wilson, J. R. (1979). Familial resemblance for specific cognitive abilities. *Behavior Genetics, 9*, 23–43.

De la Tourette, G. (1885). Étude sùr une affection nerveuse, caractérisée par de l'incoordination motrice accompagnée d'écolalie et de coprolalie. *Archives Neurologiques, 9*, 158–200.

Delgado-Escueta, A. V., Treiman, D. M., & Enrile-Bacsal, F. (1982). Phenotypic variations of seizures in adolescents and adults. In V. E. Anderson, W. A. Hauser, J. K. Penry, & C. F. Sing (Eds.), *Genetic basis of the epilepsies* (pp. 49–81). New York: Raven Press.

Delgado-Escueta, A. V., Wasterlain, C. C., Treiman, D. M., & Porter, R. J. (Eds.). (1982). *Status epilepticus* (Vol. 34). *Advances in Neurology.* New York: Raven Press.

DeMyer, M. (1979). *Parents and children in autism.* New York: Wiley.

Depue, R. A., & Monroe, S. M. (1978). The unipolar-bipolar distinction in the depressive disorders. *Psychological Bulletin, 85*, 1001–1029.

Depue, R. A., Slater, J. F., Wolfstetter-Kausch, H., Klein, D., Goplerud, E., & Farr, D. (1981). A behavioral paradigm for identifying persons at risk for bipolar depressive disorder: A conceptual framework and five validation studies. *Journal of Abnormal Psychology, 90*, 381–437.

Deroover, J., Fryns, J. P., Parloir, C., & Van Den Berghe, H. (1977). X-linked recessively inherited non-specific mental retardation: Report of a large family. *Annals of Genetics, 20*, 236–268.

Diamant, J. J. (1981). Similarities and differences in the approach of R. M. Reitan and A. R. Luria. *Acta Psychiatrica Scandinavica, 63*, 431–443.

Dohrenwend, B. S., & Dohrenwend, B. P. (1974). *Stressful life events.* New York: Wiley.

Doose, H., Gerken, H., Petersen, C. E., & Volzke, E. (1967). Electroencephalography of epileptic children's siblings. *Lancet, 1,* 578–579.

Drayna, D. T., Davies, K. E., Williamson, R., & White, R. L. (1983). *Construction of a linkage map of the human chromosome.* Paper presented at the 1983 meeting of the American Society of Human Genetics.

Dreger, R. (1964). A progress report on a factor analytic approach to classification in child psychiatry. In J. Jenkins & J. Cole (Eds.), *Research report no. 18.* Washington, DC: American Psychiatric Association.

Dreger, R. M. (1981). First, Second and Third-order factors from the Children's Behavioral Classification Project instrument and an attempt at rapprochement. *Journal of Abnormal Psychology, 49,* 242–260.

Drew, A. L. (1956). A neurological appraisal of familial word-blindness. *Brain, 79,* 440–460.

Dunn, H. G., Renpenning, H., Gerrard, J. W., Miller, J. R., Tabata, T., & Federoff, S. (1963). Mental retardation as a sex-linked defect. *American Journal of Mental Deficiency, 67,* 827–848.

Dunner, D. L., Fleiss, J., Addonizio, G., Fieve, R. (1976). Assortative mating in primary affective disorder. *Biological Psychiatry, 11,* 43–51.

Dupont, A. (1980). Medical results from registration of Danish mentally retarded persons. In P. Mittler (Ed.), *Frontiers of knowledge in mental retardation.* (Vol. 2): *Biomedical aspects.* Baltimore: University Park Press, 1980.

Eaves, L. J. (1969). The genetic analysis of continuous variation: A comparison of experimental designs applicable to human data. *British Journal of Mathematical and Statistical Psychology, 22,* 131–147.

Eaves, L. J. (1977). Inferring the causes of human variation. *Journal of the Royal Statistical Society,* Series A (General), *140,* 324–355.

Ebaugh, F. (1923). Neuropsychiatric sequelae of acute epidemic encephalitis in children. *American Journal of Diseases in Children, 25,* 89–97.

Eckert, E. D., Goldberg, S. C., Halmi, K. A., Casper, P. C., & Davis, J. M. (1982). Depression in anorexia nervosa. *Psychological Medicine, 12,* 115–22.

Edwards, J. H. (1963). The genetic basis of common disease. *American Journal of Medicine, 34,* 627–38.

Eeg-Olofsson, O., Safwenberg, J., & Wigertz, A. (1982). HLA and epilepsy: An investigation of different types of epilepsy in children and their families. *Epilepsia, 23,* 27–34.

Egeland, J. A., & Hostetter, A. M. (1983). Amish study, I: Affective disorders among the Amish, 1976–1980. *American Journal of Psychiatry, 140,* 56–61.

Eisenberg, L. (1968). Psychotic disorders in childhood. In R. E. Cooke & S. Lewis (Eds.), *Biologic basis of pediatric practice.* New York: McGraw-Hill.

Eisenberg, L. (1972). The classification of childhood psychosis reconsidered. *Journal of Autism and Childhood Schizophrenia, 2,* 338–42.

Eisenthal, S., Hartford, T., & Solomon, L. (1972). Premorbid adjustment, paranoid-nonparanoid status, and chronicity in schizophrenic patients. *Journal of Nervous and Mental Disease, 155,* 227–231.

Elandt-Johnson, R. C. (1971). *Probability models and statistical methods in genetics.* New York: Wiley.

Elston, R. C., & Campbell, M. A. (1970). Schizophrenia: Evidence for the major gene hypothesis. *Behavioral Genetics, 1,* 3.

Elston, R. C., & Namboodiri, K. K. (1977). Family studies of schizophrenia. In *Proceedings of the 41st Session of the International Statistical Institute.*

Elston, R. C., & Stewart, J. (1971). A general model for the genetic analysis of pedigree data. *Human Heredity, 21,* 523.

Elston, R. C., & Yelverton, K. C. (1975). General models for segregation analysis. *American Journal of Human Genetics*, 27, 31–45.

Endicott, J., & Spitzer, R. L. (1978). A diagnostic interview: The Schedule for Affective Disorders and Schizophrenia. *Archives of General Psychiatry*, 35, 837–844.

Endicott, J., Spitzer, R. L., Fleiss, J. L., Cohen, J. et al. (1976). The Global Assessment Scale: A procedure for measuring overall severity of a psychiatric disturbance. *Archives of General Psychiatry*, 33, 766–771.

Eren, M., & Disteche, C. (1983). *Behavioral phenotype of a fragile X syndrome: Relationship between frequency of marker X, mental retardation and verbal disability.* Paper presented at the 1983 meeting of the American Society of Human Genetics.

Erlenmeyer-Kimling, L., Cornblatt, B., & Fleiss, J. (1979). High-risk research in Schizophrenia *Psychiatric Annals*, 9, 79–102.

Erlenmeyer-Kimling, L., & Paradowski, W. (1966). Selection and schizophrenia. *American Naturalist*, 100, 651–665.

Escalante, J. A., Grunspun, H., & Frota-Passod, W. (1971). Severe sex-linked mental retardation. *Journal de Génétique Humaine*, 19, 137–140.

Eshkevari, H. S. (1977). Early infantile autism in monozygotic twins. *Journal of Autism and Developmental Disorders*, 9, 155–209.

Essen-Möller, E. (1941). Psychiatrische Untersuchungen an einer Serie von Zwillingen. *Acta Psychiatrica Scandinavica*, Suppl. 23, 187–191.

Extein, I., Pottash, A. L. C., & Gold, M. S. (1982). The TRH test in depressive and manic-depressive illness. In E. Usdin & I. Hanin (Eds.), *Biological markers in psychiatry and neurology*. New York, Pergamon Press.

Extein, I., Pottash, A. L. C., Gold, M. S., & Cowdry, R. W. (1982). Using the protirelin test to distinguish mania from schizophrenia. *Archives of General Psychiatry*, 39, 77–81.

Eysenck, H. J. (1964). *Crime and personality*. London: Routledge.

Eysenck, H. J. (1977). *Crime and personality* (3rd ed.). London: Granada.

Eysenck, H., & Eysenck, S. B. G. (1977). *The Eysenck Personality Inventory*. Kent, England: Hodder & Stoughton Educational Ltd.

Eysenck, H. J., Wakefield, J. A., & Friedman, A. F. (1983). Diagnosis and clinical Assessment, the DSM-III. In M. R. Rosenzweig & L. W. Porter (Eds.), *Annual Review of Psychology, 34*.

Falconer, D. S. (1960). *An introduction to quantitative genetics*. New York: Ronald.

Falconer, D. S. (1965). The inheritance of liability to certain diseases, estimated from the incidence among relatives. *Annals of Human Genetics*, 29, 51.

Farber, S. L. (1981). *Identical twins reared apart*. New York: Basic Books.

Federal Register Volume 5. (1977). Section 121a: U.S. Public Law 94-142, p. 9.

Feighner, J. P., Robbins, E., & Guze, S. B. Woodruff, R., Winokur, G. & Munoz, R. (1972). Diagnostic criteria for use in psychiatric research. *Archives of General Psychiatry*, 26, 57–63.

Fein, R. (1958). *Economics of mental illness: A report to the staff director, Jack R. Ewalt* (Monograph No. 2, Joint Commission on Mental Illness and Health). New York: Basic Books.

Finucci, J. M. (1978). Genetic considerations in dyslexia. In H. R. Myklebust (Ed.), *Progress in learning disabilities* (Vol. 4). New York: Grune & Stratton.

Fischer, M. (1971). Psychoses in the offspring of schizophrenic monozygotic twins and their normal cotwins. *British Journal of Psychiatry*, 118, 43–52.

Fischer, M., Harvald, B., & Hauge, M. (1969). A Danish twin study of schizophrenia. *British Journal of Psychiatry*, 115, 981–990.

Fish, B. (1977). Neurobiological antecedents of schizophrenia in children: Evidence for an inherited, congenital neurointegrative defect. *Archives of General Psychiatry, 34,* 1297–1313.

Flor-Henry, P. (1976). Epilepsy and psychopathology. In H. Granville-Grossman (Ed.), *Recent advances in clinical psychiatry.* Edinburgh: Churchill-Livingstone.

Flor-Henry, P., Fromm-Ausch, D., & Tapper, M. (1981). A neuropsychological study of the stable syndrome of hysteria. *Biological Psychiatry, 16,* 601–626.

Foch, T. T., DeFries, J. C., McClearn, G. E., & Singer, S. M. (1977). Familial patterns of impairment in reading disability. *Journal of Educational Psychology, 69,* 316–329.

Fölling, A. (1934). Uber Ausscheidung von Phenylbrenztraubensaure in den Harn als Stoffwechselanomalie in Verbindung mit Imbezillitat. [On excretion of phenylpyruvic acid in the urine as a metabolic anomaly in connection with imbecility]. *Zeitschrift für Physiologische Chemie, 227,* 169.

Folstein, S., & Rutter, M. (1977). Genetic influences and infantile autism. *Nature, 265,* 726–728. (a)

Folstein, S., & Rutter, M. (1977). Infantile autism: A genetic study of 21 twin pairs. *Journal of Child Psychology and Psychiatry, 18,* 297–32. (b)

Ford, C. E., Jones, K. W., Polani, P. E., De Almeida, J. C., & Briggs, J. H. (1959). A sex-chromosome anomaly in a case of gonadal dysgenesis (Turner's syndrome). *Lancet, 1,* 711.

Ford, F. R. (1973). *Diseases of the nervous system in infancy, childhood and adolescence* (6th ed.). Springfield, IL: C. C Thomas.

Fowler, R. C., Tsuang, M. T., Cadoret, R. J., Monnelly, E. & McCabe, M. (1974). A clinical and family comparison of paranoid and non-paranoid schizophrenics. *British Journal of Psychiatry, 124,* 346–35.

Fried, K., & Sanger, R. (1973). Possible linkage between Xg and the locus for a gene causing mental retardation with or without hydrocephalus. *Journal of Medical Genetics, 10,* 17–18.

Friedmann, J. K. (1974). A diallel analysis of the genetic underpinnings of mouse sleep. *Physiology and Behavior, 12,* 169–175.

Friedmann, J. K., & Webb, W. (1970). Genetic determinants of the sleep response. *Psychophysiology, 7,* 340.

Fryers, T. (1981). Measuring trends in prevalence and distribution of severe mental retardation. In B. Cooper (Ed.), *Assessing the handicaps and needs of mentally retarded children.* New York: Academic Press.

Fulker, D., Eysenck, S. B. G., & Zuckerman, M. (1980). A genetic and environmental analysis of sensation seeking. *Journal of Research in Personality, 1,* 261–281.

Fuller, J. L. (1975). Independence of inherited susceptibility to spontaneous and primed audiogenic seizures in mice. *Behavior Genetics, 5,* 1–8.

Galioto, G. B., & Bonaccorsi, P. *Il fattore constituzionale del trauma acuatico individuato sperimentalmente nella diversa concentrazione di melania nella stria vascolare.* Cited in Crifo, 1973.

Ganda, O. P., & Soeldner, S. S. (1977). Genetic, acquired and related factors in the etiology of diabetes mellitus. *Archives of Internal Medicine, 137,* 461–469.

Garrod, A. E. (1909). *Inborn errors of metabolism.* London: Oxford University Press.

Gershon, E. S. (1980). Nonreplication of linkage to X chromosome markers in bipolar illness. *Archives of General Psychiatry, 37,* 1200.

Gershon, E. S., Mark, A., Cohen, N., Belizon, N., Baron, M., & Knobe, K. E. (1975). Transmitted factors in the morbid risk of affected disorders: A controlled study. *Journal of Psychiatric Research, 12,* 283–299.

Gershon, E. S., Targum, S. D., & Matthysse, S. & Bunney, W. E. (1979). Color blindness not closely linked to bipolar illness: Report of a new pedigree series. *Archives of General Psychiatry, 36,* 1423–1430.

Gershon, E. S., Hamovit, J., Guroff, J. J., Dibble, E., Leckman, J. F., Sceery, W., Targum, S. D., Nurnberger, J. I., Goldin, L. R., & Bunney, W. E. (1982). A family study of schizoaffective, bipolar I, bipolar II, unipolar and normal control probands. *Archives of General Psychiatry, 39,* 1157–1167. (a)

Gershon, E. S., Hamovit, J. R., Schreiber, J. L., Dibble, E. D., Kaye, W., Nurnberger, J. I., Jr., Andersen, A. & Ebert, M. (1982). *Anorexia nervosa and major affective disorders associated in families.* Paper presented at the Annual Meeting of the American Psychopathological Association, New York. (b)

Geyer, H. (1973). Uber den Schlaf von Zwillingen. *Zeitschrift Abstamm,* 1937, 73, 524.

Gillberg, C., & Schaumann, H. (1982). Social class and infantile autism. *Journal of Autism and Developmental Disorders, 12,* 223–228.

Giraud, F., Ayme, S., Mattei, J. F., & Mattei, M. G. (1976). Constitutional chromosome breakage. *Human Genetics, 34,* 125–136.

Gladstein, K., Lange, K., & Spence, M. A. (1978). A goodness of fit test for the polygenic threshold model. *American Journal of Medical Genetics, 2,* 7.

Glassman, A. H., Kantor, S. J., & Shostak, M. (1975). Depression, delusions, and drug response. *American Journal of Psychiatry, 132,* 716–718.

Glueck, S., & Glueck, E. T. (1939). *Five hundred criminal careers.* New York: Knopf.

Glueck, S., & Glueck, E. (1940). *Juvenile delinquents grow up.* New York: Commonwealth Fund.

Glueck, S., & Glueck, E. (1974). *Of delinquency and crime: A panorama of search and research.* Springfield, IL: C. C Thomas.

Goldberg, D. P. (1972). *The detection of psychiatric illness by questionnaire.* London: Oxford University Press.

Goldberg, H. K., & Schiffman, G. S. (1972). *Dyslexia: Problems of reading disabilities.* New York: Grune & Stratton.

Golden, C. J., Purisch, A. D., & Hammeke, T. A. (1979). *The Luria-Nebraska Neuropsychological Battery: A manual for clinical and experimental use.* Lincoln: University of Nebraska Press.

Golden, C. J., Hammeke, T. A., Purisch, A. D., Berg, R. A., Moses, J. A., Newlin, D. B., Wilkening, G. N., & Puence, A. E. (1982). *Item interpretation of the Luria-Nebraska Neuropsychological Battery.* Lincoln: University of Nebraska Press.

Goldin, L. R., Gershon, E. S., Lake, C. R., Murphy, D. L., McGinnis, M., & Sparkes, R. S. (1982). Segregation and linkage studies of plasma dopamine-beta-hydroxylase (DBH), erythrocyte catechol-o-methyltransferase (COMT), and platelet monoamine oxidase (MAO): Possible linkage between the ABO locus and a gene controlling DBH activity. *American Journal of Human Genetics, 34,* 250–262.

Goldin, L. R., Gershon, E. S., Targum, S. D., Sparkes, P. S., & McGinnis, M. (1983). Segregation analyses in families of patients with bipolar, unipolar, and schizoaffective mood disorders. *American Journal of Human Genetics, 35,* 274–287.

Goldin, L. R., Cox, N. J., Pauls, D. L., Gershon, E. S., and Kidd, K. K. (1984). The detection of major loci by segregation and linkage analysis: A simulation study. *Journal of Genetic Epidemiology, 1,* 285–296.

Goodman, R. M. (Ed.). (1970). *Genetic disorders of man.* Boston: Little, Brown.

Goodwin, D. W., Schulsinger, F., Hermansen, L., Guze, S. B., & Winokur, G. (1973). Alcohol problems in adoptees raised apart from alcoholic biological parents. *Archives of General Psychiatry, 28,* 238–243.

Goodwin, D. W., Schulsinger, F., Moller, N., Hermansen, L., Winokur, G., & Guze, S. B.

(1974). Drinking problems in adopted and non-adopted sons of alcoholics. *Archives of General Psychiatry, 31,* 164–169.

Goodwin, D. W., Schulsinger, F., Hermansen, L., Guze, S. B., & Winokur, G. (1975). Alcoholism and the hyperactive child syndrome. *Journal of Nervous and Mental Disease, 160,* 349–353.

Goodwin, D. W., Schulsinger, F., & Knop, J. (1977). Psychopathology in adopted and non-adopted daughters of alcoholics. *Archives of General Psychiatry, 34,* 1005–1009.

Göring, M. H. (1910). Ein hysterischer Schwindler. *Zeitschrift fur die Gesamte Neurologie und Psychiatrie, 1,* 251.

Gottesman, I. I., & Shields, J. (1972). *Schizophrenia and genetics: A twin study vantage point.* New York: Academic Press.

Gottesman, I. I., & Shields, J. (1982). *Schizophrenia: The enigmatic puzzle.* New York: Cambridge University Press.

Gough, H., & Heilbrun, A. B. (1965). *The Adjective Checklist manual.* Palo Alto, CA: Consulting Psychologists Press.

Graham, J. R. (1977). *The MMPI: A Practical Guide.* New York: Oxford University Press.

Greden, J. F. (1982). The dexamethasone suppression test: An established biological marker of melancholia. In E. Usdin & I. Hanin (Eds.), *Biological markers in psychiatry and neurology* New York: Pergamon Press.

Greene, R. L. (1980). *The MMPI, an interpretive manual.* New York: Grune & Stratton.

Griffing, B. (1956). Concept of general and specific combining ability in relation to diallele crossing system. *Austrian Journal of Biological Science, 9,* 463–493.

Grove, W. M. (1982). Psychometric detection of schizotypy. *Psychological Bulletin, 92,* 27–38.

Gruneberg, H. (1952). *The genetics of the mouse.* The Hague: Martinus Nyhoff.

Guilleminault, C., Carskadon, M., & Dement, W. C. (1974). On the treatment of rapid eye movement narcolepsy. *Archives of Neurology, 30,* 90–93.

Gull, W. W. (1874). Anorexia nervosa (Apepsia hysteria, anorexia hysteria). *Transactions of the Clinical Society of London, 7,* 22.

Gusella, J. F., Wexler, N. S., Conneally, M. P., Naylor, S. L., Anderson, M., Tanzi, R. E., Watkins, P. C., Ottina, K., Wallace, M. R., Sakaguchi, A. Y., Young, A. B., Shoulson, I., Bonilla, E., and Martin, J. B. (1983). A polymorphic DNA marker genetically linked to Huntington's disease. *Nature, 306,* 234–238.

Guze, S. B., Goodwin, D. W., & Crane, J. B. (1970). A psychiatric study of the wives of convicted felons: An example of assortative mating. *American Journal of Psychiatry, 126,* 115–118.

Guze, S. B., Woodruff, R. A., & Clayton, P. J. (1971). Hysteria and antisocial behavior: Further evidence of an association. *American Journal of Psychiatry, 127,* 957–960.

Hagnell, O., & Kreitman, N. (1974). Mental illness in married pairs in a total population. *British Journal of Psychiatry, 125,* 203–302.

Hall, D. J., Baldwin, J. A., & Robertson, N. C. (1971). Mental illness in married pairs: Problems in estimating incidence. In J. A. Baldwin (Ed.), *Aspects of the epidemiology of mental illness: studies in record linkage* (pp. 115–134). Boston: Little, Brown.

Hallgren, B. (1950). Specific dyslexia: A clinical and genetic study. *Acta Psychiatrica et Neurologica Scandinavica,* Suppl. 65.

Hallgren, B. (1960). Nocturnal enuresis in twins. *Acta Psychiatrica et Neurologica Scandinavica, 35,* 73–90.

Hallstrom, T. (1972). Night terror in adults through 3 generations. *Acta Psychiatrica Scandinavica, 48,* 350–52.

Hamilton, M. (1959). The assessment of anxiety by rating. *British Journal of Medical Psychology, 32,* 50–55.

Hamilton, M. (1960). A rating scale for depression. *Journal of Neurology, Neuro-surgery and Psychiatry, 23;* 56.

Hanson, D. R., & Gottesman, I. I. (1976). The genetics, if any, of infantile autism and childhood schizophrenia. *Journal of Autism and Childhood Schizophrenia, 6,* 209–233.

Hanzawa, M. (1957). Elektroencephalogram bei Zwillingen. In S. Osato & I. Awano (Eds.), *Genetische Studien an Twillingen. A. Morphologischer Teil. Acta Geneticae Medicae, 6,* 283–366.

Hare, E. H., & Shaw, G. K. (1965). The patient's spouse and concordance on neuroticism. *British Journal of Psychiatry, 111,* 102–103.

Hare, E., Price, J., & Slater, E. (1971). Age distribution of schizophrenia and neurosis: Findings in a national sample. *British Journal of Psychiatry, 119,* 445–458.

Harris, E. L., Noyes, R., Crowe, R. R., & Chandhry, D. R. (1983). A family study of agoraphobia. *Archives of General Psychiatry, 40,* 1061–1064.

Harris, H., & Hirschhorn, K. (Eds.). (1972). *Advances in human genetics* (Vol. 3). New York: Plenum Press.

Harrison, C. J., Jack, E. M., Allen, T. D., & Harris, R. (1983). The fragile X: a scanning electron microscope study. *Journal of Medical Genetics, 20,* 280–285.

Harrison, R. M., & Taylor, D. C. (1976). Childhood seizures: A 25 year follow-up social and medical prognosis. *Lancet, 1,* 948–951.

Harvey, J., Judge, C., & Wiener, S. (1977). Familial X-linked mental retardation with an X chromosome abnormality. *Journal of Medical Genetics, 14,* 46–50.

Hassanyeh, R., Eccleston, T., & Davison, K. (1981). Rating of anxiety, depression and vulnerability: The development of a new rating scale (the Anxiety and Depression Scale). *Acta Psychiatrica Scandinavica, 64,* 301–313.

Hathaway, S. R., & McKinley, J. C. (1940). A multiphasic personality schedule (Minnesota): I. Construction of the schedule. *Journal of Psychology, 10,* 249–254.

Hauser, S. L., DeLong, G. R., & Rosman, N. P. (1975). Pneumographic findings in the infantile autism syndrome. A correlation with temporal lobe disease. *Brain, 98,* 667–688.

Hauser, W. A. (1978). Epidemiology of epilepsy. *Advances in Neurology, 19,* 313–339.

Heber, R. (1959). A manual on terminology and classification in mental retardation. *American Journal of Mental Deficiency, 64.*

Helperin, S. L. (1945). A clinico-genetic study of mental defect. *American Journal of Mental Deficiency, 50.*

Helweg-Larsen, P., Hoffmeyer, H., Kieler, J., Thaysen, E. H., Thaysen, J. H., Thygesen, P., & Wulff, M. H. (1952). Famine disease in German concentration camps, complications and sequels. *Acta Psychiatrica et Neurologica Scandinavica,* Suppl. 83.

Helzer, J. E., & Winokur, G. (1974). A family interview study of male manic depressives. *Archives of General Psychiatry, 31,* 73–77.

Henry, K. R. (1967). Audiogenic seizure susceptibility induced in C57BL/6J mice by prior auditory exposure. *Science, 158,* 938–940.

Hermann, K. (1959). *Reading disability: A medical study of word-blindness and related handicaps.* Springfield, IL: C. C Thomas.

Hermann, K., & Norrie, E. (1958). Is congenital word-blindness an hereditary type of Gerstmann's syndrome? *Psychiatria et Neurologia, 136,* 59–73.

Herschel, M. (1978). Dyslexia revisited, a review. *Human Genetics, 40,* 115–134.

Heston, L. L. (1966). Psychiatric disorders in foster home reared children of schizophrenic mothers. *British Journal of Psychiatry, 112,* 819–825.

Heston, L. L. (1970). The genetics of schizophrenic and schizoid disease. *Science, 167*, 249–256.

Hexter, W., & Yost, H. T. (1976). *The science of genetics*. Englewood Cliffs, NJ: Prentice-Hall.

Hirschfield, R. M. A., & Klerman, G. L. (1979). Personality attributes and affective disorders. *American Journal of Psychiatry, 136*, 67–70.

Hodge, S. E., Morton, L. A., Tideman, S., Kidd, K. K., & Spence, M. A. (1979). Age of onset correction available for linkage analysis (LIPED). *American Journal of Human Genetics, 31*, 761.

Hodges, K., Kline, J., Stern, L., Cytryn, L., & McKnew, D. (1981). The development of a child assessment interview for research and clinical use. *Journal of Abnormal Child Psychology, 10*, 173–189.

Hodges, K., McKnew, D., Cytryn, L., & Kline, J. (1982). The Child Assessment Schedule (CAS) Diagnostic Interview: A report on reliability and validity. *Journal of the Academy of Child Psychiatry, 21*, 468–473.

Hoffeditz, E. L. (1934). Family resemblances in personality traits. *Journal of Social Psychology, 5*, 214–227.

Hoffer, A., & Osmond, H. (1961). A card sorting task helpful in making psychiatric diagnoses. *Journal of Neuropsychiatry, 2*, 306–330.

Holden, J., Beckett, J., Mulligan, L., Phillips, A., Simpson, N., Partington, M., Hamerton, J., Wang, H. S., Donald, L., & White, B. (1983). *A search for restriction fragment length polymorphism (RFLPs) linked to the fragile-X form of X-linked mental retardation.* A paper presented at the 1983 meeting of the American Society of Human Genetics.

Holmes, T., & Rahe, R. H. (1967). The Social Adjustment Rating Scale. *Journal of Psychosomatic Research, 11*, 213.

Holzinger, K. J. (1929). The relative effect of nature and nurture influences on twin differences. *Journal of Educational Psychology, 20*, 241–248.

Horn, J. L., Green, M., Carney, R., & Erickson, M. T. (1975). Bias against genetic hypotheses in adoption studies. *Archives of General Psychiatry, 32*, 1365–1367.

Horowitz, M., Schaefer, C., Hiroto, D., Wilner, N., & Levin, B. (1977). Life event questionnaires for measuring presumptive stress. *Psychosomatic Medicine, 39*, 413–431.

Hough, R. L., Fairbank, D. T., & Garcia, A. (1976). Problems in the ratio measurement of life stress. *Journal of Health and Social Behavior, 17*, 70–82.

Hough, R. L., Fairbank, D. T., & Wainer, H. *The scaling of life change impacts across culturally heterogeneous groups.* Unpublished report.

Housman, D., Kidd, K. K., & Gusella, J. L. (1982). Recombinant DNA approach to neurological disorders. *Trends in Neurosciences, 5*, 320.

Howie, P. M. (1981). Intrapair similarity in frequency of disfluency in monozygotic and dizygotic twin pairs containing stutterers. *Behavior Genetics, 11*, 227–238.

Hoy, E., Weiss, G., Minde, K., & Cohen, N. (1978). The hyperactive child at adolescence: Emotional, social and cognitive functioning. *Journal of Abnormal Child Psychology, 6*, 311–24.

Hsia, D. Y., Troll, W., & Knox, W. E. (1956). Detection by phenylalanine tolerance tests of heterozygous carriers of phenylketonuria. *Nature, 178*, 1239–1240.

Hubert, N. C., Wacha, T. D., Peters-Martin, P., & Gandour, M. J. (1982). The study of early temperament. *Child Development, 53*, 571–600.

Hudson, W. W. (1982). *Clinical measurement package.* Homewood, IL: The Dorsey Press.

Hudson, J. I., Laffer, P. S., & Pope, H. G., Jr. (1982). Bulimia related to affective disorder by family history and response to the dexamethasone suppression test. *American Journal of Psychiatry, 137,* 695–697.

Huessy, H., Cohen, S., Blair, C., & Rood, P. (1978). *Clinical explorations in adult MBD.* Paper presented at the conference on MBD in adults, Scottsdale, Arizona.

Hurst, M. W., Jenkins, C. D., & Rose, R. M. (1976). The relation of psychological stress to onset of medical illness. *Annual Review of Medicine, 27,* 301–312.

Hutchings, B., & Mednick, S. A. (1975). Registered criminality in the adoptive and biological parents of registered male criminals. In S. A. Mednick (Ed.), *Genetics, environment and psychopathology.* Amsterdam: North-Holland.

Hutchings, B., & Mednick, S. A. (1977). Criminality in adoptees and their adoptive and biological parents: A pilot study. In S. A. Mednick & K. O. Christiansen (Eds.), *Biosocial bases of criminal behavior.* New York: Gardner Press.

Ihda, S. (1961). A study of neurosis by twin method. *Psychiatria et Neurologia Japonica, 63.*

Ihilevich, D., & Gleser, G. C. (1982). *Evaluating mental health programs: The Progress Evaluation Scales.* Lexington, MA: Lexington Books.

Imlah, N. W. (1961). Narcolepsy in identical twins. *Journal of Neurology, Neurosurgery, and Psychiatry, 24,* 158–160.

Ingram, T. T. S. (1970). The nature of dyslexia. In F. A. Young & D. B. Lindsley (Eds.), *Early experience and visual information processing in perceptual and reading disorders.* Washington, DC: National Academy of Sciences.

Inouye, E. (1961). Similarity and dissimilarity of schizophrenia in twins. *Proceedings of the 3rd World Congress of Psychiatry, 1,* 524–530.

Jackson, D. N. (1967). *Personality Research Form Manual.* Port Huron, MI: Research Psychologists Press.

Jackson, D. N. (1978). Interpreter's guide to the Jackson Personality Inventory. In P. McReynolds (Ed.), *Advances in psychological assessment* (Vol. 4). San Francisco: Jossey-Bass.

Jacobs, P. A., & Strong, J. A. (1959). A case of human intersexuality having a possible XXY sex-determining mechanism. *Nature, 183,* 302.

Jacobs, P. A., Brunton, M., Melville, M. M., Brittain, R. P., & McClemont, W. F. (1965). Aggressive behavior, mental sub-normality and the XYY male. *Nature, 208,* 1351–1352.

Jacobs, P. A., Glover, T. W., Mayer, M., Fox, P., Gerrard, J. W., Dunn, H., & Herbst, D. S. (1980). X-linked mental retardation: A study of seven families. *American Journal of Medical Genetics, 7,* 471–489.

James, N. M., & Chapman, C. J. (1975). A genetic study of bipolar affective disorder. *British Journal of Psychiatry, 126,* 449–456. (a)

James, N. M., & Chapman, C. J. (1975). A genetic study of bipolar affective disorder. *British Journal of Psychiatry, 126,* 440–456. (b)

James, J. W. (1971). Frequency in relatives in an all-or-none trait. *Annals of Human Genetics, 35,* 47.

James. W. (1902). *The varieties of religious experience.* New York: Longmans.

Janz, D., & Beck-Mannagetta, G. (1982). Epilepsy and neonatal seizures in the offspring of parents with epilepsy. In V. E. Anderson, W. A. Hauser, J. K. Penry, & C. F. Sing (Eds.), *Genetic basis of the epilepsies.* New York: Raven Press.

Jefferson, J. W., & Marshall, J. R. (1981). *Neuropsychiatric features of medical disorders.* New York: Plenum Press.

Jenkins, E., Duncan, C., Brooks, J., Lele, K., Sanz, M., Nolin, S., & T. Brown. (1983). *Low frequency fragile X chromosomes in cultures from normal people.* Paper presented at the 1983 meeting of the American Society of Human Genetics.

Jenkins, R. L. (1966). Psychiatric syndromes in children and their relation to family background. *American Journal of Orthopsychiatry, 36,* 450–457.

Jervis, G. A. (1939). The genetics of phenylpyruvic oligophrenia. *Journal of Mental Science, 85,* 719.

Jervis, G. A. (1953). Phenylpyruvic oligophrenia: Deficiency of phenylalanine oxidizing system. *Proceedings of the Society for Experimental Biology and Medicine, 82,* 514.

Jervis, G. A. (1959). Studies of phenylpyruvic oligophrenia: The position of the metabolic error. *Journal of Biological Chemistry, 169.*

Jervis, G. A., Block, R. J., Bolling, D., & Kanze, L. (1940). Phenylalanine content of blood and spinal fluid in phenylpyruvic oligophrenia. *Journal of Biological Chemistry, 134.*

Jinks, L. J., & Fulker, D. W. (1970). Comparison of the biometrical genetical, MAVA, and classical approaches to the analysis of human behavior. *Psychological Bulletin, 73,* 311–349.

Johnson, D. J., & Myklebust, H. R. (1967). *Learning disabilities.* New York: Grune & Stratton.

Johnson, G. F. S., Hunt, G. E., Robertson, S., & Doran, T. J. (1982). A linkage study of manic-depressive disorder and HLA antigens, blood groups, serum proteins and red cell enzymes. *Journal of Affective Disorders, 3,* 43–58.

Johnson, W. (1959). *The onset of stuttering.* Minneapolis: University of Minnesota Press.

Jonsson, E., & Nilsson, T. (1968). Alkoholkonsumtion hos monozygota och dizygota tvillingpar. *Nordisk Hygienisk Tidskrift, 49,* 21.

Juberg, R. C., & Massidi, I. (1980). A new form of X-linked mental retardation with growth retardation, deafness and microgenitalism. *American Journal of Human Genetics, 32,* 714–722.

Juda, A. (1949). The relationship between highest mental capacity and psychiatric abnormalities. *American Journal of Psychiatry, 106,* 296–307.

Juda, A. (1950). Genius and psychosis. *Journal of the American Medical Association, 144,* 692.

Juda, A. (1953). *Hochstbegabung* [High talent]. München: Urbach und Schwarzenberg.

Juel-Nielsen, N. (1964). Individual and environment: Monozygotic twins reared apart. *Acta Psychiatrica Scandinavica, 40,* 158–292.

Juel-Nielsen, N., & Harvald, B. (1958). The electroencephalogram in uniovular twins brought up apart. *Acta Genetica, 8,* 57–64.

Jung, C. G. (1923). *Psychological types.* New York: Harcourt Brace.

Kaffman, M. (1962). Enuresis amongst kibbutz children. *Journal of the Medical Association of Israel, 63,* 251–253.

Kaij, L. (1960). *Alcoholism in twins.* Stockholm: Almqvist & Wiksell.

Kaiser-McCaw, B., Hecht, F., Cadlen, J. D., & Moore, B. C. (1980). Letter to the editor: Fragile X-linked mental retardation. *American Journal of Medical Genetics, 7,* 503–506.

Kales, A., Paulson, M., Jacobsen, A., & Kales, J. D. (1966). Somnambulism: Psychophysiological correlates. *Archives of General Psychiatry, 14,* 595–604.

Kales, A., Soldatos, C., Caldwell, A., Kales, J., Humphrey, F., Charney, D., & Schweitzer,

P. (1980). Somnambulism: Clinical characteristics & personality patterns, *Archives of General Psychiatry, 37,* 1410–1420. (a)

Kales, J., Kales, A., Soldatos, C., Caldwell, A., Charney, D., & Martin, E. (1980). Night terrors. *Archives of General Psychiatry, 37,* 1413–1417. (b)

Kales, A., Soldatos, C. R., Bixler, E. O., Ladda, R. L., Charney, D. S., Weber, G., & Schweitzer, P. K. (1980). Hereditary factors in sleepwalking and night terrors. *British Journal of Psychiatry, 137,* 111–118. (c)

Kallmann, F. J. (1938). *The genetics of schizophrenia.* New York: J. J. Augustin.

Kallmann, F. (1946). Genetic theory of schizophrenia: An analysis of 691 schizophrenic twins. *American Journal of Psychiatry, 103,* 309–332.

Kallmann, F. J. (1954). Genetic principles in manic-depressive psychoses. In P. Hoch & J. Zubin (Eds.) *Depression.* New York: Grune & Stratton.

Kallmann, F. J., & Mickey, J. S. (1946). Genetic concepts and folie à deux. *Journal of Heredity, 37,* 298–305.

Kallmann, F. J., & Roth, B. (1956). Genetic aspects of preadolescent schizophrenia, *American Journal of Psychiatry, 112,* 599–606.

Kan, Y. W., & Dozy, A. M. (1978). Polymorphism of DNA sequence adjacent to human B-globin structural gene: Relationship to sickle mutation. *Proceedings of the National Academy of Science, 75,* 5631.

Kanner, L. (1943). Autistic disturbances of affective contact. *The Nervous Child, 2,* 217–250.

Kaplan, B. (1964). *The inner world of mental illness.* New York: Harper & Row.

Karlsson, J. L. (1966). *The biologic basis of schizophrenia.* Springfield, IL: C. C Thomas.

Karlsson, J. L. (1973). An Icelandic family study of schizophrenia. *British Journal of Psychiatry, 123,* 549–554.

Karlsson, J. L. (1981). Genetics of intellectual variation in Iceland. *Hereditas, 95,* 283–288.

Kay, D. W. K. (1964). The genetics of stuttering. In G. Andrews & M. Harris (Eds.), *The syndrome of stuttering* (Clinics in Developmental Medicine, No. 17). London: Heinemann.

Kendler, K. S., Gruenberg, A. M., & Strauss, J. S. (1981). An independent analysis of the Copenhagen sample of the Danish Adoption Study of Schizophrenia. I. The relationship between anxiety disorder and schizophrenia. *Archives of General Psychiatry, 38,* 973–977. (a)

Kendler, K. S., Gruenberg, A. M., & Strauss, J. S. (1981). An independent analysis of the Copenhagen sample of the Danish Adoption Study of Schizophrenia. II. The relationship between schizotypal personality disorder and schizophrenia. *Archives of General Psychiatry, 38,* 982–984. (b)

Kendler, K. S., Gruenberg, A. M., & Strauss, J. S. (1981). An independent analysis of the Copenhagen sample of the Danish Adoption Study of Schizophrenia. III. The relationship between paranoid psychosis (delusional disorder) and the schizophrenic spectrum disorders. *Archives of General Psychiatry, 38,* 985–987. (c)

Kendler, K. S., Gruenberg, A. M., & Strauss, J. S. (1982). An independent analysis of the Copenhagen sample of the Danish Adoption Study of Schizophrenia. V. The relationship between childhood social withdrawal and adult schizophrenia. *Archives of General Psychiatry, 39,* 1257–1261.

Kessler, S. (1975). Extra chromosomes and criminality. In R. Fieve, D. Rosenthal, & H. Brill (Eds.), *Genetic research in psychiatry.* Baltimore: Johns Hopkins University Press.

Kessler, S., Guilleminault, C., & Dement, W. C. (1974). A family study of 50 REM narcoleptics. *Acta Neurologica Scandinavica, 50,* 503–512.

Kety, S., Rosenthal, D., Wender, P. H., & Schulsinger, F. (1968). The types and prevalence of mental illness in the biological and adoptive families of adopted schizophrenics. In D. Rosenthal & S. S. Kety (Eds.), *The transmission of schizophrenia.* Oxford: Pergamon Press.

Kety, S. S., Rosenthal, D., & Wender, P. H. (1978). The biological and adoptive families of adopted individuals who became schizophrenic: Prevalence of mental illness and other characteristics. In L. C. Wynne (Ed.), *The nature of schizophrenia.* New York: Wiley.

Kidd, K. K. (1975). On the possible magnitudes of selective forces maintaining schizophrenia in the population. In R. Fieve, D. Rosenthal, & H. Brill (Eds.), *Genetic research in psychiatry.* Baltimore: Johns Hopkins University Press.

Kidd, K. K. (1977). A genetic perspective on stuttering. *Journal of Fluency Disorders, 2,* 259–269.

Kidd, K. K. (1979). Empiric recurrence risks and models of inheritance: Part II. In C. J. Epstein, C. R. Curry, S. Packman, S. Sherman, & B. D. Hall (Eds.), *Genetic counseling: Risks, communication and decision making.* New York: Alan R. Liss.

Kidd, K. K. (1980). Genetic models of stuttering. *Journal of Fluency Disorders, 5,* 187–201.

Kidd, K. K., & Gladstein, K. (1980). Alternative models for genetic analyses of complex human traits. In M. Melnick, D. Bixler, & E. Shields (Eds.), *Progress in clinical and biological research. Vol. 46: Etiology of cleft lip and cleft palate.* New York: Alan R. Liss.

Kidd, K. K., & Matthysse, S. W. (1978). Research designs for the study of gene–environment interactions in psychiatric disorders: Report of an FFRP panel. *Archives of General Psychiatry, 35,* 925.

Kidd, K. K., & Spence, M. A. (1976). Genetic analysis of pyloric stenosis suggesting a specific maternal effect. *Journal of Medical Genetics, 13,* 290.

Kidd, K. K., Bernoco, D., Carbonara, A. O., Daneo, V., Steiger, U., & Ceppellini, R. (1978). Genetic analyses of HLA associated diseases: The "illness susceptible" gene frequency and sex ratio in ankylosing spondylitis. In J. Dasset & A. Svejgaard (Eds.), *HLA and disease.* Copenhagen: Munksgaard.

Kidd, K. K., Prusoff, B. A., & Cohen, D. J. (1980). Familial pattern of Gilles de la Tourette syndrome. *Archives of General Psychiatry, 37,* 1336–1339.

Kidd, K. K., Egeland, J. A., Molthan, L., Pauls, D. L., Kruger, S. D., & Messner, K. H. (1984). Amish study IV. Genetic linkage study of bipolar pedigrees. *American Journal of Psychiatry, 41,* 1042–1048.

Kiloh, L., & Garside, R. (1963). The independence of neurotic depression and endogenous depression. *British Journal of Psychiatry, 109,* 451–463.

Kissin, B., & Hanson, M. (1982). The bio-psycho-social perspective in alcoholism. In J. Solomon (Ed.), *Alcoholism and clinical psychiatry.* New York: Plenum Press.

Klerman, G. L. (1982). Prevention of alcoholism. In J. Solomon (Ed.), *Alcoholism and Clinical Psychiatry.* New York: Plenum Press.

Knox, W. E. (1974). Phenylketonuria. In J. B. Stanbury, J. B. Wyngaarden, & D. S. Frederickson (Eds.), *The metabolic basis of inherited disease* (2nd ed.). New York: McGraw-Hill.

Kobasa, S. C. (1979). Stressful life events, personality and health: An inquiry into hardiness. *Journal of Personality and Social Psychology, 37,* 1–11.

Koch, G. (1967). Epilepsien. In H. Becker (Ed.), *Human-genetik: Ein kurzes Handbuch in funf Banden* (Vol. 5/2). Stuttgart: Thieme.

Kohlbeg, L., LaCrosse, J., & Ricks, D. (1972). The predictability of adult mental health from childhood behavior. In B. Wolman (Ed.), *Manual of child psychopathology*. New York: McGraw-Hill.

Kolvin, I. (1971). Psychoses in children—a comparative study. In M. Rutter (Ed.), *Infantile autism: Concepts, characteristics and treatment*. London: Churchill-Livingstone.

Kolvin, I., Wolff, S., Barber, L. M., Tweddic, E. G., Garside, R., Scott, D. M., & Chambers, S. (1975). Dimensions of behavior in infant school children. *British Journal of Psychiatry, 126*, 114–126.

Kovacs, M., & Beck, B. T. (1977). An empirical-clinical approach towards a definition of childhood depression. In J. G. Schalterbrandt & A. Raskin (Eds.), *Depression in childhood: Diagnosis, treatment and conceptual models*. New York: Raven Press.

Krabbe, E., & Magnussen, G. (1942). On narcolepsy: I. Familial narcolepsy. *Acta Psychiatrica et Neurologica, 17*, 149–173.

Kraepelin, E. (1896). *Psychiatrie, Ein Lehrbuch für Studierende und Arzte*. Leipzig: Barth.

Kraepelin, E. (1919). *Dementia praecox and paraphrenia* (R. M. Barclay, trans.). Edinburgh: Livingstone.

Kraepelin, E. (1921). *Manic-depressive insanity and paranoia* (R. M. Barclay, trans.). Edinburgh: Livingstone.

Kranz, F. (1937). Untersuchungen an Zwillingen in Fürsorgeerziehunganstalten. *Zeitschrift für induktive Abstammungs—Vererbungslehre, 73*, 508–512.

Kraulis, W. (1931). Zur Vererbung der hysterischen Reaktionsweise. *Zeitschrift für die gesamte Neurologie und Psychiatrie, 136*, 174.

Kravitz, K., Skolnick, M., Cannings, C., Carmelli, D., Baty, B., Amos, B., Johnson, A., Mendell, N., Edwards, C., & Cartwright, G. (1979). Genetic linkage between hereditary hemochromatosis and HLA. *American Journal of Human Genetics, 31*, 601.

Kreitman, N. (1964). The patient's spouse. *British Journal of Psychiatry, 110*, 159–173.

Kringlen, E. (1967). *Heredity and environment in the functional psychoses*. London: Heinemann Medical.

Kringlen, E. (1968). *An epidemiological-clinical twin study on schizophrenia: The transmission of schizophrenia*. New York: Pergamon Press.

Krishef, C. H. (1982). *An introduction to mental retardation*. Springfield, IL: C. C Thomas.

Krohn, A. (1978). *Hysteria: The elusive neurosis* (Psychological Issues Monograph 45-46). New York: International Universities Press.

Kudo, A., Ito, K., & Tanaka, K. (1972). Genetic studies on inbreeding in some Japanese populations. X. The effects of parental consanguinity on psychometric measurements, school performances and school attendance in Shizuoka school children. *Japanese Journal of Human Genetics, 17*, 231–248.

Kunkel, L., Lalande, M., Aldridge, J., Flint, A., & Latt, S. (1983). *A large insert X chromosome specific library for the identification of RFLP haplotypes*. Paper presented at the 1983 meeting of the American Society of Human Genetics.

Kurth, W. (1967). *Genie, Irrsinn and Ruhm* (6th ed. reworked and expanded of original by Wilhelm Lange-Eichbaum). München: E. Reinhardt.

Lachar, D., Gdowski, C. L., & Snyder, D. K. (1982). Broad-band dimensions of psychopathology: Factor scales for the Personality Inventory for Children. *Journal of Consulting and Clinical Psychology, 50,* 634–642.

Lalouel J.-M., Rao, D. C., Morton, N. E., & Elston, R. C. (1983). A unified model for complex segregation analysis. *American Journal of Human Genetics, 35,* 939.

Landis, C., & Bolles, M. M. (1950). *Textbook of abnormal psychology.* New York: Macmillan.

Landis, C., & Mettler, F. A. (1964). *Varieties of psychopathological experience.* New York: Holt, Rinehart & Winston.

Lange, J. (1929). *Verbrechen als Schicksal: Studien an kriminellen Zwillingen* [Crime as fate: Studies of criminal twins]. Leipzig: Thieme.

Lange, K., & Elston, R. C. (1976). Extensions to pedigree analysis: I. Likelihood calculations for simple and complex pedigrees. *Human Heredity, 26,* 337.

Lange, K., Westlake, J., Spence, M. A. (1976).Extensions to pedigree analysis: II. Recurrence risk calculation under the polygenic threshold model. *Human Heredity, 26,*

Lange-Eichbaum, W. *Genie, Irrsinn und Ruhm: Genie Mythes und Pathographie des Geistes* [*Genius, insanity and fame: The myth of genius and the pathological description of genius*]. Basel: E. Reinhardt.

Langfeldt, G. (1956). *Acta Psychiatrica Scandinavica,* Suppl. 110.

Leckman, J., & Gershon, E. (1976). A genetic model of narcolepsy. *British Journal of Psychiatry, 128,* 276–279.

Leckman, J. F., Gershon, E. S., McGinniss, M. H., Targum, S. D., & Dibble, E. D. (1979). New data do not suggest linkage between the Xg blood group and bipolar illness. *Archives of General Psychiatry, 36,* 1436–1441.

Leckman, J. F., Weissman, M. M., Prusoff, B. A., Caruso, K. A., Merikangas, K. R., Pauls, D. L., & Kidd, K. K. (1984). Subtypes of depression: Family study perspective. *Archives of General Psychiatry, 41,* 833–838. (a)

Leckman, J. F., Caruso, K. A., Prusoff, B. A., Weissman, M. M., Merikangas, K. R., & Pauls, D. L. (1984). Appetite disturbance and excessive guilt in major depression: Use of family study data to define depressive subtypes. *Archives of General Psychiatry, 41,* 839–844. (b)

Lefkowitz, M. M., & Burton, N. (1978). Childhood depression: A critique of the concept. *Psychological Bulletin, 85,* 716–726.

Lefkowitz, M. M., Eron, L. D., Walder, L. O., & Huesmann, L. R. (1977). *Growing up to be violent: A longitudinal study of the development of aggression.* New York: Pergamon Press.

Legras, A. M. (1933). Psychose und Kriminalitat bei Zwillingen. *Zeitschrift für die gesamte Neurologie und Psychiatrie, 144,* Parts 1 and 2.

Lehrke, R. G. (1974). X-linked mental retardation and verbal disability. *Birth Defects, 12,* 1–100.

Lejeune, J., Gautier, M., & Turpin, R. (1959). Étude des chromosomes somatiques de neuf enfants mongoliens. *Comptes Rendus des Séances de l'Academie des Sciences,* Paris, *248,* 1721–1722.

Lenneberg, E. H. (1967). *Biological foundations of language.* New York: Wiley.

Lennox, W. G., & Jolly, D. (1954). Seizures, brain waves and intelligence tests of epileptic twins. In D. Hooker & C. C. Hare (Eds.), *Genetics and the inheritance of integrated neurological and psychiatric patterns. Proceedings of the Association for Research in Nervous and Mental Disease, 33,* 325–345.

Lennox, W. G., Gibbs, F. A., & Gibbs, E. L. (1945). The brain wave pattern: An hereditary trait, evidenced from 74 normal twins. *Journal of Heredity, 36,* 233–243.

Lennox, W., & Jolly, D. (1954). Seizures, brain waves and intelligence: Tests of Epileptic brains. In W. Lennox & D. Jolly (Eds.), *Genetics and the inheritance of integrated neurological and psychiatric patterns.* Baltimore: Williams & Witkins.

Leonard, K. (1957). *Aufteilung der endogenen Psychosen.* Berlin: Akademie Verlag.

Lewine, R. R. (1981). Sex differences in schizophrenia: Timing or subtypes. *Psychological Bulletin, 90*, 432–44.

Lewinsohn, P. M., & Talkington, J. (1979). Studies on the measurement of unpleasant events and relations with depression. *Applied Psychological Measurement, 3*, 83–101.

Lewitter, F., DeFries, J. C., & Elston, R. C. (1980). Genetic models of reading disability. *Behavior Genetics, 10*, 9–30.

Lieber, C. S. (1972). Metabolism of ethanol and alcoholism: Racial and acquired factors. *Annals of Internal Medicine, 76*, 326–327.

Linna, S. L., Koivisto, M., & Herva, R. (1980). Chromosomal etiology of mental retardation: A survey of 1,000 mentally retarded patients. In P. Mittler (Ed.), *Frontiers of knowledge in mental retardation* (Vol. 2): *Biomedical aspects.* Baltimore: University Park Press.

Ljungberg, L. (1957). Hysteria—a clinical, prognostic and genetic study. *Acta Psychiatrica et Neurologica Scandinavica, 32*, Suppl. 112.

Lloyd, C. (1980). Life events and depressive disorder reviewed. I. Events as pre-disposing factors. *Archives of General Psychiatry, 37*, 529–535. (a)

Lloyd, C. (1980). Life events and depressive disorder reviewed. II. Events as precipitating factors. *Archives of General Psychiatry, 37*, 541–548. (b)

Loeber, R., & Dishion, T. (1983). Early predictors of male delinquency: A review. *Psychological Bulletin, 94*, 68–99.

Lombroso, C. (1887). *L'homme criminel.* Paris: Alcan.

Loney, J., & Milich, R. (1981). Hyperactivity, inattention, and aggression in clinical practice. In M. Wolraich & D. D. Routh (Eds.), *Advances in behavioral pediatrics* (Vol. 2). Greenwich, CT: JAI Press.

Lopez, R. E. (1965). Hyperactivity in twins. *Canadian Psychiatric Association Journal, 10*.

Lorr, M., Klett, C. J., & McNair, D. M. (1963). *Syndromes of psychosis.* New York: Macmillan.

Lorr, M., Klett, C. J., McNair, D. M., & Lasky, J. J. (1963). *Inpatient multi-dimensional psychiatric scale: Manual.* Palo Alto, CA: Psychological Press.

Lorr, M. (1974). Assessing psychotic behavior by IMPS. *Modern problems in Pharmacopsychiatry, 1*, 50–63.

Losowsky, M. S. (1944). Hereditary mental defect showing the pattern of sex influence. *Journal of Mental Deficiency Research, 48*, 60–62.

Lowe, T. L., Tanaka, K. Seashore, M. R., Young, J. G., & Cohen, D. J. (1980). Detection of phenylketonuria in autistic and psychotic children. *Journal of the American Medical Association, 243*, 126–128.

Luborsky, L. (1962). Clinicians' judgments of mental health: A proposed scale. *Archives of General Psychiatry, 7*, 407–417.

Lubs, H. A. (1969). A marker X chromosome. *American Journal of Human Genetics, 21*, 231–244.

Lubs, H. A., & Walknowska, J. (1977). New chromosomal syndromes and mental retardation. In P. Mittler (Ed.), *Research to practice in mental retardation* (Vol. 3): *Biomedical aspects.* Baltimore: University Park Press.

Lucas, A., Rodin, E., & Simson, C. (1965). Neurological assessment of children with early school problems. *Developmental Medicine and Child Neurology, 7,* 145–149.

Luchsinger, R., & Arnold, C. E. (1965). *Voice, speech and language.* Belmont, CA: Wadsworth.

Luxenberger, H. (1930). Psychiatrisch-neurologische Zwillingspathologie. *Zentralblatt für die gesamte Neurologie und Psychiatrie, 56,* 145–181.

Lykken, D. T., Tellegen, A., & Thorkelson, K. A. (1974). Genetic determination of EEG frequency spectra. *Biological Psychology, 1,* 245–259.

Lykken, D. T., Tellegen, A., & Iacono, W. G. (1982). EEG spectra in twins: Evidence for a neglected mechanism of genetic determination. *Physiological Psychology, 10,* 60–65.

Lyon, M. F. (1961). Gene action in the X-chromosome of the mouse (*Mus musculus L.*). *Nature, 190,* 372–373.

Maas, J. W., Koslow, S. H., Davis, J. M., Katz, M. M., Mendels, J. H., Robins, E., Stokes, A., & Bowden, C. L. (1980). Biological component of the NIMH Clinical Research Branch Collaborative Program on the Psychobiology of Depression: I. Background and theoretical considerations. *Psychological Medicine, 10,* 759–776.

MacMahon, B. (1978). Epidemiological approaches to family resemblance. In N. Morton, & C. Chung (Eds.), *Genetic epidemiology.* New York: Academic Press.

Mahanand, D., Wypych, M., & Calcagno, P. (1976). Serum zinc and copper levels in autistic patients and matched controls. In M. Coleman (Ed.), *The autistic syndromes.* Amsterdam: North-Holland.

Malec, J. (1978). Neuropsychological assessment of schizophrenia versus braindamage: A review. *Journal of Nervous and Mental Disease, 166,* 507–516.

Marsh, B., Yen, P., Mohandas, T., & Shapiro, L. J. (1983). *Isolation of human X chromosome DNA clones homologous to coding sequences.* Paper presented at the meeting of the American Society of Human Genetics.

Marshall, W., & Ferguson, J. (1939). Hereditary word blindness as a defect of selective attention. *Journal of Nervous and Mental Ability, 89,* 164–173.

Martin, J. P., & Bell, J. (1943). A pedigree of mental defect showing sex linkage. *Journal of Neurology and Psychiatry, 6,* 154–157.

Mash, E. J., & Terdal, L. G. (Eds.) (1981). *Behavioral assessment of childhood disorders.* New York: Guilford Press.

Matheny, A. P., & Dolan, A. B. (1974). A twin study of genetic influence in reading achievement. *Journal of Learning Disabilities, 7,* 99–102.

Matthews, A. M., Gelder, M. G., & Johnston, D. W. (1981). *Agoraphobia, nature and treatment.* New York: Gilford Press.

Matthysse, S. W., & Kidd, K. K. (1976). Estimating the genetic contribution to schizophrenia. *American Journal of Psychiatry, 133,* 185–191.

Mattei, M. G., Mattei, J. F., Vidal, I., & Giraud, F. (1981). Expression in lymphocyte and fibroblast culture of the fragile X-chromosome—a new technical approach. *Human Genetics, 59,* 166–169.

Mattis, S., French, J. H., & Rapin, I. (1975). Dyslexia in children and young adults: Three independent neuropsychological syndromes. *Developmental Medicine and Child Neurology, 17,* 150–163.

Maxson, S. C., & Cowen, J. S. (1976). Electroencephalographic correlates of the audiogenic seizure response of inbred mice. *Physiology and Behavior, 16,* 623–629.

McClearn, G. E. (1973). The genetic aspects of alcoholism. In P. G. Bourne & R. Fox (Eds.), *Alcoholism: Progress in research and treatment.* New York: Academic Press.

McClearn, G. E., & DeFries, J. C. (1973). *Introduction to behavioral genetics.* San Francisco: Freeman.

McCullough, J. M. (1978). Phenylketonuria: A balanced polymorphism in Europe? *Journal of Human Evolution, 7,* 231–237.

McDevitt, S. C., & Carey, W. B. (1978). The measurement of temperament in 3–4 year old children. *Journal of Child Psychology and Psychiatry, 19,* 245–253.

McInnes, R. G. (1937). Observations on heredity in neurosis. *Proceedings of the Royal Society of Medicine, 30,* 895–904.

McKusick, V. A. (1978). *Mendelian inheritance in man: Catalogs of autosomal dominant, autosomal recessive, and X-linked phenotypes* (5th ed.). Baltimore: Johns Hopkins University Press.

McMenemey, W. H. (1970). Alois Alzheimer and his disease. In G. E. W. Wolstenholme & M. O'Connor (Eds.), *Alzheimer's disease and related conditions* (pp. 5–9). London: J. & A. Churchill.

McQuaid, P. E. (1975). Infantile autism in twins. *British Journal of Psychiatry, 127,* 530–534.

Mednick, S. A., & Schulsinger, F. (1968). Some premorbid characteristics related to breakdown in children with schizophrenic mothers. In D. Rosenthal & S. S. Kety (Eds.), *The transmission of schizophrenia.* Oxford: Pergamon Press.

Mednick, S. A., & Volavka, J. (1980). Biology and crime. In N. Morris & M. Tonry (Eds.), *Crime and justice: An annual review of research* (Vol. 11). Chicago: University of Chicago Press.

Mednick, S. A., Pollock, V., Volavka, J., & Gabrielli, W. F. (1982). Biology and violence. In M. E. Wolfgang & N. A. Weiner (Eds.), *Criminal violence.* Beverly Hills: Sage Publications.

Mednick, S. A., Gabrielli, W. F., & Hutchings, B. (1983). Genetic influences in criminal behavior: Some evidence from an adoption cohort. In K. T. VanDusen & S. A. Mednick (Eds.), *Prospective studies of crime and delinquency.* Hingham, MA: Martinus Nyhoff.

Mellsop, G. (1972). Psychiatric patients seen as children and adults: Childhood predictors of adult illness. *Journal of Child Psychology and Psychiatry, 13,* 91–101.

Mendell, N. R., & Spence, M. A. (1979). Empiric recurrence risks and models of inheritance: Part I. In C. J. Epstein, C. R. Curry, S. Packman, S. Sherman, & B. D. Hall (Eds.), *Genetic counseling: Risks, communication and decision making.* New York: Alan R. Liss.

Mendlewicz, J., & Rainer, J. D. (1974). Morbidity risk and genetic transmission in manic-depressive illness. *American Journal of Human Genetics, 26,* 692–701.

Mendlewicz, J., & Rainer, J. D. (1977). Adoption study supporting genetic transmission in manic-depressive illness. *Nature, 268,* 327–329.

Mendlewicz, J., Fleiss, J. L., & Fieve, R. R. (1972). Evidence for X-linkage in the transmission of manic-depressive illness. *Journal of the American Medical Association, 222,* 1624–1627.

Mendlewicz, J., Fleiss, J. L., & Fieve, R. R. (1975). Linkage studies in affective disorders: The Xg blood group and manic-depressive illness. In R. Fieve, D. Rosenthal, & H. Brill (Eds.), *Genetics and psychopathology.* Baltimore: Johns Hopkins University Press.

Mendlewicz, J., Linkowski, P., Guroff, J. J., & Van Praag, H. M. (1979). Color blindness linkage to bipolar manic-depressive illness: New evidence. *Archives of General Psychiatry, 36,* 1442–1447.

Mendlewicz, J., Linkowski, P., & Wilmotte, J. (1980). Linkage between glucose-6-phosphate dehydrogenase deficiency and manic depressive psychosis. *British Journal of Psychiatry, 137,* 337–342.

Merikangas, K. R. (1982). Assortative mating for psychiatric disorders and psychological traits. *Archives of General Psychiatry, 39,* 1173–1180.

Merikangas, K. R., Leckman, J. F., Prusoff, B. A., Pauls, D. L., & Weissman, M. M. (1985). Familial transmission of depression and alcoholism. *Archives of General Psychiatry, 42,* 367–372.

Meryash, D. L., Szymanski, L. S., & Gerald, P. S. (1982). Infantile autism associated with the fragile X syndrome. *Journal of Autism and Developmental Disorders, 12,* 295–302.

Metrakos, J. D., & Metrakos, K. (1960). Genetics of convulsive disorders. I. Introduction, problems, methods and base lines. *Neurology, 10,* 228–240.

Metrakos, K., & Metrakos, J. D. (1961). Genetics of convulsive disorders. II. Genetic and electro-encephalographic studies in centrencephalic epilepsy. *Neurology, 11,* 474–483.

Meyer-Gross, W., Slater, E., & Roth, M. (1969). *Clinical psychiatry* (3rd ed.). London: Bailliera, Tindall and Cassell.

Michael-Smith, H., Morgenstern, M., & Karp, E. (1969). *Dyslexia in four siblings.* Paper presented at the meeting of the American Orthopsychiatric Association.

Miner, G. D. (1973). The evidence of genetic components in the neuroses: A review. *Archives of General Psychiatry, 29,* 111–118.

Mirowsky, J., & Wheaton, B. (1970). *A comparison of factor structures for a sample of life change events in four populations.* Unpublished report.

Mirsky, A. F. (1969). Neuropsychological bases of schizophrenia. *Annual Review of Psychology, 20,* 321–348.

Mischel, W. (1968). *Personality and assessment.* New York: Wiley.

Mischel, W. (1971). *Introduction to personality.* New York: Holt, Rinehart & Winston.

Mitsuda, H. (1965). The concept of atypical psychoses from the aspect of clinical genetics. *Acta Psychiatrica Scandinavica. 41,* 372–377.

Mitsuda, H., Sakai, T., & Kobayashi, J. (1967). A clinico-genetic study on the relationship between neurosis and psychosis. *Bulletin of the Osaka Medical School, 12,* 27–35.

Moor, L. (1967). Niveau intellectuel et polygonosomie: Confrontation du caryotype et due niveau mental de 374 malades dont le caryotype comporte un exces de chromosomes X ou Y [Intellectual level and polyploidy: A comparison of karyotype and intelligence of 374 patients with extra X or Y chromosomes]. *Revue de Neuropsychiatrie Infantile, 15,* 325–348.

Morgan, H. G., & Russell, G. F. M. (1975). Value of family background in clinical features as predictors of long-term outcome in anorexia nervosa: Four-year follow-up study of 41 patients. *Psychological Medicine, 5,* 355–71.

Morihisa, J. M., Duffy, F. H., & Wyatt, R. J. (1982). Topographic analysis of computer processed electroencephalography in schizophrenia. In E. Usdin & I. Hanin (Eds.), *Biological markers in psychiatry and neurology.* New York: Pergamon Press.

Morris, H. H. Jr., Escoll, P. J., & Wexler, R. (1956). Aggressive behavior disorders of childhood: A follow-up study. *American Journal of Psychiatry, 112,* 991–997.

Morrison, J. R., & Stewart, M. A. (1971). A family study of the Hyperactive Child syndrome. *Biological Psychiatry, 3,* 189–195.

Morrison, J. R., & Stewart, M. A. (1973). The psychiatric status of the legal families of adopted hyperactive children. *Archives of General Psychiatry, 28,* 888–891.

Morrison, J. R., & Stewart, M. (1974). Bilateral inheritance as evidence for polygenicity in the hyperactive child syndrome. *Journal of Nervous and Mental Diseases, 158,* 226–228.

Morton, L. A., & Kidd, K. K. (1979). Likelihood analysis of high-density pedigrees of stuttering. *Behavior Genetics, 9,* 470A. (Abstract)

Morton, N. E. (1955). Sequential test for the detection of linkage. *American Journal of Human Genetics, 7,* 277–318.

Morton, N. E. (1956). The detection and estimation of linkage between the genes for elliptocytosis and the Rh blood type. *American Journal of Human Genetics, 8,* 80–96.

Morton, N. E., & MacLean, C. J. (1974). Analysis of family resemblance. III. Complex segregation analysis of quantitative traits. *American Journal of Human Genetics, 26,* 489.

Morton, N. E., Yee, S., & Lew, R. (1971). Complex segregation analysis. *American Journal of Human Genetics, 23,* 602.

Mosher, L. R., Pollin, W., & Stabenau, J. P. (1971). Families with identical twins discordant for schizophrenia: Some relationships between identification, thinking styles, psychopathology and dominance-submissiveness. *British Journal of Psychiatry, 118,* 29–42.

Murray, H. A. (1938). *Explorations in personality.* New York: Oxford University Press.

Myrianthopoulos, N. C. (1966). Huntington's chorea. *Journal of Medical Genetics, 3,* 298–314.

Nachtsheim, H. (1939). Krampfbereitschaft und Genotypus. I. Die Epilepsie der weissen Wiener Kaninchen. *Zeitschrift für Menschliche Vererbungs und Konstitutionslehre, 22,* 791–810.

Naidoo, S. (1972). *Specific dyslexia.* New York: Wiley.

Nance, W. E., Corey, L. A. (1976). Genetic models for the analysis of data from families of identical twins. *Genetics, 83,* 811.

Nance, W. E., & Corey, L. A. (1977, March). Letter to the editor. *Genetics, 85.*

National Center for Health Statistics. (1971). *Report number 108, Series 11.* Washington, DC: Department of Health, Education, and Welfare.

Neale, J. M., & Oltmanns, T. F. (1980). *Schizophrenia.* New York: Wiley.

Neel, J. V., Schull, W. J., Yamamoto, M., Uchida, S., Yanabe, T., & Fujiki, N. (1970). The effects of parental consanguinity and inbreeding in Hirado, Japan. II. Physical development, tapping rate, blood pressure, intelligence quotient, and school performance. *American Journal of Human Genetics, 22,* 263–286.

Nelson, J. C., & Charney, D. A. (1980). Primary affective disorder criteria and the endogenous-reactive distinction. *Archives of General Psychiatry, 37,* 786–793.

Nelson, K., & Ellenberg, J. (1978). Prognosis in children with febrile seizures. *Pediatrics, 61,* 720–722.

Nelson, S. E., Hunter, N., & Walter, M. (1945). Stuttering in twin types. *Journal of Speech Disorders, 10,* 335–343.

Newell, T. G. (1969). Three biometrical genetic analyses of activity in the mouse. *Journal of Comparative and Physiological Psychology, 70,* 34–47.

Nielsen, K. B., Tommerup, N., Poulsen, H., & Mikkelsen, M. (1981). X-linked mental retardation with fragile X: A pedigree showing transmission by apparently unaffected males and partial expression in female carriers. *Human Genetics, 59,* 23–25.

Nogami, Y. & Yabana, F. (1977). On kibarashi-gui (binge-eating). *Folia Psychiatrica et Neurologica Japonica, 31,* 159–66.

Nomura, Y., & Segawa, M. (1979). Gilles de la Tourette syndrome in Oriental children. *Brain Development, 2,* 103–111.

Noyes, R., Clancy, J., & Crowe, R. (1978). The familial prevalence of anxiety neurosis. *Archives of General Psychiatry, 35,* 1057–1059.

Nuechterlein, K. H., Soli, S. D., Garmezy, N., Devine, V. T., & Schaefer, S. M. (1981). A classification system for research in childhood psychopathology: Part II. Validation research examining converging descriptions from the parent and from the child. In B. A. Maher & W. B. Maher (Eds.), *Progress in experimental personality Research* (Vol. 10, 163–202). New York: Academic Press.

Nurnburger, J. (1981). *Genetics of affective disorders.* Paper presented at the meeting of the American Society of Human Genetics.

Omenn, G. (1973). Genetic approaches to the syndrome of minimal brain dysfunction. *Annals of the New York Academy of Sciences, 205,* 212–23.

Ornitz, E. M., & Ritvo, E. R. (1976). The syndrome of autism: A critical review. *The American Journal of Psychiatry, 133,* 609–621.

O'Rourke, D. H., Gottesman, I. I., Suarez, B. K., Rice, J., & Reich, T. (1982). Refutation of the general single-locus model for the etiology of schizophrenia. *American Journal of Human Genetics, 34,* 630–649.

Orton, S. T. (1937). *Reading, writing and speech problems in children.* New York: W. W. Norton.

Ott, J. (1976). A computer program for linkage analysis of general human pedigrees. *American Journal of Human Genetics, 28,* 528.

Ovenstone, I. M. K. (1973). The development of neurosis in the wives of neurotic men: II. Marital role functions and marital tension. *British Journal of Psychiatry, 122,* 711–717.

Overall, J. E., & Gorham, D. R. (1962). The brief psychiatric rating scale. *Psychological Reports, 10,* 799–812.

Overall, J. E. (1982). Determinants of alcohol abuse in a psychiatric population: A two-dimensional model. *Applied Psychological Measurement, 6,* 213–218.

Parker, N. (1966). Twin relationships and concordance for neurosis. *Proceedings of 4th World Congress of Psychiatry, 2,* 1112.

Partanen, J. K., Brun, T., & Markkanen, M. (1966). *Inheritance of drinking behavior: A study on intelligence, personality and use of alcohol in adult twins.* Helsinki: The Finnish Foundation for Alcohol Studies (mo. 14).

Pasamanick, B., & Knobloch, H. (1960). Brain damage and reproductive casualty. *American Journal of Orthopsychiatry, 30,* 298–305.

Pauls, D. L., Noyes, R., & Crowe, R. R. (1979). The familial prevalence in second degree relations of patients with anxiety neurosis (panic disorders). *Journal of Affective Disorders, 1,* 279–285.

Pauls, D. L., Bucher, K. D., Crowe, R. R., & Noyes, R. (1980). A genetic study of panic disorder pedigrees. *American Journal of Human Genetics, 32,* 639–644.

Pauls, D. L., Cohen, D. J., Heimbuch, R., Detlor, J., & Kidd, K. K. (1981). Familial pattern and transmission of Gilles de la Tourette syndrome and multiple tics. *Archives of General Psychiatry, 38,* 1091–1093.

Pauls, D. L., Kruger, S. D., Leckman, J. F., Cohen, D. J., & Kidd, K. K. (1984). The risk of Tourette's syndrome and chronic multiple tics among relatives of Tourette's syndrome patients obtained by direct interview. *Journal of the American Academy of Child Psychiatry, 23:* 134–137.

Paulson, G., & Allen, N. (1970). The nervous system. In R. M. Goodman (Ed.), *Genetic disorders of man.* Boston: Little, Brown.

Paykel, E. S. (1979). Predictors of treatment response. In E. S. Paykel & A. Coppen (Eds.), *Psychopharmacology of affective disorders* (pp. 193–220). New York: Oxford University Press.

Payne, T. W. (1970). Disorders of thinking. In C. G. Costello (Ed.), *Symptoms of psychopathology.* New York: Wiley.

Pearson, J. S., & Kley, I. B. (1957). On the application of genetic expectancies as age-specific base rates on the study of human behavior disorders. *Psychological Bulletin, 54,* 406–420.

Peckham, C. (1973). A national study of child development. *Proceedings of the Royal Society of Medicine, 66,* 701–704.

Penfield, W., & Erickson, T. C. (1941). *Epilepsy and cerebral localization.* Springfield, IL: C. C. Thomas.

Penrose, L. S. (1935). The detection of autosomal linkage in data which consist of pairs of brothers and sisters of unspecified parentage. *Annals of Eugenics, 6,* 133.

Penrose, L. S. (1938). *A clinical and genetic study of 1280 cases of mental defect (Colchester Survey).* Medical Research Council Report No. 229. London: Her Majesty's Stationery Office.

Penrose, L. S. (1953). The general purpose sib-pair linkage test. *Annals of Eugenics, 18,* 120–124.

Penrose, L. S., & Smith, G. F. (1966). *Down's anomaly.* London: J. & A. Churchill.

Perley, M. G., & Guze, S. (1962). Hysteria—the stability and usefulness of clinical criteria. *New England Journal of Medicine, 266,* 421–426.

Perris, C. (1966). A study of bipolar (manic-depressive) and unipolar recurrent depressive psychoses. *Acta Psychiatrica Scandinavica,* Suppl. 194.

Petersen, I., & Akesson, H. O. (1968). EEG studies of siblings of children showing 14 and 6 per second positive spikes. *Acta Genetique, 18,* 163–169.

Peterson, D. R. (1961). Behaviour problems in middle childhood. *Journal of Consulting Psychology, 25,* 205–209.

Peterson, M., & Torrey, E. (1976). Viruses and other infectious agents as behavioral teratogens. In M. Coleman (Ed.), *The autistic syndromes.* Amsterdam: North-Holland.

Pierce, C. M., & Lipcon, H. H. (1956). Somnambulism. Electroencephalographic studies and related findings. *U.S. Armed Forces Medical Journal, 7,* 1419.

Pollak, J. M. (1978). Obsessive-compulsive personality: A review. *Psychological Bulletin, 86,* 225–241.

Pollin, W. (1976). Genetic and environmental determinants of neurosis. In A. R. Kaplan (Ed.), *Human behavior genetics.* Springfield, IL: C. C Thomas.

Pond, D. A., Ryle, A., & Hamilton, M. (1963). Marriage and neurosis in a working class population. *British Journal of Psychiatry, 109,* 592–598.

Posen, C. M., & Van Bogaert, L. (1959). Neuropathologic observations in phenylketonuria. *Brain, 82,* 1.

Pratt, R. T. C. (1967). *The genetics of neurological disorders.* London: Oxford University Press.

Prechtl, H., & Stemmer, C. (1962). The choreiform syndrome in children. *Developmental Medicine and Childhood Neurology, 8,* 149–59.

Price, B. (1950). Primary biases in twin studies: A review of prenatal and natal difference-producing factors in monozygotic pairs. *American Journal of Human Genetics, 2,* 293–352.

Price, R. A., Kidd, K. K., Pauls, D. L., Gershon, E. S., Prusoff, B. A., Weissman, M. M. and Goldin, L. R. (1986). Multiple threshold models for the affective disorders: The Yale-NIMH collaborative family study. *Psychiatry Research.*

Propping, P. (1977). Genetic control of ethanol action in the central nervous system: An EEG study in twins. *Human Genetics, 35,* 309–334.

Puig-Antich, J. (1982). Major depression and conduct disorder in prepuberty. *Journal of the Academy of Child Psychiatry, 21,* 118–128.

Puig-Antich, J., & Weston, B. (1963). The diagnosis and treatment of major depressive disorder in childhood. *Annual Review of Medicine, 34,* 231–245.

Purisch, A. D., Golden, C. J., & Hammeke, T. A. (1978). Discrimination of schizophrenic and brain damaged patients by a standardized version of Luria's neuro-psychological tests. *Journal of Consulting and Clinical Psychology, 46,* 1266–1273.

Pyle, R. L., Mitchell, J. E., & Eckert, E. D. (1981). Bulimia: A report of 34 cases. *Journal of Clinical Psychiatry, 42,* 60–64.

Quay, H. C. (1972). Patterns of aggression, withdrawal, and immaturity. In H. C. Quay & J. S. Werry (Eds.), *Psychopathological disorders of childhood.* New York: Wiley.

Quay, H. C., & Werry, J. S. (1979). *Psychopathological disorders of childhood* (2nd ed.). New York: Wiley.

Rabkin, J. G. (1980). Stressful life events and schizophrenia: A review of the research literature. *Psychological Bulletin, 87,* 408–425.

Rabkin, J. G., & Struening, E. L. (1976). Life events, stress and illness. *Science, 198,* 1013–1020.

Rachman, S. J. (1978). *Fear and courage.* San Francisco: W. H. Freeman.

Rachman, S. J., & Hodgson, R. H. (1980). *Obsessions and compulsions.* Englewood Cliffs, NJ: Prentice-Hall.

Rall, T. W., & Schleifer, L. S. (1980). Drugs effective in the therapy of the epilepsies. In L. S. Goodman & A. Gilman (Eds.), *The pharmacological basis of therapeutics* (6th ed.). New York: Macmillan.

Rao, D. C., Morton, N. E., & Yee, S. (1976). Resolution of cultural and biological inheritance by path analysis. *American Journal of Human Genetics, 28,* 228.

Rao, D. C., Morton, N. E., Gottesman, I. I., & Lew, R. (1981). Path analysis of qualitative data on pairs of relatives: Application to schizophrenia. *Human Heredity, 31,* 325–332.

Reed, E. W., & Reed, S. C. (1965). *Mental retardation.* Philadelphia: Saunders.

Reich, T., James, J. W., Morris, C. A. (1972). The use of multiple thresholds in determining the mode of transmission of semi-continuous traits. *Annals of Human Genetics, 36,* 163.

Reich, T., Winokur, G., & Mullaney, J. (1975). The transmission of alcoholism. In R. R. Fieve, D. Rosenthal, & H. Brill (Eds.), *Genetic research in psychiatry.* Baltimore: Johns Hopkins University Press.

Reich, T., Rice, J., Cloninger, C. R., Wette, R., & James, J. (1979). The use of multiple thresholds and segregation analysis in analyzing the phenotypic heterogeneity of multifactorial traits. *Annals of Human Genetics, 42,* 371.

Reich, T., Rice, J., & Cloninger, C. R. (1981). The detection of a major locus in the presence of multifactorial variation. In E. Gershon, S. Matthysse, R. D. Cairanello, & X. O. Breakfield (Eds.), *Genetic strategies in psychobiology and psychiatrv.* Pacific Grove, CA: Boxwood Press.

Reid, E. C. (1910). Autopsychology of the manic-depressive. *Journal of Nervous and Mental Disease, 37,* 606–620.

Reisby, N., Gram, L. F., Bech, P., Sihm, F., Krautwald, O., Elley, J., Ortmann, J., & Christiansen, J. (1979). Plasma levels and clinical effects. *Communications in Psychopharmacology, 3,* 341–351.

Reitan, R. M., & Davison, L. A. (Eds.). (1974). *Clinical neuropsychology: Current status and applications.* New York: Wiley.

Reite, M., & Zimmerman, J. (1978). Magnetic phenomena of the central nervous system. *Annual Review of Biophysics and Bioengineering, 7,* 167–188.

Renpenning, H., Gerrard, J. W., Zaleski, W. A., & Tabata, T. (1962). Familial sex-linked mental retardation. *Canadian Medical Association Journal, 87,* 954–956.

Rice, J., Cloninger, C. R., & Reich, T. (1978). Multifactorial inheritance with cultural transmission and assortative mating. I. Description and basic properties of the unitary models. *American Journal of Human Genetics, 30,* 618.

Richards, B. W., Sylvester, P. E., & Brooker, C. (1981). Fragile X-linked mental retardation: The Martin-Bell syndrome. *Journal of Mental Deficiency Research, 25,* 253–256.

Rimland, B. (1964). *Infantile autism.* New York: Appleton-Century-Crofts.

Rimland, B. (1971). The differentiation of childhood psychoses: An analysis of checklists for 2218 psychotic children. *Journal of Autism and Childhood Schizophrenia, 1,* 161–174.

Roberts, J. A., & Fraser, I. (1952). The genetics of mental deficiency. *Eugenics Review, 44,* 71–83.

Roberts, R. E., & Vernon, S. W. (1983). The Center for Epidemiologic Studies Depression Scale: Its use in a community sample. *American Journal of Psychiatry, 140,* 41–46.

Robins, L. N. (1966). *Deviant children grow up.* Baltimore: Williams & Wilkins.

Robins, L. (1972). Follow-up studies of behavior disorders in children. In H. L. Quay & J. S. Werry (Eds.), *Psychopathological disorders in childhood.* New York: Wiley.

Robins, L. (1978). Sturdy childhood predictors of adult antisocial behaviors: A replication from longitudinal studies. *Psychological Medicine, 8,* 611–622.

Robins, L. N., Helzer, J. E., Weissmann, M. M., Orvaschel, H., Gruenberg, E., Burke, J. D., & Regier, D. A. (1984). Lifetime prevalence of specific psychiatric disorders in three sites. *Archives of General Psychiatry, 41,* 949–958.

Rodin, E., Lucas, A., & Simson, C. (1963). A study of behavior disorders in children by means of general purpose computers. *Proceedings of the Conference on Data Acquisition and Processing in Biological Medicine.* Oxford: Pergamon Press.

Rodin, E. A., & Whelan, J. L. (1960). Familial occurrence of focal temporal electroencephalographic abnormalities. *Neurology, 10,* 542–545.

Rojas-Ramirez, J., & Tauber, E. (1970). Paradoxical sleep in two species of avian predator (Falconiformes). *Science, 167,* 1754–1755.

Rosanoff, A. J., Handy, L. M., & Plesset, I. R. (1935). The etiology of manic-depressive syndromes with special reference to their occurrence in twins. *American Journal of Psychiatry, 91,* 725–762.

Rosanoff, A. J., Handy, L. M., & Plesset, I. R. (1941). The etiology of child behavior difficulties, juvenile delinquency and adult criminals with special reference to their occurence in twins. *Psychiatric Monograph* No. 1. Department of Institutions, Sacramento, California.

Rose, R., & Ditto, W. B. (1983). A developmental-genetic analysis of common fears from early adolescence to early adulthood. *Child Development, 54,* 361–368.

Rosenthal, D. (1959). Some factors associated with concordance and discordance with respect to schizophrenia in monozygotic twins. *Journal of Nervous and Mental Disease, 129,* 1–10.

Rosenthal, D. (1960). Confusion of identity and the frequency of schizophrenia in twins. *Archives of General Psychiatry, 3,* 297–304.

Rosenthal, D. (1961). Sex distribution and the severity of illness among samples of schizophrenic twins. *Journal of Psychiatric Research, 1,* 26–36.

Rosenthal, D. (1963). Familial concordance by sex with respect to schizophrenia. *Psychological Bulletin, 59,* 401.

Rosenthal, D. (1970). *Genetic theory and abnormal behavior.* New York: McGraw-Hill.

Rosenthal, D. (1975). Discussion: The concept of subschizophrenic disorders. In R. R. Fieve, D. Rosenthal, & Brill, H. (Eds.) *Genetic Research in Psychiatry.* Baltimore: Johns Hopkins University Press.

Rosenthal, D., Wender, P. H., Kety, S. S., Schulsinger, F., Welner, J., & Ostergaard, L. (1968). Schizophrenics' offspring reared in adoptive homes. In D. Rosenthal & S. S. Kety (Eds.), *The transmission of schizophrenia* (pp. 377–391). London: Pergamon Press.

Ross, D. M. & Ross, S. A. (1976). *Hyperactivity: Research, theory, action.* New York: Wiley.

Roth, B. (1978). Narcolepsy and hypersomnia. In R. L. William & I. Caracan (Eds.), *Sleep disorders, diagnosis and treatment.* New York: Wiley. (a)

Roth, M. (1978). Diagnosis of senile and related forms of dementia. In R. Katzman, R. D. Terry, and K. L. Bick (Eds.), *Alzheimer's disease: Senile dementia and related disorders.* New York: Raven Press. (b)

Rothman, D., Sorrells, J., & Heldman, P. (1976). *A Global Assessment Scale for Children.* Oakland, CA: Alameda County Mental Health Services.

Routh, D. (1980). Developmental and social aspects of hyperactivity. In C. Wahlen & B. Henker (Eds.), *Hyperactive children: The social ecology of identification and treatment* (pp. 55–62). New York: Academic Press.

Ruckebusch, Y., & Morel, M. T. (1968). Étude polygraphique du sommeil chez le porc. *Comptes Rendus du Sociale Biologie, 162,* 1345–1354.

Rudin, E. (1953). Ein Beitrag zur Frage der Zwangskrankheit, insbesondere ihrer hereditaren Beziehungen [A contribution to the question of compulsive disorder, especially its genetic relations]. *Archiv für Psychologie und Zeitschrift der Neurologie, 191,* 14–54.

Rushton, J. P., & Chrisjohn, R. D. (1981). Extraversion, neuroticism, psychoticism and self-reported delinquency: Evidence from eight separate samples. *Personality and Individual Differences, 2,* 11–20.

Russell, G. F. M. (1979). Bulimia nervosa: An ominous variant of anorexia nervosa. *Psychological Medicine, 9,* 429–448.

Rutter, M. (1967). Psychotic disorders in early childhood. In A. Copper & A. Walk (Eds.), *Recent developments in schizophrenia.* Ashford, Kent: Headley Bros.

Rutter, M. (1968). Concepts of autism: A review of research. *Journal of Child Psychology and Psychiatry, 9,* 1–25.

Rutter, M. (1970). Autistic children: Infancy to adulthood. *Seminars in Psychiatry, 2,* 435–450.

Rutter, M. (1974). The development of infantile autism. *Psychological Medicine, 4,* 147–163.

Rutter, M. (1981). Psychological sequelae of brain damage in children. *American Journal of Psychiatry, 138,* 1533–1544.

Rutter, M. (1982). Syndromes attributed to "minimal brain dysfunction" in childhood. *American Journal of Psychiatry, 139,* 21–33. (a)

Rutter, M. (1982). Introduction. In M. Rutter (Ed.), *Scientific foundations of developmental psychology*. Baltimore: University Park Press. (b)

Rutter, M. (Ed.). (1982). *Temperamental differences in infants and young children*. Ciba Foundation Symposium No. 89. London: Pitman. (c)

Rutter, M., & Hersov, L. (Eds.). (1976). *Child psychiatry: Modern approaches*. Oxford: Blackwell Scientific Publications.

Rutter, M., Graham, P., & Yule, W. (1970). A neuropsychiatric study in childhood. *Clinics in Developmental Medicine*, No. 36, Philadelphia: Lippincott.

Rutter, M., Yule, W., & Graham, P. (1973). Enuresis and behavioural deviance: Some epidemiological considerations. In I. Kolvin, R. MacKeith, & S. R. Meadow, (Eds.), *Bladder control and enuresis* (Clinics in Development Medicine Nos. 48/49). London: Heinemann.

Ryle, A., & Hamilton, M. (1962). Neurosis in 50 married couples. *Journal of Mental Science, 108,* 265–273.

Safer, D. J. (1973). A familial factor in minimal brain dysfunction. *Behavior Genetics, 3,* 175–186.

Sandberg, A. A., Koef, G. F., Ishihara, T., & Hauschka, T. S. (1961). XYY human male. *Lancet, 2,* 488–489.

Sandberg, S., Rutter, M., & Taylor, E. (1978). Hyperkinetic disorder in psychiatric clinic attenders. *Developmental Medicine and Child Neurology, 20,* 279–99.

Sarason, S. B. (1949). *Psychological problems in mental deficiency*. New York: Harper & Row.

Sartorius, N. (1976). Classification: An international perspective. *Psychiatric Annals, 6,* 8.

Sartorius, N., Jablonsky, A., & Shapiro, R. (1977). Two-year follow-up of the patients in the WHO International Pilot Study of Schizophrenia. *Psychological Medicine, 7,* 529–541.

Satz, P., Rardin, D., & Ross, J. (1971). An evaluation of a theory of specific developmental dyslexia. *Child Development, 42,* 2009–2021.

Scarr-Salapatek, S. (1979). Twin method: Defense of a critical assumption. *Behavior Genetics, 9,* 527–542.

Schatzberg, A. F., Rothschild, A. J., Stahl, J. B., Bond, T. C., Rosenbaum, A. H., Lofgren, S. B., MacLaughlin, R. A., Sullivan, M. A., & Cole, J. O. (1983). The dexamethasone suppression test: Identification of subtypes of depression. *American Journal of Psychiatry, 140,* 88–91.

Schepank, H. (1971). Erb-und Umwelteinflusse bei 50 neurotischen Zwillingspaaren. *Zeitschrift fur Psychotherapie und medizinische Psychologie, 21,* 41–50.

Schepank, H. (1974). *Erb-und Umwelfaktoren bei Neuroses*. Berlin: Springer.

Schmettau, A. (1970). Zwei elektroencephalographische Merkmalsverbande und ihre psychologischen Korrelaten. *EEG-EMG. 1,* 169–182.

Schneider, K. (1959). *Clinical psychopathology*. New York: Grune & Stratton.

Schooler, C., & Feldman, S. E. (1967). *Experimental studies of schizophrenia*. Goleta, CA: Psychonomic Press.

Schooley, M. (1936). Personality resemblances among married couples. *Journal of Abnormal and Social Psychology, 31,* 340–347.

Schuckit, M., Goodwin, D. W., & Winokur, G. (1972). The half-sibling approach in a genetic study of alcoholism. In M. Roff, L. N. Rolins, & M. Pollack (Eds.), *Life history research in psychopathology* (Vol. 2). Minneapolis: University of Minneapolis Press.

Schull, W. J., & Neel, J. V. (1983). The effects of inbreeding on Japanese children. Test for depression called inreliable. *Science News, 123,* p. 326.

Schulsinger, F. (1972). Psychopathy: Heredity and environment. *International Journal of Mental Health, 1*, 190–206.

Scriver, C. R., & Clow, C. L. (1980). Phenylketonuria and other phenylalanine hydroxylation mutants in man. *Annual Review of Genetics, 14*, 179–202.

Seidman, L. J. (1983). Schizophrenia and brain dysfunction: An integration of recent neurodiagnostic findings. *Psychological Bulletin, 94*, 195–238.

Shapiro, A. K., & Shapiro, E. (1982). Tourette syndrome: History and present status. In A. J. Friedhoff & Thomas N. Chase (Eds.), *Gilles de la Tourette syndrome*. New York: Raven Press.

Shapiro, A., Shapiro, E., Brunn, R. & Sweet, R. (1978). *Gilles de la Tourette syndrome*. New York: Raven Press.

Shapiro, L. R., Kuhr, M. D., Wilmot, P. L., Lilienthal, E. R., & Higgs, L. C. (1982). Multiple sibling mental retardation and the impact of the fragile X chromosome. *American Journal of Human Genetics, 34*, 112A.

Shapiro, L. R., Summa, G. M., Wilmot, P. L., & E. Gloth (1983). *Screening and detection of the fragile X syndrome*. Paper presented at the 1983 meeting of the American Society of Human Genetics.

Shapiro, R. W., Ryder, I. P., Svejgaard, A., & Rafaelson, O. J. (1977). HLA antigens and manic-depressive disorders: Further evidence of an association. *Psychological Medicine, 7*, 387–396.

Shapiro, W. R. (1970). A twin study of non-endogenous depression. *Acta Jutlandica (Aarhus), 42*, 2.

Shields, J. (1962). *Monozygotic twins brought up apart and brought up together*. London: Oxford University Press.

Shields, J. (1954). Personality differences and neurotic traits in normal school children. *Eugenic Review, 45*, 213.

Shields, J. (1975). Some recent developments in psychiatric genetics. *Archive fuer Psychiatrie und Nervenkramkheitens., 220*, 347–360.

Shields, J., & Slater, E. (1971). Diagnostic similarity in twins with neuroses and personality disorders. In J. Shields & I. I. Gottesman (Eds.), *Man, mind and heredity* (Selected papers of Eliot Slater on psychiatry and genetics). Baltimore: The Johns Hopkins University Press.

Shopler, E., Reichler, R., DeVillis, R., & Daley, K. (1980). Toward objective classification of childhood autism: The Childhood Autism Rating Scale (CARS). *Journal of Autism and Developmental Disorders, 10*, 91–103.

Sigvardsson, S., Cloninger, C. R., Bohman, M., & von Knorring, A. L. (1982). Predisposition to petty criminality in Swedish adoptees. III. Sex differences and validation of the male typology. *Archives of General Psychiatry, 39*, 1248–1253.

Singer, F. M., & Merrill, C. R. (1982). Alzheimer's disease, Down's Syndrome, and aging. *Annals of the New York Academy of Sciences, 396*.

Singer, S. & Hardy-Brown, K. (1984). Selective placement in infant adoptions. In P. Sachdev (Ed.), *Adoption: Current issues and trends*. Toronto: Butterworth.

Singer, S., Stewart, M., & Pulaski, L. (1981). Minimal brain dysfunction: Differences in two groups of index cases and their relatives. *Journal of Learning Disabilities, 14*, 470–473.

Skolnick, M. H., Willard, H. F., & Menlove, L. (1984). Report of the committee on human gene mapping by recombinant DNA techniques. *Cytogenetics and Cell Genetics, 37*, 210.

Sladen, B. (1970). Inheritance of dyslexia. *Bulletin of the Orton Society, 20*, 30–40.

Sladen, B. K. (1972). Some genetic aspects of dyslexia. *Bulletin of the Orton Society, 22*, 41–53.

Slater, E. (1943). The neurotic constitution: A statistical study of two thousand neurotic soldiers. *Journal of Neurology, Neurosurgery, and Psychiatry, 6,* 1–16.

Slater, E. (1953). *Psychotic and neurotic illnesses in twins.* London: Her Majesty's Stationery Office.

Slater, E. (1958). The monogenic theory of schizophrenia. *Acta Genetica, 8.*

Slater, E. (1961). Hysteria. *Journal of Mental Science, 107.*

Slater, E. (1964). Genetical factors in neurosis. *British Journal of Psychology, 55,* 265–269.

Slater, E. (1966). Expectation of abnormality on paternal and maternal sides: A computational model. *Journal of Medical Genetics, 3,* 159–161.

Slater, E., & Cowie, V. (1971). *The genetics of mental disorders.* London: Oxford University Press.

Slater, E. & Shields, J. (1969). Genetical aspects of anxiety. In M. Lader (Ed.), *British Journal of Psychiatry,* Special Publication, No. 3. Ashford, Kent: Headley, pp. 69–71.

Slatis, H. W., & Hoene, R. E. (1961). The effect of consanguinity on the distribution of continuously variable characteristics. *American Journal of Human Genetics, 13,* 28–31.

Smart, C. (1950). *Rejoice in the lamb: A song out of bedlam.* R. Brittain (Ed.), *Poems.* Princeton, NJ: Princeton University Press.

Smeraldi, E., Negri, F., & Melica, A. M. (1977). A genetic study of affective disorders. *Acta Psychiatrica Scandinavica, 56,* 382–398.

Smeraldi, E., Negri, F., Melica, A. M., & Scorze-Smeraldi, R. (1978). HLA system and affective disorders: A sibship genetic study. *Tissue Antigens, 12,* 270–274.

Smith, A. (1975). Neuropsychological testing in neurological disorders. In W. J. Friedlander (Ed.), *Advances in Neurology* (Vol. 7). New York: Raven Press.

Smith, R. T. (1965). A comparison of socio-environmental factors in monozygotic and dizygotic twins, testing an assumption. In S. G. Vandenberg (Ed.), *Methods and goals in human behavior genetics.* New York: Academic Press.

Smith, S., Kimberling, W., Pennington, B. & Lubs, H. (1983). Specific reading disability: Identification of an inherited form through linkage analysis. *Science, 219,* 1345–1347.

Solis, S. D., Neuchterlein, K. H., Garmezy, N., Devine, V. T., & Schaefer, S. M. (1981). A classification system for research in childhood psychopathology: Part I. An empirical approach using factor and cluster analyses and conjuctive decision rules. In B. A. Maher & W. B. Maher (Eds.), *Progress in experimental personality research* (Vol. 10, 115–161). New York: Academic Press.

Solyom, L., Beck, P., Solyom, C., & Hugel, R. (1974). Some etiological factors in phobic neurosis. *Canadian Psychiatric Association Journal, 19,* 69–71.

Sours, J. A. (1963). Narcolepsy and other disturbances in the sleep-walking rhythm. A study of 115 cases with review of the literature. *Journal of Nervous and Mental Disease, 137,* 525–542.

Spitz, R. A. (1946). Anaclitic depression. In *The psychoanalytic study of the child* (Vol. 2). New York, International Universities Press.

Spitzer, R., Endicott, J., & Robins, E. (1975). Clinical criteria for psychiatric diagnoses and DSM-III. *American Journal of Psychiatry, 132,* 1187–1192. (a)

Spitzer, R., Endicott, J., & Robins, E. (1975). *Research diagnostic criteria* (Instrument No. 58). New York: New York State Psychiatric Institute. (b)

Spitzer, R., Endicott, J., & Robins, E. (1978). Research diagnostic criteria: Rationale and reliability. *Archives of General Psychiatry, 35,* 773–782.

Spitzer, R., Skodol, Andrew E., Gibbon, M., Williams, J. B. W. (1983). *Psychopathology: A case book.* New York: McGraw-Hill.

Stabenau, J. R. (1977). Early infantile autism: A genetic central nervous system disorder? *Research Communications in Psychology, Psychiatry and Behavior, 2,* 131–146.

Stafford, R. E. (1961). Sex differences in spatial visualization as evidence of sex linked inheritance. *Perceptual and Motor Skills, 13,* 300–308.

Stanbury, J. B., Wyngaarden, J. B., & Fredericksen, D. S. (Eds.). (1966). *The metabolic basis of inherited disease* (2nd ed.). New York: McGraw-Hill.

Steg, J., & Rapoport, J. (1975). Minor physical anomalies in normal, neurotic, learning disabled and severely disturbed children. *Journal of Autism and Childhood Schizophrenia, 5,* 299–302.

Stephenson, S. (1907). Six cases of congenital word blindness affecting three generations of one family. *The Ophthalmoscope, 5,* 482–484

Sterman, M., Knauss, T., Lehmann, D., & Clemente, C. (1965). Circadian sleep and waking patterns in the laboratory cat. *Electroencephalography and Clinical Neurophysiology, 19,* 509–513.

Stern, C. (1973). *Principles of Human Genetics* (3rd ed.). San Francisco: W. H. Freeman.

Stevens, J., Sachdev, K., & Milstein, V. (1968). Behavior disorders of childhood and the electroencephalogram. *Archives of Neurology, 18,* 160–164.

Stewart, M. A., DeBlois, C. S., & Cummins, C. (1980). Psychiatric disorders in the parents of hyperactive boys and those with conduct disorders. *Journal of Child Psychology and Psychiatry, 21,* 283–292.

Stewart, M., & Gath, A. (1978). *Psychological disorders of children.* Baltimore: Williams & Wilkins.

Stewart, M., & Morrison, J. (1973). Affective disorder among the relatives of hyperactive children. *Journal of Child Psychology and Psychiatry, 14,* 209–212.

Stone, A. A., & Stone, S. S. (1966). *The abnormal personality through literature.* Englewood Cliffs, NJ: Prentice-Hall.

Stott, M. (1974). *Manual to the Bristol Social Adjustment Guides.* London: Hodder & Stoughton.

Strauss, A., & Lehtinen, L. (1947). *Psychopathology and education in the brain injured child.* New York: Grune & Stratton.

Stumpfl, F. (1936). *Die Upsprunge des Verbrechens Dargestellt am Lebenslauf von Zwillingen.* London: Thieme.

Stumpfl, F. (1937). Untersuchungen an psychopathischen Zwillingen. *Zeitschrift für die Gesamte Neurologie und Psychiatrie, 158,* 480.

Suarez, B. K., Reich, T., & Trost, J. (1976). Limits of the general two-allele single locus model with incomplete penetrance. *Annals of Human Genetics, 40,* 231.

Suarez, B. K., Rice, J., & Reich, T. (1978). The generalized sib pair IBD distribution: Its use in the detection of linkage. *Annals of Human Genetics, 42,* 87–94.

Suslak, L., Shopsin, B., Silbey, E., Mendlewicz, J., & Gershon, S. (1976). Genetics of affective disorders. I. Familial incidence study of bipolar, unipolar and schizo-affective illnesses. *Neuropsychobiology, 2,* 18–27.

Sutherland, G. R. (1977). Fragile sites on human chromosomes: Demonstration of their dependence on the type of tissue culture medium. *Science, 197,* 265–266.

Sutherland, G. R. (1979). Heritable fragile sites on human chromosomes. I. Effect of composition of culture medium on expression. *American Journal of Human Genetics, 31,* 125–135. (a)

Sutherland, G. R. (1979). Heritable fragile sites on human chromosomes. II. Distribution, phenotypic effects and cytogenetics. *American Journal of Human Genetics, 31,* 136–148. (b)

Sutherland, G. R., & Ashforth, P. L. C. (1979). X-linked mental retardation with macroorchidism and the fragile site at Xq 27 or 28. *Human Genetics, 48,* 117–120.

Sward, K., & Friedman, M. B. (1935). The family resemblance in temperament. *Journal of Abnormal and Social Psychology, 30,* 256–289.

Swenson, W. M., Pearson, J. S., & Osborne, D. (1973). *An MMPI source book: Basic items, scale and pattern data on 50,000 medical patients.* Minneapolis: University of Minnesota Press.

Symmes, J. S., & Rapaport, J. L. (1972). Unexpected reading failure. *American Journal of Orthopsychiatry, 42,* 382–391.

Szasz, T. (1961). *The myth of mental illness.* New York: Harper & Row.

Taft, L. T., & Cohen, H. J. (1971). Hypsarrhythmia and infantile autism: A clinical report. *Journal of Autism and Childhood Schizophrenia, 1,* 327–336.

Targum, S. D., Gershon, E. S., Van Eerdewegh, M., & Rogentine, N. (1979). Human leucocyte antigen system not closely linked to or associated with bipolar manic-depressive illness. *Biological Psychiatry, 14,* 615–636.

Taylor, M. A., & Abrams, R. (1980). Reassessing the bipolar-unipolar dichotomy. *Journal of Affective Disorders, 2,* 195–217.

Terman, L. M., & Buttenwieser, P. (1935). Personality factors in marital compatibility. *Journal of Social Psychology, 6,* 143–171, 267–289.

Thomas, A., & Chess, S. (1977). *Temperament and development.* New York: Brunner/Mazel.

Thomas, A., Chess, S., Birch, H. G., Hertzig, M. E. and Korn, S. (1963). *Behavioral individuality in early childhood.* New York: New York University Press.

Thomas, A., Chess, S., & Birch, H. G. (1968). *Temperament and behavior disorders in children.* New York: New York University Press.

Tienari, P. (1963). Psychiatric illnesses in identical twins. *Acta Psychiatrica Scandinavica, 39,* Suppl. 171.

Tills, D., Warlow, A., Richens, A., & Laidlau, J. (1981). Genetic markers in epilepsy. *Human Heredity, 31,* 19–31.

Tjio, J. H., & Levan, A. (1956). The chromosome number of man. *Hereditas, 42,* 1–6.

Torgerson, S. (1980). Hereditary-environmental differentiation of general neurotic, obsessive, and impulsive hysterical personality traits. *Acta Geneticae Medicae Gemellologia, 29,* 193–207.

Torup, E. (1962). A follow up study of children with tics. *Acta Paediatrica, 51,* 261–268.

Trostorff, S. von. (1968). Über die hereditare Belastung bei den bipolaren und monopolaren phasischen Psychosen. *Schweizer Archiv für Neurologie und Psychiatrie, 102,* 235

Tsuang, M. T. (1978). Familial subtyping of schizophrenia and affective disorders. In R. L. Spitzer & D. F. Klein (Eds.), *Critical issues in psychiatric diagnosis.* New York: Raven Press.

Tsuang, Ming T., Fowler, R. C., Cadoret, R. J., & Monnelly, E. (1974). Schizophrenia among first-degree relatives of paranoid and non-paranoid schizophrenics. *Comprehensive Psychiatry, 15*(4), 295–301.

Tsuboi, T., & Endo, S. (1977). Incidence of seizures and EEG abnormalities among offspring of epileptic patients. *Human Genetics, 36,* 173–189.

Turner, G., & Turner, B. (1974). X-linked mental retardation. *Journal of Medical Genetics, 11,* 109–113.

Turner, G., English, B., Lindsay, D. G., & Turner, B. (1972). X-linked mental retardation without physical abnormality (Renpenning's syndrome) in sibs in an institution. *Journal of Medical Genetics, 9,* 324–330.

Turner, G., Eastmen, C., Casey, J., McLeay, A., Procopis, P., & Turner, B. (1975). X-linked mental retardation associated with macro-orchidism. *Journal of Medical Genetics, 12,* 367–371.

Turner, W. J. (1979). Genetic markers for schizotaxia. *Biological Psychiatry, 14*, 177–206.

Turner, W. J., & King, S. (1983). BPD-2 an autosomal dominant form of bipolar affective disorder. *Biological Psychiatry, 18*, 63–88.

Uchida, I. A., & Joyce, E. M. (1982). Activity in the fragile X in heterozygous carriers. *American Journal of Human Genetics, 34*, 286–293.

U.S. Department of Health, Education & Welfare. (1975). *Vital Statistics of the United States*. Rockville, Md: Public Health Service.

U.S. Department of Health, Education & Welfare. (1976). *Vital Statistics of the United States*. Rockville, Md: Public Health Service.

U.S. Department of Health, Education & Welfare. (1980). *Statistical Abstracts of the United States*. Washington, D.C. Government Printing Office.

Usdin, E., & Hanin, I. (Eds.). (1982). *Biological markers in psychiatry and neurology*. New York: Pergamon Press.

Van Den Berghe, H., Deroover, J., Parloir, C., & Fryns, J. P. (1978). X-linked non-specific mental retardation. *Clinical Genetics, 13*, 106.

Van Den Berghe, H., Fryns, J. P., Parloir, C., Deroover, J., & Keulemans, M. (1980). Genetic causes of severe mental handicap: Preliminary data from a University of Leuven study. In P. Mittler (Ed.), *Frontiers of knowledge in mental retardation* (Vol. 2): *Biomedical aspects*. Baltimore: University Park Press.

Van Twyver, H. B., & Allison, T. (1970). Sleep in the opossum (Didelphis marsupialis). *Electroencephalography and Clinical Neurophysiology, 29*, 181–186.

Van Valkenburg, C., Lowry, M., Winokur, G., & Cadoret, R. (1977). Depression spectrum disease versus pure depressive disease: Clinical, personality and course differences. *Journal of Nervous and Mental Disease, 165*(5), 341–347.

Vandenberg, S. (1969). Contributions of twin research to psychology. In M. Manosevitz, G. Lindzey, & D. Thiessen (Eds.), *Behavioral genetics: Method and research*. New York: Appleton-Century-Crofts.

Vandenberg, S. G. (1972). Assortative mating, or who marries whom? *Behavior Genetics, 2*, 127–157.

Vandenberg, S. G. (1976). Twin Studies. In A. R. Kaplan (Ed.), *Human behavior genetics*, Springfield, IL: Charles C Thomas.

Veith, I. (1965). *Hysteria, the history of a disease*. Chicago: University of Chicago Press.

Vellutino, F. R. (1980). *Dyslexia: Theory and research*. Cambridge, MA: M.I.T. Press.

Vogel, F. (1958). *Uber die Erblichkeit des normalen Elektroencephalogramms: Vergleichende Untersuchungen an ein-und zwei-eiigen Zwillingen*. Stuttgart: Thieme.

Vogel, F. (1965). "14 and 6/s positive spikes" im Schlaf EEG von jugendlichen ein-und zwei-eiigen Zwillingen. *Human Genetics, 1*, 290–291.

Vogel, F. (1970). The genetic basis of the normal human electroencephalogram. *Humangenetik, 10*, 91–114.

Vogel, F., & Gotze, W. (1959). Familienuntersuchungen zur Genetik des normalen Elektroencephalogramms. *Deutsche Zeitschrift fur Nervenheilkundes, 178*, 668–700.

Vogel, F., & Helmbold, W. (1959). Koppelungsdaten für zwei wahrscheinlich einfach mendelnde EEG Merkmale des Menschen. *Zeitschrift für Menschliche Vererbungs- und Konstitutionslehre, 35*, 28.

Vogel, F. & Kruger, J. (1967). Multifactorial determination of genetic affections. In *Proceedings of the Third International Congress of Human Genetics*. Baltimore: Johns Hopkins University Press.

Vogel, F., Schalt, E., & Kruger, J. (1979). The electroencephalogram (EEG) as a research tool in human behavior genetics: Psychological examinations in healthy males with various inherited EEG variants. I. Rationale of the study, material, methods, heritability of test parameters. *Human Genetics, 47,* 1–45. (a)

Vogel, F., Schalt, E., & Kruger, J. (1979). The electroencephalogram (EEG) as a research tool in human behavior genetics: Psychological examinations in healthy males with various inherited EEG variants. II. Results. *Human Genetics, 47,* 47–80. (b)

Vogel, F., Schalt, E., & Kruger, J. (1979). The encephalogram (EEG) as a research tool in human behavior genetics: Psychological examinations in healthy males with various inherited EEG variants. III. Interpretation of the results. *Human Genetics, 47,* 81–111. (c)

Volavka, J., Mednick, S. A., Sergeant, J., & Rasmussen, L. (1977). EEGs of XYY and XXY men found in a large birth cohort. In S. A. Mednick & K. O. Christiansen (Eds.), *Biosocial bases of criminal behavior.* New York: Gardner Press.

Von Grieff, H., McHugh, P. R., & Stokes, P. (1975). *The familial history in sixteen males with bipolar manic-depressive disorder.* Paper presented at 63rd Annual Meeting, American Psychiatric Association, New York.

Wainer, H., Fairbank, D. T., & Hough, R. L. (1978). Predicting the impact of simple and compound life change events. *Applied Psychological Measurement, 2,* 311–320.

Waldron, S. (1976). The significance of childhood neurosis for adult mental health. *American Journal of Psychiatry, 133,* 532–538.

Waldrop, M., & Halverson, C. (1971). Minor physical anomalies: Their incidence and relation to behavior in a normal and deviant sample. In R. Smart, Jr. & M. Smart (Eds.), *Readings in development and relationships.* New York: Macmillan.

Waldrop, M. F., Pedersen, F. A., & Bell, R. (1968). Minor physical anomalies and behavior in preschool children. *Child Development, 39,* 391–394.

Walker, H. (1976). Incidence of minor physical anomalies in autistic patients. In M. Coleman (Ed.), *The autistic syndromes.* Amsterdam: North-Holland.

Walker, H. (1977). Incidence of minor physical anomaly in autism. *Journal of Autism and Childhood Schizophrenia, 7,* 165–178.

Warren, R. J., Karduck, W. A., Bussaratid, S., Stewart, M. A., & Sly, W. S. (1971). The hyperactive child syndrome. *Archives of General Psychiatry, 24,* 161–162.

Watson, P. (1981). *Twins, an uncanny relationship.* New York: The Viking Press.

Watt, N. F., Stolorow, R. D., Lubensky, A., & McClelland, D. (1970). School adjustment and behavior of children hospitalized for schizophrenia as adults. *American Journal of Orthopsychiatry, 40,* 637–657.

Watt, N. F., Fryer, J. H., Lewine, R. R. J., & Prentky, R. A. (1979). Toward longitudinal conceptions of psychiatric disorder. In B. A. Maher & W. B. Maher (Eds.), *Progress in experimental personality research* (Vol. 9). New York: Academic Press.

Webb, W. B. (1970). Individual differences in sleep length. In E. Hartmann (Ed.), *Sleep and dreaming.* Boston: Little, Brown.

Webb, W. B., & Friedmann, J. K. (1971). Attempts to modify the sleep patterns of the rat. *Physiology and Behavior, 6,* 459–460.

Weinberger, D. R., & Wyatt, R. J. (1982). Cerebral ventricular size: A biological marker for subtyping chronic schizophrenia. In E. Usdin & I. Hanin (Eds.), *Biological markers in Psychiatry and Neurology.* New York: Pergamon Press.

Weiss, G., Hechtman, L., & Perlman, T. (1978). Hyperactives as young adults: School, employer and self-rating scales obtained during ten-year follow-up evaluation. *American Journal of Orthopsychiatry, 48,* 438–445.

Weissman, M. M., Gershon, E., Kidd, K. K., Prusoff, B. A., Leckman, J. F., Dibble, E., Hamovitt, J., Thompson, W. D., Pauls, D. L., & Guroff, J. J. (1984). Psychiatric disorders in the relatives of probands with affective disorders. *Archives of General Psychiatry, 41,* 13–21. (a)

Weissman, M. M., Prusoff, B. A., & Merikangas, K. R. (1984). Is delusional depression related to bipolar disorder? *American Journal of Psychiatry, 41,* 892–893. (b)

Weitkamp, L. R., Purdue, L. H., & Huntzinger, R. S. (1980). Genetic marker studies in a family with unipolar depression. *Archives of General Psychiatry, 37,* 1187–1192.

Weitkamp, L. R., Stancer, H. C., Persad, E., Flood, C., & Guttormsen, S. (1981). Depressive disorders and HLA: A gene on chromosome 6 that can affect behavior. *The New England Journal of Medicine, 305,* 1301–1306.

Weitzman, E. D. (1981). Sleep and its disorders. *Annual Review of Neuroscience, 4,* 381–417.

Welner, Z., Welner, A., Stewart, M. A., Palkes, H., & Wish, E. (1977). A controlled study of siblings of hyperactive children. *Journal of Nervous and Mental Disease, 165,* 110–117.

Wender, P. H., Rosenthal, D., & Kety, S. S. (1968). A psychiatric assessment of the adoptive parents of schizophrenics. In D. Rosenthal & S. S. Kety (Eds.), *The transmission of schizophrenia.* London: Pergamon Press.

Wender, P., Rosenthal, D., Rainer, J., Greenhill, L., & Sarlin, B. (1977). Schizophrenics' adopting parents: Psychiatric status. *Archives of General Psychiatry, 34,* 777–799.

Werry, J. S. (1972). Organic factors in childhood psychology. In H. Quay & J. Werry (Eds.), *Psychopathological Disorders of Childhood.* New York: Wiley.

West, D. J., & Farrington, D. P. (1977). *The delinquent way of life.* London: Heinemann Educational.

Wiggins, J. S. (1966). Substantive dimensions of self-report in the MMPI item pool. *Psychological Monographs, 80* (22, Whole No. 630).

Willerman, L. (1973). Activity level and hyperactivity in twins. *Child Development, 44,* 288–293.

Willoughby, R. R. (1927). Family similarities in mental test abilities. *Genetic Psychology Monograph, 2,* 235–275.

Wilson, J. R., DeFries, J. C., McClearn, G. E., Vandenberg, S. G., Johnson, R. C., & Rashad, M. N. (1975). Cognitive abilities: Use of family data as a control to assess sex and age differences in two ethnic groups. *International Journal of Aging and Human Development, 6,* 261–276.

Wilson, R. S. (1978). Synchronies in mental development: An epigenetic perspective. *Science, 202,* 939–948.

Wilson, R. S., Brown, A. M., & Matheny, A. P. (1971). Emergence and persistence of behavioral differences in twins. *Child Development, 42,* 1381–1398.

Wilson, R. S., Garron, D. C., & Klawans, H. L. (1978). Significance of genetic factors in Gilles de la Tourette syndrome: A review. *Behavior Genetics, 8,* 503–510.

Wing, J. K. (Ed.). (1966). *Early childhood autism: Clinical, educational and social aspects.* Elmsford, NY: Pergamon Press.

Wing, J. K. (Ed.). (1978). *Schizophrenia, toward a new synthesis.* New York: Grune & Stratton.

Wing, J. K., Cooper, J. E., & Sartorius, N. (1974). *The measurement and classification of psychiatric symptoms. An instruction manual for the PSE and Catego Program.* London: Cambridge University Press.

Wing, L., & Gould, J. (1978). Systematic recording of behaviors and skills of retarded and psychotic children. *Journal of Autism and Childhood Schizophrenia, 8,* 79.

Winokur, G. (1975). Heredity in the affective disorders. In E. Anthony & T. Benedek (Eds.), *Depression in human existence.* Boston: Little, Brown.

Winokur, G., & Clayton, P. (1967). Family history studies: II. Sex differences and alcoholism in primary affective illness. *British Journal of Psychiatry, 113*, 973. (a)

Winokur, G., & Clayton, P. (1967). Family history studies: I. Two types of affective disorders separated according to genetic and clinical factors. In J. Wortis (Ed.), *Recent advances in biological psychiatry* (Vol. 9). New York: Plenum Press. (b)

Winokur, G., & Pitts, F. M. (1965). Affective disorder: VI. A family history study of prevalences, sex differences and possible genetic factors. *Journal of Psychiatric Research, 3*, 113.

Winokur, G., & Tanna, V. (1969). Possible role of X-linked dominant factor in manic-depressive disease. *Diseases of the Nervous System, 30*, 89.

Winokur, G., Clayton, P., & Reich, T. (1969). *Manic depressive illness*. St. Louis: C. V. Mosby.

Winokur, G., Cadoret, R., Dorzab, J., & Baker, M. (1971). Depressive disease: A genetic study. *Archives of General Psychiatry, 29*, 135–144.

Winokur, G., Tsuang, M. T., & Crowe, R. R. (1982). The Iowa 500: Affective disorder in relatives of manic and depressed patients. *American Journal of Psychiatry, 139*, 209–212.

Wirt, R. D., & Lachar, D. (1981). The Personality Inventory for Children: Development and Clinical Applications. In P. McReynolds (Ed.), *Advances in psychological assessment* (Vol. 5). San Francisco: Jossey-Bass.

Wirt, R. D., Lachar, D., Klinedinst, J. K., & Seat, P. D. (1977). *Multidimensional description of child personality: A manual for the Personality Inventory for Children*. Los Angeles: Western Psychological Services.

Wirt, R. D., Seat, P. D., & Broen, W. E. Jr. (1977). *The Personality Inventory for Children*. Los Angeles: Western Psychological Services.

Witkin, H. A., Mednick, S. A., Schulsinger, F., Bakkestrom, E., Christiansen, K. O., Goodenough, D. R., Hirschhorn, K., Lundsteen, C., Owen, D. R., Philip, J., Rubin, D. B., & Stocking, M. (1977). Criminality, aggressiveness and intelligence among XYY and XXY men. In S. A. Mednick & K. O. Christiansen (Eds.), *Biosocial bases of criminal behavior*. New York: Gardner Press.

Wittenborn, J. R. (1955). *Psychiatric rating scales*. New York: Psychological Corporation.

Wittenborn, J. R. (1962). The dimensions of psychoanalysis. *Journal of Nervous and Mental Disorders, 134*, 117–128.

Wolf, C. (1967). An experimental investigation of specific language disability. *Bulletin of the Orton Society, 17*, 32–38.

Wolff, G., Hameister, H., & Roper, H. H. (1978). X-linked mental retardation: Transmission of the trait by an apparently unaffected male. *American Journal of Medical Genetics, 2*, 217–224.

Woodruff, R. A., Guze, S. B., Clayton, P. J., & Carr, D. (1973). Alcoholism and depression. *Archives of General Psychiatry, 28*, 97–100.

Woodruff, R., Goodwin, D., & Guze, S. (1974). *Psychiatric diagnosis*. New York: Oxford University Press.

Wooley, C. F. (1976). Where are the diseases of yesteryear? DaCosta's syndrome, soldier's heart, the effort syndrome, neurocirculatory asthenia, and the mitral valve prolapse syndrome. *Circulation, 53*, 749–751.

World Health Organization. (1973). *Report of the international pilot study of schizophrenia*. Geneva: World Health Organization.

World Health Organization. (1977). *Manual of the international statistical classification of diseases, injuries and causes of death*. 9th. revision, Geneva: World Health Organization.

World Health Organization. (WHO) (1979). *Schizophrenia, an international follow-up study.* New York: Wiley.

Yoshimasu, S. (1961). The criminological significance of the family in the light of the studies of criminal twins. *Acta Criminologica Medica Legal Japonica, 27,* 117–141.

Yoss, R. E., & Daly, D. D. (1960). Narcolepsy. *Medical Clinics of North America, 44,* 953–968.

Young, J. K. (1975). A possible neuroendocrine basis of two clinical syndromes: Anorexia nervosa and the Kleine-Levin syndrome. *Physiological Psychology, 3,* 322–330.

Yunis, J. J. (1976). High resolution of human chromosomes. *Science, 191,* 1268–1270.

Záhálková, M., Vrzal, V., & Kloboukova, E. (1972). Genetical investigations in dyslexia. *Journal of Medical Genetics, 9,* 48–52.

Zajonc, R., & Markus, G. B. (1976). Birth order and intellectual development. *Psychological Review, 82,* 74–88.

Zausmer, R. C. M. (1954). Treatment of tics in childhood. *Archives of Disease in Childhood, 29,* 537–542.

Zazzo, R. (1960). *Les jumeaux, le couple et la personne* [Twins, the pair and the individual]. Paris: Presses Universitaires de France, 1960.

Zerbin-Rudin, E. (1967). Endogene psychosen. In P. E. Becker (Ed.), *Hummangenetik: Ein kurzes Handbuch in finf Banden* (Vol. 2). Stuttgart: Theime.

Zerbin-Rudin, E. (1969). Zur Genetik der depressiver Erkrankungen. In H. Hippius & H. Selback (Eds.) *Das depressive Syndrom.* Munich: Urban und Schwartzenberg.

Zilborg, G. (1941). *A history of medical psychology.* New York: W. W. Norton.

Zubin, J., & Spring, B. (1977). Vulnerability: A new view of schizophrenia. *Journal of Abnormal Psychology, 86,* 103–126.

Zubin, J., & Steinhauer, S. (1981). How to break the logjam in schizophrenia: A look beyond genetics. *Journal of Nervous and Mental Disease, 169,* 477–492.

Zuckerman, M. (1979). *Sensation seeking: Beyond the optimal level of arousal.* Hillsdale, NJ: Lawrence Erlbaum.

Zung, W. K., & Wilson, W. P. (1967). Sleep and dream patterns in twins. In J. Wortis (Ed.), *Recent advances in biological psychiatry* (Vol. 9). New York: Plenum Press.

Zurif, E. B., & Carson, G. (1970). Dyslexia in relation to cerebral dominant temporal analysis. *Neuropsychologia, 8,* 351–361.

Zvolsky, P. (1973). A contribution to questions of genetics of mood disorders. *Acta Universitatis Carolinae, 19,* 541–557.

INDEX